NUTRITION IN DERMATOLOGY

An Evidence-Based Guide

NUTRITION IN DERMATOLOGY

An Evidence-Based Guide

Editors

Sqn Ldr (Dr) Aseem Sharma MD DNB MBA FAGE FMUHS
Chief Dermatologist
Skin Saga Centre for Dermatology, Mumbai
Maharashtra State Liaison, Fever Rash Surveillance, World Health Organization
Ex-Assistant Professor of Dermatology, LTMMC & GH, Mumbai
Honorary Secretary, IADVL Maharashtra
Mumbai, Maharashtra, India

Abhishek De MD FAGE SCE(Dermatology)
FRCP(Edinburgh) FAAD PhD (Schl)
Consultant Dermatologist, Aesthetician and Laser Surgeon
Associate Professor, Calcutta National Medical College
Associate Editor, Indian Journal of Dermatology
Associate Editor, Indian Journal of Skin Allergy
Member of American Academy of Dermatology
Member of the International Society of Dermatology
Member of the European Academy of Dermatology and Venereology
Fellows of the Academy of General Education
Member of SIG Biologics and Small Molecule Immunomodulators
Member of SIG Psoriasis
Honorary Secretary, Skin Allergy Research Society of India
Kolkata, West Bengal, India

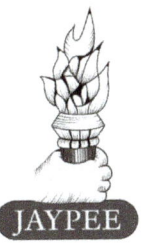

JAYPEE BROTHERS MEDICAL PUBLISHERS

The Health Sciences Publisher

New Delhi | London

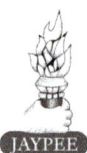 **Jaypee Brothers Medical Publishers (P) Ltd**

Headquarters
EMCA House
23/23-B, Ansari Road, Daryaganj
New Delhi 110 002, India
Landline: +91-11-23272143, +91-11-23272703
+91-11-23282021, +91-11-23245672
E-mail: jaypee@jaypeebrothers.com

Corporate Office
Jaypee Brothers Medical Publishers (P) Ltd.
4838/24, Ansari Road, Daryaganj
New Delhi 110 002, India
Phone: +91-11-43574357
Fax: +91-11-43574314
E-mail: jaypee@jaypeebrothers.com

Overseas Office
JP Medical Ltd.
83, Victoria Street, London
SW1H 0HW (UK)
Phone: +44-20 3170 8910
Fax: +44(0)20 3008 6180
E-mail: info@jpmedpub.com

Website: www.jaypeebrothers.com
Website: www.jaypeedigital.com

© 2025, Jaypee Brothers Medical Publishers

The views and opinions expressed in this book are solely those of the original contributor(s)/author(s) and do not necessarily represent those of editor(s) or publisher of the book.

All rights reserved. No part of this publication may be reproduced, stored or transmitted in any form or by any means, electronic, mechanical, photocopying, recording or otherwise, without the prior permission in writing of the publishers.

All brand names and product names used in this book are trade names, service marks, trademarks or registered trademarks of their respective owners. The publisher is not associated with any product or vendor mentioned in this book.

Medical knowledge and practice change constantly. This book is designed to provide accurate, authoritative information about the subject matter in question. However, readers are advised to check the most current information available on procedures included and check information from the manufacturer of each product to be administered, to verify the recommended dose, formula, method and duration of administration, adverse effects and contraindications. It is the responsibility of the practitioner to take all appropriate safety precautions. Neither the publisher nor the author(s)/editor(s) assume any liability for any injury and/or damage to persons or property arising from or related to use of material in this book.

This book is sold on the understanding that the publisher is not engaged in providing professional medical services. If such advice or services are required, the services of a competent medical professional should be sought.

Every effort has been made where necessary to contact holders of copyright to obtain permission to reproduce copyright material. If any have been inadvertently overlooked, the publisher will be pleased to make the necessary arrangements at the first opportunity.

Inquiries for bulk sales may be solicited at: jaypee@jaypeebrothers.com

Nutrition in Dermatology: An Evidence-Based Guide / *Aseem Sharma, Abhishek De*

First Edition: **2025**

ISBN: 978-93-5696-775-5

Contributors

Abhishek De MD FAGE SCE(Dermatology) FRCP(Edinburgh) FAAD PhD (Schl)
Consultant Dermatologist, Aesthetician and Laser Surgeon
Associate Professor, Calcutta National Medical College
Associate Editor, Indian Journal of Dermatology
Associate Editor, Indian Journal of Skin Allergy
Member of American Academy of Dermatology
Member of the International Society of Dermatology
Member of the European Academy of Dermatology and Venereology
Fellows of the Academy of General Education
Member of SIG Biologics and Small Molecule Immunomodulators
Member of SIG Psoriasis
Honorary Secretary, Skin Allergy Research Society of India
Kolkata, West Bengal, India

Sqn Ldr (Dr) Aseem Sharma MD DNB MBA FAGE FMUHS
Chief Dermatologist
Skin Saga Centre for Dermatology, Mumbai
Maharashtra State Liaison, Fever Rash Surveillance, World Health Organization
Ex-Assistant Professor of Dermatology, LTMMC & GH, Mumbai
Honorary Secretary, IADVL Maharashtra
Mumbai, Maharashtra, India

Geetanjali Shetty MBBS MD DDV FCPS
Founder and Medical Director for Revitalis Skin & Hair Clinic, Mumbai
Faculty at Trichology Update National Faculty at iDoc Academy
Fellow of the Royal Society of Public Health
Fellow of the American Academy of Dermatology (FAAD)
Mumbai, Maharashtra, India

Jaishree Sharad MBBS DDV IFAAD Fellowship in Lasers(Bangkok) Fellowship in Cosmetic Dermatology(USA)
Director, Skinfinitii Aesthetic Skin and Laser Clinic
Associate Editor, Journal of Cosmetic Dermatology
Joint Secretary, Association of Cutaneous Surgeons (India)
International Mentor, American Society of Dermatologic Surgery
Mumbai, Maharashtra, India

Madhulika Mhatre MBBS MD(Gold Medalist) FRGUHS(Aesthetic Dermatology) FIADVL(Trichology)
Director and Consultant Dermatologist
Skin Saga Centre for Dermatology
Mumbai, Maharashtra, India

Rajat Kandhari MBBS MD MSc
Chief Dermatologist
Dr Kandhari's Skin and Dental Clinic
New Delhi, India

Rajesh Mikkilineni MBBS MS(General Surgery) MCh(Plastic Surgery)
Director
Dr Sculpt Aesthetic Clinic (Svakruthi Aesthetic Pvt Ltd)
Bengaluru, Karnataka, India

Rasya Dixit MBBS MD
Medical Director
Dr Dixit Cosmetic Dermatology
Bengaluru, Karnataka, India

Rohit Batra MBBS MD
Director
DermaWorld Skin Clinic
New Delhi, India

Sachin Varma MBBS MD(SKIN & VD) FAGE FAAD(USA)
Chief Dermatologist and Cosmetologist
Skinvita Clinic, Kolkata
Member of the International Society of Dermatology (USA)
Member of the European Academy of Dermatology and Venereology
Kolkata, West Bengal, India

Preface

"More than skin deep"

While the cosmetology industry has long thrived on a narrative of external solutions, the realm of dermatology is evolving, acknowledging the undeniable truth, that true skin health is also a function of the right nutrition. This is a paradigm shift that recognizes our bodies as integrated ecosystems and explains why some respond and others do not. The radiance of our skin and the vitality of our hair serve as external mirrors of our internal health and while these signs are often attributed to genetics or external care routines, they are, in fact, profoundly influenced by a significant factor: nutrition, which plays on epigenetics and actual gene expression, as documented in various studies.

"Nutrition in Dermatology: An Evidence-Based Guide" takes you through the pivotal role that nutrition plays in the realm of skin and hair function and maintenance. This book is not merely an exploration of vanity; it is an exploration of the fundamental and intricate connections between what we consume and the canvas that is our skin.

Drawing from a wealth of scientific research and expert insights, we will explore the effects that the foods we eat have on our skin and hair. From micronutrients like vitamins, minerals, and antioxidants to macronutrients like protein and fatty acids, the significance of these nutritional elements will be translated to dermatological practices, shedding light on their impact on our body.

This book underscores the profound implications of nutrition in preventing and managing various dermatological concerns and conditions. It is a guide for dermatologists seeking well-rounded interventions for promoting our skin's intrinsic mechanisms for protecting itself. And all of it is backed by data stratified into good evidence, moderate evidence, and poor evidence, which can give the reader the prowess to make an informed decision.

As we traverse the chapters, we will encounter not just a compilation of data, but a comprehensive understanding of nutrition's impact on cellular regeneration, inflammation modulation, and hormone regulation, which is ushering in a new era of patient care because gone are the days when we negate the role of nutrition in body processes and push it under a rug.

Aseem Sharma
Abhishek De

Acknowledgments

The completion of this volume has been made possible through the concerted efforts of numerous individuals whose expertise and dedication have been invaluable.

We are profoundly indebted to our esteemed colleagues in the field of dermatology whose collaboration has significantly enhanced the scientific rigor of this work. We wish to express our deepest appreciation for their expert insights.

We extend our sincere gratitude to Mr Akshay Pai and his team at Nutrova for their diligent work and unwavering commitment to scientific excellence. The research contributions of Dr Meghna Motwani, Ms Kasturi Deorukhkar, and Ms Nikita Kochrekar were particularly crucial to the successful completion of this project.

Furthermore, we acknowledge with gratitude the contributions of Mr Suvajit Sinha and Ms Fashutana Patel, for project management and design inputs.

It is our sincere hope that this work will serve as a valuable contribution to the scientific literature in the field of dermatology and prove beneficial to researchers, clinicians, and students alike.

Aseem Sharma
Abhishek De

Scale for Evidence Level

EVIDENCE LEVEL	STUDY PARAMETERS	
+	Case study (noncomparative observational study)	Observational study Association with $n \leq 30$ subjects
++	In vitro proof-of-concept Proof of mechanism	Observational study Association with $n \geq 30$ subjects Confounding factors considered
+++	Interventional study $n < 30$ subjects Proof-of-concept	In vivo animal model with evidence-based hypotheses
++++	Interventional study $n \geq 30$ subjects or sample is representative placebo-controlled Baseline values recorded Only clinical measurements	Observational study $n \geq 100$ subjects or the sample size is representative Confounding factors considered
+++++	Interventional study $n \geq 30$ subjects Placebo-controlled Randomized double-blind or single-blind crossover Clinical and instrumental measurements	Meta-analysis of several studies with confounding factors considered

Abbreviations

ADI	:	Acceptable Daily Intake
AI	:	Adequate Intake
AR	:	Average Requirement
BCAA	:	Branched-chain Amino Acids
BMI	:	Body Mass Index
DRI	:	Dietary Reference Intake
DRV	:	Dietary Reference Value
EAR	:	Estimated Average Requirement
EFSA	:	European Food Safety Authority
FAO	:	Food and Agriculture Organization
FDA	:	Food and Drug Administration
FSSAI	:	Food Safety and Standards Authority of India
GOED	:	Global Organization for EPA (eicosapentaenoic acid) and DHA (docosahexaenoic acid) Omega-3s
HDL	:	High-density Lipoprotein
ICMR-NIN	:	Indian Council of Medical Research-National Institute of Nutrition
IOC	:	Institute of Coaching
IOM	:	Institute of Medicine
IU	:	International Unit
LDL	:	Low-density Lipoprotein
LOAEL	:	Lowest-observed-adverse-effect Level
MED	:	Minimal Erythema Dose
NIH	:	National Institutes of Health
NOAEL	:	No-observed-adverse-effect Level
OSL	:	Observed Safe Level
RDA	:	Recommended Dietary Allowance
ROS	:	Reactive Oxygen Species
TEWL	:	Transepidermal Water Loss
UL	:	Tolerable Upper Intake Level
UV	:	Ultraviolet
WHO	:	World Health Organization

Contents

Section 01: Vitamins

01	Vitamin A and β-carotene *Aseem Sharma*	02
02	Vitamins B1, B2, and B5 *Rohit Batra*	11
03	Niacin (Vitamin B3) *Rohit Batra*	23
04	Vitamins B6, B9, and B12 *Rohit Batra*	32
05	Biotin (Vitamin B7) *Abhishek De*	47
06	Vitamin C *Sachin Varma*	54
07	Vitamin D *Sachin Varma*	65
08	Vitamin E *Sachin Varma*	74
09	Vitamin K *Sachin Varma*	87

Section 02: Minerals

10	Iron *Rasya Dixit*	98
11	Zinc *Rasya Dixit*	105
12	Magnesium *Abhishek De*	117
13	Calcium *Abhishek De*	127
14	Selenium *Abhishek De*	135
15	Copper *Rasya Dixit*	148
16	Iodine *Abhishek De*	154

Section 03: Protein and Peptides

17	Protein *Rajat Kandhari*	164
18	Collagen Peptides *Rajat Kandhari*	176
19	Hyaluronic Acid *Aseem Sharma*	192
20	Lactoferrin and Colostrum *Aseem Sharma*	200

Section 04: Fatty Acids

21	Omega-3 Fatty Acids *Madhulika Mhatre*	212
22	Omega-6 Fatty Acids *Madhulika Mhatre*	221
23	Phytoceramides *Madhulika Mhatre*	228

Section 05: Antioxidants and Enzymes

24	Non-provitamin A Carotenoids *Rajat Kandhari*	236
25	Glutathione *Geetanjali Shetty*	251
26	Coenzyme Q10 *Geetanjali Shetty*	259
27	Alpha Lipoic Acid *Geetanjali Shetty*	267
28	Polyphenols *Rajesh Mikkilineni*	274
29	Phytoestrogens *Rajesh Mikkilineni*	286

Section 06: Probiotics and Prebiotics

30	Prebiotics and Synbiotics *Jaishree Sharad*	298
31	Probiotics *Jaishree Sharad*	308
	INDEX	319

SECTION 01

Vitamins

1. Vitamin A and β-carotene — *Aseem Sharma*
2. Vitamins B1, B2, and B5 — *Rohit Batra*
3. Niacin (Vitamin B3) — *Rohit Batra*
4. Vitamins B6, B9, and B12 — *Rohit Batra*
5. Biotin (Vitamin B7) — *Abhishek De*
6. Vitamin C — *Sachin Varma*
7. Vitamin D — *Sachin Varma*
8. Vitamin E — *Sachin Varma*
9. Vitamin K — *Sachin Varma*

Nutrition in Dermatology

01

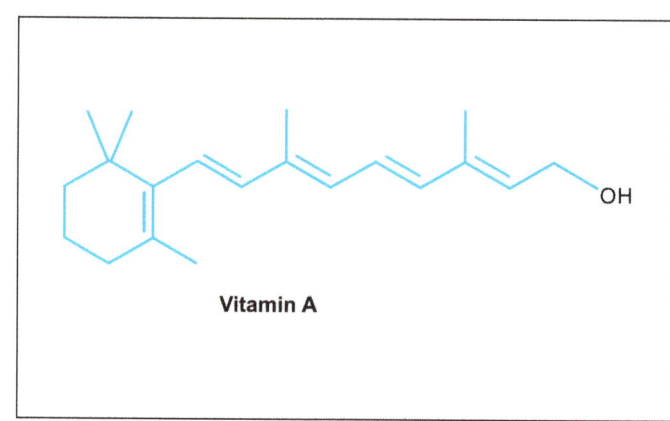

Retinol

Vitamin A and β-carotene

✍ Aseem Sharma

CONTENTS

VITAMIN A AND β-CAROTENE: NUTRIENT SNAPSHOT

- ▶ REQUIREMENT IN THE INDIAN CONTEXT | 03
- ▶ ACTIVE FORMS | 04
- ▶ SAFETY AND DOSAGE | 04
- ▶ CLINICAL CONDITIONS | 05
- ▶ SUPPLEMENTATION | 07

INTRODUCTION | 08

DIGESTION, ABSORPTION AND STORAGE | 08

MECHANISM OF ACTION | 08

KEY TOPICS

- ANTI-AGING
- CHRONIC DERMATITIS
- CHRONIC HAND ECZEMA
- PHOTOAGING/UV-INDUCED ERYTHEMA

Nutrient Snapshot

▶ **REQUIREMENT IN THE INDIAN CONTEXT**

- Vitamin A is a fat-soluble vitamin required for normal growth and development, maintenance of healthy mucosal membranes, reproductive health, immunity, and vision.[1] Vitamin A refers to a family of compounds found as preformed vitamin A (retinol) in animal products and as provitamin A carotenoids in fruit and vegetables. Retinol, retinal, retinoic acid (RA), and related compounds are known as retinoids.

- In dermatology, retinoids are commonly known for their anti-aging and anti-acne properties, and often feature in topical applications. From a nutritional perspective, vitamin A is involved in the growth and differentiation of cells, thereby contributing to every single process and more. Other than preformed vitamin A, the carotenoid, β-carotene is also converted into vitamin A. β-carotene is the most abundant provitamin A carotenoid in the human diet, and it serves as a UV protector and an antioxidant in skin.

- Vitamin A deficiency continues to be a major public health concern in India for children and pregnant women, despite the implementation of a program for vitamin A supplementation for over four decades. Thus, food staples, like milk and oil, have been recently fortified with vitamin A.[1]

- Being a fat-soluble vitamin, vitamin A is stored in the body. So humans can go months without it and not show any symptoms of deficiency. Vegetarians, especially vegans, rely on the conversion of provitamin A carotenoids in fruit and vegetables as their source of vitamin A, which is not very efficient in the body.[2] An unplanned vegan diet may require fortification or supplementation to meet their vitamin A needs.[3]

- While the benefits of vitamin A sufficiency cannot be overstated, an excess can be equally harmful. Supplementation with vitamin A and provitamin A carotenoids must be given with caution and complement dietary intake, especially as fortification increases, in low-risk groups for deficiency. However, given that subclinical deficiency is very prevalent in India,[4] the benefits of vitamin A on general skin and hair health can be maintained by ensuring sufficiency while remaining within recommended doses.

ACTIVE FORMS

ACTIVE FORMS	SUPPLEMENT SOURCES	SALIENT FEATURES
• Retinoic acid • Retinal • Retinol • Retinyl esters	Synthetic form	These are preformed vitamin A, so it can be readily used instead of β-carotene. These may be preferred as the bioavailability of provitamin A carotenoids vary.
β-carotene	Synthetic form Dunaliella salina (microalgae) Blakeslea trispora (fungus)	Provitamin A form: The conversion rate of β-carotene to retinol (active form) in our body varies from 3.6–28: 1 by weight, i.e., 3.6–28 μg β-carotene is equal to 1 μg retinol.[5] The dose administered affects carotenoid conversion. The higher the intake, the lower the conversion. Vitamin A status of the individual also affects carotenoid conversion. The higher the status, the lower the conversion.[6]

SAFETY AND DOSAGE

GENERAL REQUIREMENTS	
Indian recommendations	**Vitamin A:** RDA: Male—1000 μg or Female—840 μg EAR: Male— 460 μg or Female—390 μg TUL: 3000 μg β-carotene: RDA or upper limit is not established for β-carotene. FSSAI allows the use of β-carotene in the nutraceutical supplement but has not stated any permitted range for the same.[6]
Global recommendations and limits	**Vitamin A:** NIH-RDA(M/F): 900 μg/700 μg Average requirements (AR): Male—570 μg retinol activity equivalent (RAE)/day, Female—490 μg RAE/day NOAEL: 3000 μg and LOAEL: 10,000 μg **β-carotene:** EFSA: Exposure to β-carotene from its use as a food additive and as food supplement at a level below 15 mg/day do not cause adverse health effects adverse health effects in the general population, including heavy smokers.[7]

▶ SAFETY AND DOSAGE (Continued)

GENERAL REQUIREMENTS	
Notes:	There are no side effects of vitamin A if the dose is within the safety limits. But mega doses can lead to toxicity causing various adverse effects.[8] Vitamin A is a fat-soluble vitamin and thus needs to be taken with or after a meal. The activity of β-carotene is expressed in retinol activity equivalents (RAE): 1 RAE = 1 μg retinol = 3.6–28 μg β-carotene. Being a phytonutrient, there is no established requirement for β-carotene. However, its intake in reasonable amounts can benefit our health. High doses should be avoided. The purity of extracts may vary. Clinical data on the specific product is the best indicator of safety and efficacy.

▶ CLINICAL CONDITIONS

EVIDENCE LEVEL	CONDITION OR USE CASE	DOSAGE	BENEFIT OR MECHANISM OF ACTION
+++++	Photodamage (vitamin A)	7.5 mg, 15 mg, and 22.5 mg/day for 12 months	There was a dose-dependent beneficial effect in patients' sun-damaged skin as per karyometric features.[9]
+++	UV-induced erythema (β-carotene)	A carotenoid supplement with 25 mg total carotenoids and a combination of the carotenoid supplement and vitamin E (335 mg α-tocopherol) were given daily for 12 weeks.	Level of vitamin E and β-carotene increased in plasma. Erythema was significantly diminished after week 8, and erythema suppression was greater with the combination of carotenoids and vitamin E than with carotenoids alone.[10]
+++	UV protection (β-carotene)	30 mg of natural carotenoids containing 29.4 mg of β-carotene, 0.36 mg of α-carotene was given for 24 weeks.	The minimum erythema dose increased significantly. Serum lipid peroxidation was inhibited in a dose-dependent manner.[11]

▶ CLINICAL CONDITIONS (Continued)

EVIDENCE LEVEL	CONDITION OR USE CASE	DOSAGE	BENEFIT OR MECHANISM OF ACTION
+++	Inflammation caused by UV exposure (β-carotene)	Mice were fed a diet supplemented with 0.5% β-carotene for 1 month	After feeding, mice were subjected to O_3 exposure. β-carotene downregulated the induction of proinflammatory markers such as tumor necrosis factor-alpha (TNF-α), macrophage inflammatory protein-2 (MIP-2), and inducible nitric oxide synthase (iNOS), and markers of oxidative stress, heme-oxygenase-1 (HO-1).[12]
+++	Anti-aging (β-carotene)	30 or 90 mg/day of β-carotene for 90 days	β-carotene improved facial wrinkles and elasticity only in the low-dose group, whilst also increasing procollagen synthesis, and reducing a marker of DNA oxidation, 8-hydroxy-2'-deoxyguanosine. The minimal erythema dose decreased significantly only in the high-dose group.[13]
++	Anti-aging (β-carotene)	The in vitro mesenchymal stem cells (MSCs) were induced by H_2O_2 with β-carotene, followed by feeding of 0.5 mg β-carotene to mice.	The in vitro experiment revealed that β-carotene could relieve the aging of MSCs, as shown by a series of aging marker molecules such as p16 and p21. β-carotene appeared to inhibit aging by regulating the KAT7-p15 signalling axis. The in vivo experiment revealed that β-carotene treatment significantly down-regulated the aging level of tissues and organs.[14]

▶ SUPPLEMENTATION

	BASIS	**WHAT TO LOOK OUT FOR**
Supplementation form	Retinyl acetate (preformed) Retinyl palmitate (preformed) β-carotene (provitamin A) Combination of preformed and provitamin A.[15]	Form of vitamin A is mentioned on the label. If vitamin A is in β-carotene form, then some brands say the source on the packaging.
Administration form	A multivitamin formulation or a stand-alone vitamin A in the form of capsules, tablets, syrups, gummies and powders.	The form is mentioned on the packaging.
Purity considerations	1 μg retinol = 3.33 IU[6]	The dose is normally mentioned in IU or μg.
Patient considerations	Vegetarians may need to check whether the product is vegetarian as sometimes vitamin A can be sourced from an animal origin. Preferably taken after a meal as the fat in the meal will help to facilitate absorption. Individuals who consume over 30 mg β-carotene daily for prolonged periods of time have been found to have high levels of β-carotene in the blood and skin (hypercarotenodermia) and may develop a yellowing of the skin that is not considered a health problem. It is reversible on reduction of intake.[16]	Products sold in the Indian market have a logo to declare whether a product is vegetarian or nonvegetarian.
Safety considerations	The safety limit for vitamin A is 3,000 μg/day. Chronic supplementation of preformed vitamin A can have negative effects on bone mineral density and liver abnormalities.[6,17] β-carotene use has been associated with increasing the risk of tobacco-related cancers (≥ 20 mg/day of β-carotene; in current smokers).[18] High doses of vitamin A has a potent teratogenic effect and is therefore contraindicated during pregnancy.	Vitamin A serum levels need to be checked while recommending mega doses of either vitamin A or β-carotene. The amount mentioned on the nutrition label should not exceed RDA. If a product meets 100% RDA, long-term use must be monitored (as vitamin A is provided from the diet as well).

INTRODUCTION

Vitamin A is important for normal vision, gene expression, reproduction, embryonic development, growth, and immune function. Vitamin A comprises a family of two sources for vitamin A: preformed vitamin A (retinol and retinyl esters) and provitamin A carotenoids. Preformed vitamin A is found in foods from animal sources, including dairy products, eggs, fish, and organ meats. Provitamin A carotenoids are plant pigments that the body converts into vitamin A in the intestine. The main provitamin A carotenoids in the human diet are β-carotene, α-carotene, and β-cryptoxanthin.[15]

Adequate consumption of vitamin A is necessary for the maintenance of healthy skin and hair. It is involved in the regulation of cell growth and differentiation, thereby affecting skin maintenance and repair, hair growth and even immunity.[19] Because it affects the skin and hair in a dose-dependent manner, too much or too little has deleterious effects.[20] For example, vitamin A deficiency can lead to follicular hyperkeratosis, atrophy of the sebaceous gland,[19] increased susceptibility to skin infection and inflammation.[21]

Retinol can be converted by the body to retinal, which can, in turn, be irreversibly oxidized to RA, the form of vitamin A known to regulate gene transcription. This is catalyzed by retinol dehydrogenases, which function as gatekeepers to limiting the creation of RA. Retinaldehyde reductases also prevent toxicity by converting retinal back to retinol.[20] Yet toxicity can be an issue through unnecessary supplementation of high doses. Due to its teratogenicity, potential for toxicity, and long half-life, strict monitoring under the care of a medical provider is prudent.

DIGESTION, ABSORPTION AND STORAGE

Digestion and Absorption

- Intestinal absorption of preformed vitamin A occurs following the processing of retinyl esters to retinol in the lumen of the small intestine.

- A small percentage of dietary retinoids is converted to RA in intestinal cells.

- Absorbed β-carotene is converted to retinal or RA. Some β-carotene is deposited in the skin.

- As the amount of ingested preformed vitamin A increases, its absorbability remains high (70–90%), whereas with carotenoids, absorption efficiency decreases as dose increases.[22]

- Vitamin A and carotenoid absorption is improved with fats.

Storage

- Vitamin A compounds are predominantly stored in the liver in the form of retinyl esters (e.g., retinyl palmitate or stearate). When appropriate, retinyl esters are hydrolyzed to generate all-trans-retinol, which binds to retinol binding protein (RBP) before being released in the bloodstream bound to the protein, transthyretin.[23]

- Retinyl esters in chylomicrons also help deliver vitamin A to extrahepatic tissues.[23]

MECHANISM OF ACTION

Beta-carotene that is deposited in skin can absorb UV radiation, thereby preventing UV-damage, and acts as an antioxidant. It also affects the color of skin. β-carotene that is converted to vitamin A has the same mechanism of action as preformed vitamin A (stated below).

01 | Cell Growth and Differentiation

RA diffuses into the cell nucleus where it regulates more than 500 genes by binding and activating heterodimers of the retinoic acid receptor (RAR)/retinoid X receptor (RXR), which activates or represses target genes. This is how it affects the growth and differentiation of keratinocytes, fibroblasts and melanocytes. It also affects keratin expression, and stimulates fibroblasts for collagen and elastin production, and inhibits the activity of metalloproteinases which are responsible for degradation of the extracellular matrix.[20]

02 | Modulation of the Hair Cycle

Vitamin A is important for healthy hair; since both too much or too little retinyl esters leads to alopecia.[19] High-level of dietary retinyl esters results in a greater percentage of hair follicles in refractory telogen, and vice versa. Vitamin A regulates hair follicle stem cell activity through BMP and Wnt signaling pathways.[24]

03 | Modulation of Skin's Immunity

As part of the innate immune system, toll-like receptors in skin cells respond to pathogens and cell damage by inducing a proinflammatory immune response which includes increased RA production. RA promotes the production of antimicrobial peptides, resistin and cathelicidin, by epidermal keratinocytes.[21,25] Fat-soluble vitamins appear to be of particular importance for the expression of lipophilic skin antimicrobial proteins. Vitamin D also plays a role in cathelicidin production.[21,26]

04 | Modulation of Sebaceous Glands

Vitamin A is required for the maintenance of sebaceous glands. A deficiency can result in atrophy of the gland. Excess RA also inhibits sebaceous gland function, as is exploited in the treatment of acne. It decreases the activity of enzymes involved in lipogenesis, and reduces sebocyte growth and differentiation.[19] Furthermore, the effect of vitamin A on keratinization and immune cells makes it a suitable treatment of acne, given the primary pathophysiological factors leading to acne include increased sebum production, altered growth and differentiation of follicular keratinocytes, bacterial colonization of the follicle by *P. acnes*, and inflammatory and immune reactions.

▶ REFERENCES

1. Arlappa N. Vitamin A supplementation policy: A shift from universal to geographical targeted approach in India considered detrimental to health and nutritional status of under 5 years children. Eur J Clin Nutr. 2023;77(1):1-6.
2. Weber D, Grune T. The contribution of β-carotene to vitamin A supply of humans. Mol Nutr Food Res. 2012;56(2):251-8.
3. Weikert C, Trefflich I, Menzel J, Obeid R, Longree A, Dierkes J, et al. Vitamin and Mineral Status in a Vegan Diet. Dtsch Arztebl Int. 2020;117(35–36):575-82.
4. Akhtars, Ahmed A, Randhawa MA, Atukorala S, Arlappa N, Ismail T, et al. Prevalence of Vitamin A Deficiency in South Asia: Causes, Outcomes, and Possible Remedies. J Health Popul Nutr. 2013;31(4):413-23.
5. Tang G. Bioconversion of dietary provitamin A carotenoids to vitamin A in humans. Am J Clin Nutr. 2010;91(5):1468S-73S.
6. National Institute of Nutrition Indian Council of Medical Research. Recommended Dietary Allowances and Estimated Average Requirements for Indians – 2020. [Online] Available from https://www.nin.res.in/RDA_Full_Report_2020.html.
7. EFSA Panel on Food Additives and Nutrient Sources added to Food (ANS). Statement on the safety of β-carotene use in heavy smokers. EFSA Journal. 2012;10(12):2953.
8. McEldrew EP, Lopez MJ, Milstein H. Vitamin A. PMID: 29493984. Treasure Island (FL): StatPearls Publishing, 2024.
9. Alberts D, Ranger-Moore J, Einspahr J, Saboda K, Bozzo P, Liu Y, et al. Safety and efficacy of dose-intensive oral vitamin A in subjects with sun-damaged skin. Clin Cancer Res. 2004;10(6):1875-80.
10. Stahl W, Heinrich U, Jungmann H, Sies H, Tronnier H. Carotenoids and carotenoids plus vitamin E protect against ultraviolet light-induced erythema in humans. Am J Clin Nutr. 2000;71(3):795-8.
11. Lee J, Jiang S, Levine N, Watson RR. Carotenoid supplementation reduces erythema in human skin after simulated solar radiation exposure. Proc Soc Exp Biol Med. 2000;223(2):170-4.
12. G Valacchi, A Pecorelli, M Mencarelli, E Maioli, PA Davis. Beta-carotene prevents ozone-induced proinflammatory markers in murine skin. Toxicol. Ind. Health., 2009;25(4-5):241-7.
13. Cho S, Lee DH, Won CH, Kim SM, Lee S, Lee MJ, et al. Differential effects of low-dose and high-dose beta-carotene supplementation on the signs of photoaging and type I procollagen gene expression in human skin in vivo. Dermatology. 2010;221(2):160-71.
14. Zheng WV, Wang Xu, Yaqin Li, Jie Qin, Zhou T, Li D, et al. Anti-aging effect of β-carotene through regulating the KAT7-P15 signaling axis, inflammation and oxidative stress process. Cell Mol Biol Lett. 2022;27(1):86.
15. Fact Sheet for Health Professionals. Vitamin A and Carotenoids [Online]. Available from: https://ods.od.nih.gov/factsheets/VitaminA-HealthProfessional/
16. Ch Bayerl. Beta-carotene in dermatology: does it help? Acta Dermatovenerol Alp Pannonica Adriat. 2008;17(4):160-2, 164-6.
17. Ronis JJ, Pedersen KB, Watt J. Adverse effects of nutraceuticals and dietary supplements. Annu Rev Pharmacol Toxicol. 2018;58:583-601.
18. Middha P, Weinstein SJ, Männistö S, Albanes D, Mondul AM. β-Carotene Supplementation and Lung Cancer Incidence in the Alpha-Tocopherol, Beta-Carotene Cancer Prevention Study: The Role of Tar and Nicotine. Nicotine Tob Res. 2018;21(8):1045-50.
19. Everts HB. Endogenous retinoids in the hair follicle and sebaceous gland. Biochim Biophys Acta. 2012;1821(1):222-9.
20. VanBuren CA, Everts HB. Vitamin A in Skin and Hair: An Update. Nutrients. 2022;14(14):2952.
21. Harris TA, Gattu S, Propheter DC, Kuang Z, Bel S, Ruhn KA, et al. Resistin-like Molecule α Provides Vitamin-A-Dependent Antimicrobial Protection in the Skin. Cell Host & Microbe. 2019;25(6):777-88.

22. Novotny JA, Harrison DJ, Pawlosky R, Flanagan VP, Harrison EH, Kurilich AC. β-Carotene Conversion to Vitamin A Decreases As the Dietary Dose Increases in Humans. The Journal of Nutrition. 2010;140(5):915.
23. Carazo A, Macáková K, Matoušová K, Krčmová LK, Protti M, Mladěnka P. Vitamin A Update: Forms, Sources, Kinetics, Detection, Function, Deficiency, Therapeutic Use and Toxicity. Nutrients. 2021;13(5):1703.
24. Suo L, VanBuren C, Hovland ED, Kedishvili NY, Sundberg JP, Everts HB. Dietary Vitamin A Impacts Refractory Telogen. Front Cell Dev Biol. 2021;571474.
25. Liggins MC, Zhang LJ, Dokoshi T, Gallo RL. Retinoids Enhance the Expression of Cathelicidin Antimicrobial Peptide during Reactive Dermal Adipogenesis. J Immunol. 2019;203(6):1589-97.
26. Schröder JM., Seeing Is Believing: Vitamin A Promotes Skin Health through a Host-Derived Antibiotic. Cell Host Microbe. 2019;25(6):769-70.

02

Vitamins B1, B2, and B5

Vitamins B1, B2, and B5

Rohit Batra

CONTENTS

VITAMINS B1, B2, AND B5: NUTRIENT SNAPSHOT
- REQUIREMENT IN THE INDIAN CONTEXT | 12
- ACTIVE FORMS | 13
- SAFETY AND DOSAGE | 13
- CLINICAL CONDITIONS | 14
- SUPPLEMENTATION | 18

INTRODUCTION | 20

DIGESTION, ABSORPTION AND STORAGE | 20

MECHANISM OF ACTION | 20

KEY TOPICS
- ACNE BLEMISHES
- ACNE VULGARIS
- COLLAGEN SYNTHESIS
- HAIR AGING
- HAIR FOLLICLE GROWTH
- HAIR LOSS
- TELOGEN EFFLUVIUM
- UV PROTECTION
- WOUND HEALING

Nutrient Snapshot

▶ **REQUIREMENT IN THE INDIAN CONTEXT**

- Three of the B-vitamins, thiamine (vitamin B1), riboflavin (vitamin B2) and pantothenic acid (vitamin B5) are essential to many biological reactions and are required to convert food to energy.

- Thiamine, occurs mainly in its enzymatic forms, which play a role in carbohydrate and fat metabolism. Riboflavin is a catalyst for redox reactions. Pantothenic acid is a precursor in the synthesis of coenzyme A, which is essential to many biochemical reactions, especially those involving fatty acid metabolism.

- They are found in a variety of foods, but they are also lost by food storage and processing. In India, an overall insufficiency of B-complex vitamins has been reported based on nonspecific symptoms. Their requirement may be higher in patients with metabolic disorders such as diabetes,[1] obesity, with malabsorption issues, and alcohol abuse.[2]

- Dietary supplements of these vitamins are mostly available in combination with other nutrients in multivitamin/multimineral products. They are often used for general wellness as these processes likely affect all aspects of wellness. In dermatology, the use of multivitamin/multimineral products are used for hair growth or prevent hair loss, and can also be added to skin care therapies.

- It is important to note that these vitamins are beneficial only in cases of hypovitaminosis or specific states associated with functional lack of the vitamin. It is advisable to use recommended doses to achieve sufficiency.

▶ ACTIVE FORMS

ACTIVE FORMS	SUPPLEMENT SOURCES	SALIENT FEATURES
B1: Thiamine pyrophosphate	Synthetic	High blood levels of thiamine can be achieved rapidly with oral supplementation.[3] Thiamine hydrochloride is used in liquids because of its high solubility, whereas the low hygroscopicity of thiamine mononitrate makes it better suited for use in dry products.[4]
B2: Riboflavin	Synthetic	Compared to other B-vitamins, vitamin B2 does not accumulate in the body after stopping supplementation, and must be acquired regularly from the diet or supplements.[5]
B5: Pantothenic acid	Synthetic calcium pantothenate or other salts	The bioavailability of pantothenic acid in various forms is not studied.[6]

▶ SAFETY AND DOSAGE

GENERAL REQUIREMENTS	
Indian recommendations	**RDA 2020:** B1 – Male: 1.4–2.3 mg, Female: 1.4–2.2 mg/day B2 – Male: 2.0–3.2 mg, Female: 1.9–3.1 mg/day B5 – Adequate intake (AI): 5 mg/day The TUL for these vitamins has not been established.
Global recommendations and limits	**NIH RDA:** B1 – Male: 1.2 mg, Female: 1.1 mg B2 – Male: 1.3 mg, Female: 1.1 mg B5 – Adequate intake (AI): 5 mg/day
	EFSA: B1 – Dietary reference value (DRV): Male (19–65 years): 1.2-1.3 mg, Female (19–65 years): 1 mg/ day[7,8] B2 – Average requirement (AR): 1.3 mg/day[8,9] B5 – Adequate intake (AI): 5 mg/day[8,10]

▶ SAFETY AND DOSAGE (Continued)

GENERAL REQUIREMENTS	
Notes:	Little or no toxicity has been associated with dietary and supplemental forms of these vitamins. Therefore, the TUL has not been established.
	In the absence of clinical signs of deficiencies, the RDAs of vitamins B1, B2, and B5 should be used, even though they are water-soluble. Additional dosage may either lead to imbalances between B-vitamins, and are unlikely to offer any additional benefit.
	Oral contraceptives (containing estrogen and progestin) and diuretics may increase the requirement of vitamins B1, B2, and B5. However, this has not been clinically validated to date.[11] Long term use of antidepressants, other drugs and alcohol may also affect their status. Taking a daily multivitamin should provide sufficiency of these vitamins.
	A derivative of vitamin B5, pantethine, has lipid-lowering activity, and may be used synergistically with statins and niacin.[12]

▶ CLINICAL CONDITIONS

EVIDENCE LEVEL	CONDITION OR USE CASE	DOSAGE	BENEFIT OR MECHANISM OF ACTION
+++	Wound healing (vitamin B1)	Rats were divided into three dietary groups and fed either a thiamine-deficient diet, a thiamine-deficient diet supplemented with 1 mg thiamine-HCl or a thiamine-deficient diet supplemented with 3 mg thiamine-HCl.	The changes observed in the wounded skin of rats demonstrated an involvement of thiamine in wound repair and scar development.[13]
+++	Wound healing (vitamin B2)	Mice either ingested a control diet, riboflavin deficient diet or food restricted weight-matched diet.	A lower tensile strength was observed in the riboflavin-deficient rats. The data suggest that alteration in collagen content and its maturity at the incision wound of the rat's skin may be responsible.[14]

▶ CLINICAL CONDITIONS (Continued)

EVIDENCE LEVEL	CONDITION OR USE CASE	DOSAGE	BENEFIT OR MECHANISM OF ACTION
+++	Wound healing (vitamin B5)	Rabbits were injected with pantothenic acid (20 mg/kg body weight/24 hours) for 3 weeks and compared to a control group. Deficient animals were fed with a pantothenate free diet for 3 weeks.	This animal study suggests that pantothenic acid induces an accelerating effect of the normal healing process. The mechanism responsible for this improvement is increase in cellular multiplication during the first postoperative period.[15]
++	Collagen synthesis (vitamin B5)	Keratinocytes and fibroblasts were cultured with or without pantothenic acid supplemented medium.	The depletion of pantothenic acid from the culture medium suppressed keratinocyte proliferation and promoted differentiation. The pantothenic acid depletion decreased the synthesis of keratinocyte growth factor and procollagen in fibroblasts, thus suggesting that pantothenic acid is essential for maintaining keratinocyte proliferation and differentiation.[16]
++	UV protection (vitamin B5)	Human epidermal keratinocytes were incubated with the oral formulation: L-cystine, thiamine, calcium D-Pantothenate and folic acid in vitro.	This study demonstrated that L-cystine and thiamine are essential for keratinocyte metabolism and proliferation. The formulation prevented UV-induced reduction in metabolic activity.[17]

▶ **CLINICAL CONDITIONS** (*Continued*)

EVIDENCE LEVEL	CONDITION OR USE CASE	DOSAGE	BENEFIT OR MECHANISM OF ACTION
+++	Acne vulgaris (vitamin B5)	Subjects were administered two tablets twice a day for 12 weeks. Each four-tablet dose of the study agent contained 2.2 g of pantothenic acid.	There was a mean reduction in total lesion count in the pantothenic acid group vs. placebo at week 12. The mean reduction in inflammatory lesions was also reduced and Dermatology Life Quality Index (DLQI) scores were lower at week 12 in the pantothenic acid group versus placebo.[18]
+++	Acne blemishes (B complex vitamins)	Subjects ingested a dietary supplement (two tablets) containing B1:1.5 mg, B2: 1.7 mg, B3: 20 mg, B6: 2 mg, B9: 400 µg, B12: 6 µg, biotin: 300 µg, B5: 2.2 g and L-carnitine: 733.3 mg twice a day for 8 weeks	The administration of the supplement significantly reduced global facial blemishes.[19]
+++	Telogen effluvium (vitamin B1 and B5)	Supplement containing L-cystine 20 mg, keratin 20 mg, medicinal yeast 100 mg, calcium pantothenate 60 mg, thiamine nitrate 60 mg, PABA 20 mg. One capsule 3 times a day for 6 months.	The treatment showed improvement and normalization of the mean anagen hair rate within 6 months of the treatment. The appearance of hair growth in the global photographic assessment was better in the treatment group than placebo.[20]

▶ CLINICAL CONDITIONS (Continued)

EVIDENCE LEVEL	CONDITION OR USE CASE	DOSAGE	BENEFIT OR MECHANISM OF ACTION
+++	Hair loss (vitamin B5)	Subjects were divided into four groups: Group 1 took zinc sulfate (50 mg elemental zinc) + calcium pantothenate (100 mg) twice a week. Group 2 and 3 ingested either one zinc capsule/ B5 tablet once a day. Group 4 had to apply 2% minoxidil solution twice daily in the scalp. Study period was 4 months	The increase in primary hair count and thickness was the same in all the groups, compared to baseline. Hair density increments were more obvious in the minoxidil group, and hair thickness increments were more obvious in pantothenate group. Participants' satisfaction was 85% in the combination therapy, which was more than other groups. Based on this, the combination of zinc sulfate and calcium pantothenate, when administered intermittently, could be a good choice for hair loss control in its initial stages.[21]
++	Hair follicle growth (vitamin B5)	Mink hair follicles (HFs) and dermal papilla (DP) cell culture were treated with 0, 10, 20, 40 µg/mL pantothenic acid in vitro.	The in vitro study demonstrates the pantothenic acid stimulates growth of hair follicle cells and dermal papillae cell proliferation.[22]
++	Aging-related changes in hair (vitamin B5)	Human hair follicle cells, including dermal papilla cells (hDPCs) and outer root sheath cells (hORSCs) were treated with D-panthenol in vitro.	The in vitro study suggests that the hair growth stimulating activity of D-Panthenol was exerted by increasing the cell viability, suppressing the apoptotic markers, and elongating the anagen phase in hair follicles.[23]

▶ CLINICAL CONDITIONS (Continued)

EVIDENCE LEVEL	CONDITION OR USE CASE	DOSAGE	BENEFIT OR MECHANISM OF ACTION
++	Wound healing (B-complex vitamins)	Vitamins B and C were tested individually or in combination on their ability to promote the proliferation and migration of human skin fibroblasts and keratinocytes in vitro.	A reduction in initial wound area was achieved by several combinations of vitamins, compared to untreated control. The expression of the cell migration marker, CXCR4 increased in fibroblasts with the vitamin combination.[24]

▶ SUPPLEMENTATION

	BASIS	WHAT TO LOOK OUT FOR
Supplementation form	B1: Thiamine chloride hydrochloride Thiamine mononitrate B2: Riboflavin Riboflavin 5'- phosphate sodium B5: Calcium pantothenate Sodium pantothenate D-Panthenol DL-Panthenol	The form of vitamin B used in the product is stated on the ingredients list of the product packaging.
Administration form	Capsules, tablets, gummies, soft gels, syrups, powders, chewable tablets, sublingual, strips	N/A
Purity considerations	Synthetic vitamins normally have >99% purity.	N/A
Patient considerations	It is suggested to take vitamin B2 with the meal. Normally antibiotic use increases the demand of nutrients. However, B-complex vitamins (like vitamin B5) should not be taken alongside antibiotics (e.g., tetracycline) as there may be competitive inhibition. A gap of a few hours should suffice.	

▶ SUPPLEMENTATION (Continued)

	BASIS	WHAT TO LOOK OUT FOR
Safety considerations	The lack of toxicity of B1 may be explained by the rapid decline in the absorption of thiamine at intakes above 5 mg. The Food and Nutrition Board (Institute of Medicine) suggests that despite the lack of evidence of adverse effects, excessive intakes of thiamine could have adverse effects.[24] There are no known adverse effects of consuming these B vitamins, however, it is recommended to exercise caution in case of exceeding the RDA dose.[25] Oral intakes of vitamin B5 above 5 mg may lower its efficacy of absorption. Some individuals taking large doses (e.g., 10 g/day) develop mild diarrhea and gastrointestinal distress, but the mechanism for this effect is not known.[6,26]	There has been some apprehension for several decades about how harmless generous doses of these vitamins are, thus it is advised to not exceed the RDA as it may lead to non-specific side effects.[27]
Other considerations	B1 has contraindicated in certain chemotherapy drugs which increase thiamine metabolism.[24]	Individuals with clinical conditions and on medication are advised to seek doctor's consultation before starting any nutritional supplementation.

▶ INTRODUCTION

The two major contributors to cellular aging are accumulation of DNA damage, and the resulting mitochondrial dysfunction. By supporting key enzymatic reactions for energy production by mitochondria, B-vitamins can help deter the changes that occur with cellular aging.

Inside the cell, vitamin B1 or thiamine is transformed into its active form called thiamine pyrophosphate (TPP), which requires the presence of magnesium and adenosine triphosphate (ATP; cellular energy). TPP serves as an important cofactor in various reactions for the metabolism of carbohydrates and branched-chain amino acids. It is essential for other cellular processes, including the synthesis of nucleic acid precursors, myelin, and neurotransmitters (like acetylcholine), as well as antioxidant defences.[26]

Riboflavin or vitamin B2 is an integral component of two enzymes, flavin mononucleotide (FMN) and flavin-adenine dinucleotide (FAD). These flavoproteins function as a catalyst for redox reactions in numerous metabolic pathways and in cellular energy production. They are also involved in synthesis of coenzyme A, coenzyme Q10, heme, pyridoxal 5-phosphate (active form of vitamin B6), and various hormones.[26]

Pantothenic acid or vitamin B5 is essential for the synthesis of coenzyme A (CoA) and acyl-carrier protein (ACP), both of which are required for fat metabolism. CoA is also involved in processing carbohydrates and proteins and for synthesis of fatty acids, cholesterol, acetylcholine, bile acids, and others. It also plays a role in regulation of metabolism and gene expression.[26]

▶ DIGESTION, ABSORPTION AND STORAGE

Digestion and Absorption

- Following ingestion, absorption of these B-vitamins occurs mainly in the small intestine, at lower concentrations by an active, carrier-mediated system, and at higher concentrations, by passive diffusion.[28,29]

- The absorption of these B vitamins can be influenced by factors such as the presence of other nutrients (like fat and protein) and individual variations.

Storage

- Like all B vitamins, these are water soluble, and the body does not store them.

▶ MECHANISM OF ACTION

These vitamins are involved in the conversion of food to energy, and so they are required for a number of processes that maintain skin, and consequently, hair health.

01 | Anti-inflammatory Action and Promoting Skin Barrier

By virtue of their role in lipid metabolism, vitamin B1, B2, and B5 are involved in barrier function.

- By supporting the breakdown of fatty acids, they regulate the production of lipid mediators, such as prostaglandins and leukotrienes, which are involved in inflammation.

- These vitamins are involved in the availability of fatty acids and sphingosine for ceramide synthesis.

- They are required for regulating immunity. Their deficiencies lead to pro-inflammatory responses (increase in IL-1, IL-8, TNF-α, NF-κB), disturbance of our gut's tight junction proteins and antioxidant enzymes, and aberrant antibody responses.[30]

- Vitamin B2 participates in the production of glutathione, an antioxidant that helps protect cells from oxidative stress.

- Vitamin B5 may regulate epidermal barrier function through proliferation and differentiation of keratinocytes via CoA metabolism.[31] It is often used for acne vulgaris and photoprotection. This is relevant in wound healing and various dermatosis. An improvement in elasticity and hydration has been reported with topical use of vitamin B5.[32]

02 | Promoting Hair Growth

These vitamins are not directly linked to hair growth but are available in many supplements for the same. This is because they are required for mitochondrial respiration – the production of ATP – which is essential for the rapidly growing cells in the hair follicle. Mitochondrial dysfunction, associated with aging, is thought to be a driving force for hair thinning and many types of hair loss.

Furthermore, vitamin B2 helps convert tryptophan to niacin, which converts vitamin B6 to its active, coenzyme form, pyridoxal 5′-phosphate. Studies have found that a deficiency of vitamin B2 can result in alopecia.[33]

▶ REFERENCES

1. Thornalley PJ, Babaei-Jadidi R, Al Ali H, Rabbani N, Antonysunil A, Larkin J, et al. High prevalence of low plasma thiamine concentration in diabetes linked to a marker of vascular disease. Diabetologia. 2007;50(10):2164-70.
2. Marrs C, Lonsdale D. Hiding in Plain Sight: Modern Thiamine Deficiency. Cells. 2021;10(10):2595.
3. Smithline HA, Donnino M, Greenblatt DJ. Pharmacokinetics of high-dose oral thiamine hydrochloride in healthy subjects. BMC Clinical Pharmacology. 2012;12:4.
4. Voelker A, Miller J, Running CA, Taylor LS, Mauer LJ. Chemical stability and reaction kinetics of two thiamine salts (thiamine mononitrate and thiamine chloride hydrochloride) in solution. Food Res Int. 2018;112:443-56.
5. Lindschinger M, Tatzber F, Schimetta W, Schmid I, Lindschinger B, Cvirn G, et al. A Randomized Pilot Trial to Evaluate the Bioavailability of Natural versus Synthetic Vitamin B Complexes in Healthy Humans and Their Effects on Homocysteine, Oxidative Stress, and Antioxidant Levels. Oxid Med Cell Longev. 2019:6082613.
6. Fact Sheet for Health Professionals. Pantothenic Acid [Online]. Available from: https://ods.od.nih.gov/factsheets/PantothenicAcid-HealthProfessional/
7. EFSA Panel on Dietetic Products, Nutrition and Allergies (NDA), Turck D, Bresson JL, Burlingame B, Dean T, Fairweather-Tait S, et al. Dietary reference values for thiamin. EFSA Journal. 2016;14(12):e04653.
8. Overview on Tolerable Upper Intake Levels as derived by the Scientific Committee on Food (SCF) and the EFSA Panel on Dietetic Products, Nutrition and Allergies (NDA). | European Food Safety Authority. 2024.
9. EFSA Panel on Dietetic Products, Nutrition and Allergies (NDA), Turck D, Bresson JL, Burlingame B, Dean T, Fairweather-Tait S, et al. Dietary Reference Values for riboflavin. EFSA Journal. 2017;15(8):e04919.
10. EFSA Panel on Dietetic Products, Nutrition and Allergies (NDA). Scientific Opinion on Dietary Reference Values for pantothenic acid. EFSA Journal. 2014;12(2):3581.
11. Lewis CM, King JC. Effect of oral contraceptives agents on thiamin, riboflavin, and pantothenic acid status in young women. Am J Clin Nutr. 1980;33(4):832-8.
12. Evans M, Rumberger JA, Azumano I, Napolitano JJ, Citrolo D, Kamiya T. Pantethine, a derivative of vitamin B5, favorably alters total, LDL and non-HDL cholesterol in low to moderate cardiovascular risk subjects eligible for statin therapy: a triple-blinded placebo and diet-controlled investigation. Vasc Health Risk Manag. 2014:10:89-100.
13. Alvarez OM, Gilbreath RL. Effect of dietary thiamine on intermolecular collagen cross-linking during wound repair: a mechanical and biochemical assessment. J Trauma. 1982;22(1):20-4.
14. R Lakshmi, AV Lakshmi, MS Bamji. Skin wound healing in riboflavin deficiency. Biochem Med Metab Biol. 1989;42(3):185-91.
15. M Aprahamian, A Dentinger, C Stock-Damgé, JC Kouassi, JF Grenier. Effects of supplemental pantothenic acid on wound healing: experimental study in rabbit. Am J Clin Nutr. 1985;41(3):578-89.
16. Kobayashi D, Kusama M, Onda M, Nakahata N. The effect of pantothenic acid deficiency on keratinocyte proliferation and the synthesis of keratinocyte growth factor and collagen in fibroblasts. J Pharmacol Sci. 2011;115(2):230-4.
17. Hengl T, Herfert J, Soliman A, Schlinzig K, Trüeb RM, Abts HF. Cystine-thiamin-containing hair-growth formulation modulates the response to UV radiation in an in vitro model for growth-limiting conditions of human keratinocytes. J Photochem Photobiol B. 2018:189:318-25.
18. Yang M, Moclair B, Hatcher V, Kaminetsky J, Mekas M, Chapas A, et al. A Randomized, Double-Blind, Placebo-Controlled Study of a Novel Pantothenic Acid-Based Dietary Supplement in Subjects with Mild to Moderate Facial Acne. Dermatol Ther (Heidelb). 2014;4(1):93-101.
19. Capodice JL. Feasibility, Tolerability, Safety and Efficacy of a Pantothenic Acid Based Dietary Supplement in Subjects with Mild to Moderate Facial Acne Blemishes. JCDSA. 2012;2(3):132-5.
20. Lengg N, Heidecker B, Seifert B, Trueb RM. Dietary supplement increases anagen hair rate in women with telogen effluvium: result of a double-blind, placebo-controlled trail. Therapy. 2007;4(1):59-65.
21. Siavash M, Tavakoli F, Mokhtari F. Comparing the Effects of Zinc Sulfate, Calcium Pantothenate, Their Combination and Minoxidil Solution Regimens on Controlling Hair Loss in Women: A Randomized Controlled Trial. J Res Pharm Pract. 2017;6(2):89-93.
22. Wang Z, Nan W, Si H, Wang S, Zhang H, Li G. Pantothenic acid promotes dermal papilla cell proliferation in hair follicles of American minks via inhibitor of DNA Binding 3/Notch signaling pathway. Life Sci. 2020;252:117667.
23. Shin JY, Kim J, Choi YH, Kang NG, Lee S. Dexpanthenol Promotes Cell Growth by Preventing Cell Senescence and Apoptosis in Cultured Human Hair Follicle Cells. Curr Issues Mol Biol. 2021;43(3):1361-73.

24. Fact Sheet for Health Professionals. Thiamin. Available from: https://ods.od.nih.gov/factsheets/Thiamin-HealthProfessional/
25. Fact Sheet for Health Professionals. Riboflavin. Available from: https://ods.od.nih.gov/factsheets/Riboflavin-HealthProfessional/
26. Hrubša M, Siatka T, Nejmanová I, Vopršalová M, Krčmová LK, Matoušová K, et al. Biological Properties of Vitamins of the B-Complex, Part 1: Vitamins B1, B2, B3, and B5. Nutrients. 2022;14(3):484.
27. Jasvinder Chawla, David Kvarnberg. Hydrosoluble vitamins. Handb Clin Neurol. 2014:120:891-914.
28. Folate I of M (US) SC on the SE of DRI and its P on, Vitamins OB, Choline A. Riboflavin. In: Dietary Reference Intakes for Thiamin, Riboflavin, Niacin, Vitamin B6, Folate, Vitamin B12, Pantothenic Acid, Biotin, and Choline. National Academies Press (US); 1998.
29. Dietary Reference Intakes for Thiamin, Riboflavin, Niacin, Vitamin B6, Folate, Vitamin B12, Pantothenic Acid, Biotin, and Choline - NCBI Bookshelf.
30. Mikkelsen K, Apostolopoulos V. Vitamin B1, B2, B3, B5, and B6 and the Immune System. In: Mahmoudi M, Rezaei N, editors. Nutrition and Immunity. Cham: Springer International Publishing. 2019. pp. 115–25.
31. Kelly GS. Pantothenic acid. Monograph. Altern Med Rev. 2011;16(3):263-74.
32. Ebner F, Heller A, Rippke F, Tausch I. Topical use of dexpanthenol in skin disorders. Am J Clin Dermatol. 2002;3(6):427-33.
33. Almohanna HM, Ahmed AA, Tsatalis JP, Tosti A. The Role of Vitamins and Minerals in Hair Loss: A Review. Dermatol Ther (Heidelb). 2018;9(1):51-70.

Nutrition in Dermatology

03

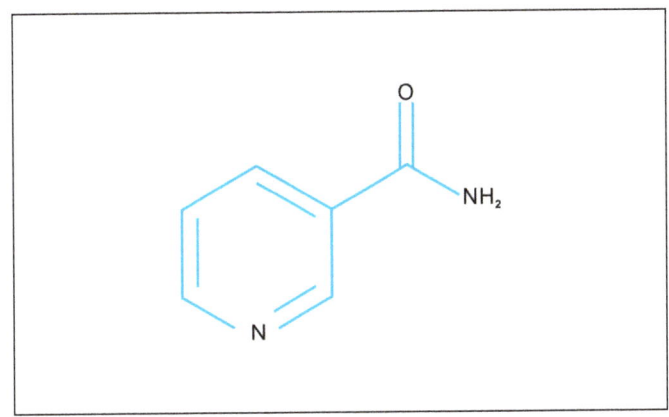

Niacinamide

Niacin (Vitamin B3)

✍ Rohit Batra

CONTENTS

NIACIN (VITAMIN B3): NUTRIENT SNAPSHOT
- ▶ REQUIREMENT IN THE INDIAN CONTEXT | 24
- ▶ ACTIVE FORMS | 25
- ▶ SAFETY AND DOSAGE | 25
- ▶ CLINICAL CONDITIONS | 26
- ▶ SUPPLEMENTATION | 29

INTRODUCTION | 30
DIGESTION, ABSORPTION AND STORAGE | 30
MECHANISM OF ACTION | 30

KEY TOPICS
- ACNE VULGARIS
- CELLULAR AGING
- CUTANEOUS PIGMENTATION
- PHOTOAGING
- PHOTOIMMUNOSUPPRESSION
- ROSACEA
- SKIN BARRIER FUNCTION
- SKIN CANCER
- WOUND HEALING

Nutrient Snapshot

▶ **REQUIREMENT IN THE INDIAN CONTEXT**

- Living organisms derive energy from redox reactions. Dietary precursors of nicotinamide adenine dinucleotide (NAD), including nicotinic acid, nicotinamide, and nicotinamide riboside, are collectively referred to as niacin or vitamin B3. Over 400 enzymes require the niacin coenzymes, NAD and its phosphorylated form, NADP, mainly to accept or donate electrons for redox reactions, and for genome stability.

- In dermatology, topical nicotinamide is often used in the treatment of aging skin, acne vulgaris, melasma, atopic dermatitis, and rosacea, and orally administered for skin cancer.[1,2]

- Niacin is found in plant foods, particularly nuts and oil seeds, while niacinamide in animal foods. The amino acid, tryptophan, can be converted to nicotinamide in the liver, so it can satisfy the requirement for dietary niacin.[3]

- The average intake of niacin in India is believed to be nearly 10 mg/day, while the recommended dietary allowance (RDA) is approximately 11–14 mg. About 25% is thought to be lost upon cooking, so there may still be an insufficiency, but unlikely to be a serious deficiency in a standard Indian diet. This is especially true in the cases of calorie restriction and specialized diets, as niacin levels depend on energy and protein intake. While there are no adverse effects from dietary niacin, high doses from supplements can cause discomfort. However, recommended doses can help meet an insufficiency that may exist.[3]

Nutrition in Dermatology

▶ ACTIVE FORMS

ACTIVE FORMS	SUPPLEMENT SOURCES	SALIENT FEATURES
Niacin	Synthetic	B3 is absorbed well in the body. Even very high doses of niacin are almost completely absorbed.[4] Niacin is the generic name for nicotinic acid, nicotinamide, and related derivatives, such as nicotinamide riboside.
Niacin-related derivatives, such as nicotinamide mononucleotide (NMN)	Synthetic	All forms of vitamin B3, as well as NMN, are converted to NAD+, and may help combat age-related issues.

▶ SAFETY AND DOSAGE

GENERAL REQUIREMENTS		
Indian recommendations	RDA 2020: Male—14–23 mg, Female—11–18 mg/day TUL: 35 mg/day	
Global recommendations and limits	NIH RDA: Male—16 mg, Female—14 mg/day TUL: 35 mg/day	
	EFSA: Average requirement (AR)-1.3 mg /MJ* TUL: Nicotinamide-900 mg, Nicotinic acid-10 mg/day[5]	
	NOAEL: 200 mg/kg BW/day	
Notes:	1 mg of niacin is defined as 1 mg niacin equivalent (NE). Approximately 60 mg of tryptophan yields 1 mg of niacin, which is also defined as 1 mg NE.[5] In the absence of clinical signs of deficiencies, the RDAs of niacin should be prescribed, even though it is water-soluble. Niacin has a very low TUL, and megadoses may not offer any additional benefit. Niacin supplementation at RDA doses must be considered for diets with energy restriction or protein restriction.[5] 250 mg of NMN has been safely used long-term.[6]	
*Niacin requirement is strongly dependent on energy intake, so EFSA measures its units in milligrams per megajoule (MJ) of energy consumed rather than mg/day. As the conversion is 1 MJ = 239 kcal, an adult consuming 2,000 kilocalories should be consuming 10.9 mg niacin.		

▶ **CLINICAL CONDITIONS**

EVIDENCE LEVEL	CONDITION OR USE CASE	DOSAGE	BENEFIT OR MECHANISM OF ACTION
+++	Photoimmunosuppresion	Mice were fed a diet supplemented with 0%, 0.1%, 0.5%, or 1% niacin throughout the experiment and five exposures (30 minutes each) of UV irradiation per week.	This study demonstrated a dose-dependent preventive effect of oral niacin on incidence photocarcinogenesis and photoimmunosuppression. It also established the capacity of oral niacin to elevate skin NAD levels, which is known to modulate the function of DNA strand scission surveillance proteins p53 and poly(ADP-ribose) polymerase, two proteins critical in cellular responses to UV-induced DNA damage.[7]
++	Skin cancer	N/A (observational study)	The study evaluated whether total, dietary and supplemental niacin intake was associated with skin cancer risk. It supports a potential beneficial role of niacin intake in relation to squamous cell carcinoma but not to basal cell carcinoma or melanoma.[8]
+++++	Skin cancer	Subjects who had at least two nonmelanoma skin cancers in the previous 5 years received 500 mg of nicotinamide twice daily or placebo for 12 months.	At 12 months, the rate of new nonmelanoma skin cancers was lower in the nicotinamide group vs. placebo. Similar differences were found between the nicotinamide group and the placebo with respect to new basal-cell and new squamous-cell carcinomas, with lower rates with nicotinamide. The number of actinic keratoses was lower in the nicotinamide group than in the placebo group. There was no evidence of benefit seen after nicotinamide was discontinued.[9]

▶ CLINICAL CONDITIONS (Continued)

EVIDENCE LEVEL	CONDITION OR USE CASE	DOSAGE	BENEFIT OR MECHANISM OF ACTION
++	Skin barrier function	Human keratinocytes were incubated with 1–30 mM/L nicotinamide for 6 days in vitro.	The rate of ceramide biosynthesis was increased dose-dependently compared with control. The activity of serine palmitoyltransferase (SPT), the rate-limiting enzyme in sphingolipid synthesis, was increased in nicotinamide-treated cells. Nicotinamide increased not only ceramide synthesis but also free fatty acid and cholesterol synthesis.[10]
+++	UV-induced photoaging	Mice were divided into six groups and ingested supplements before and after UV radiation: *Group 1*: Placebo *Group 2*: Was exposed to UV radiation, *Group 3*: Vitamin C *Group 4*: Nicotinamide mononucleotide (NMN; 300 mg/kg) *Group 5*: Lactic acid bacteria (LAB) *Group 6*: A combination of NMN (300 mg/kg) and LAB	NMN combined with *Limosilactobacillus fermentum* improved murine skin damage caused by UVB irradiation, and the protective mechanism may be related to activation of the AMPK signaling pathway.[11]
++	Aging-related cellular changes	Fibroblasts cells from the skin of an old age female were treated with nicotinamide in vitro.	The study showed that there are changes in mitochondrial functionality with aging and that nicotinamide treatment can restore bioenergetic efficiency and capacity in older fibroblasts with an amplifying effect in younger cells.[12]

▶ CLINICAL CONDITIONS (Continued)

EVIDENCE LEVEL	CONDITION OR USE CASE	DOSAGE	BENEFIT OR MECHANISM OF ACTION
++	Cutaneous pigmentation	A coculture of keratinocyte and melanocytes model and a pigmented reconstructed epidermis (PREP) model were treated with niacinamide in vitro.	The study demonstrated that niacinamide treatment led to 35–68% inhibition of melanosome transfer in the coculture model and reduced cutaneous pigmentation in the PREP model.[13]
++	Wound healing	Dermal fibroblasts from human skin were treated with 0.31 mg/mL niacinamide, 0.10 mg/mL l-carnosine, 0.05 mg/mL hesperidin and 5.18 µg/mL Biofactor HSP® for 24 hours.	Results showed that the niacinamide-dominated formulation proved optimal in vitro. The results show that fibroblast collagen synthesis was increased alongside cellular migration and proliferation.[14]
+++	Acne vulgaris and rosacea	Subjects ingested a formulation containing nicotinamide 750 mg, zinc 25 mg, copper 1.5 mg, and folic acid 500 µg for 4–8 weeks.	Nicotinamide and zinc supplementation appears to be an effective oral therapy for the treatment of acne vulgaris and rosacea when used alone or with other topical therapies and should be considered a useful alternative approach to oral antibiotics for the treatment of acne vulgaris and rosacea.[15]
+++	Acne vulgaris	Subjects ingested 1–4 NicAzel tablets (composed of nicotinamide, azelaic acid, zinc, pyridoxine, copper, and folic acid) daily for 8 weeks (formulation not available).	Several patients demonstrated improvement over their previous acne treatment regimens after both 4 and 8 weeks of NicAzel use. At week 8, 88% of the patients experienced a visible reduction in inflammatory lesions, and 81% of the patients rated their appearance as much or moderately better compared with baseline. 76% of patients thought NicAzel was as effective as previous treatment with oral antibiotics.[16]

▶ SUPPLEMENTATION

	BASIS	WHAT TO LOOK OUT FOR
Supplementation form	• Nicotinic acid • Nicotinamide/Niacinamide • NMN (nicotinamide mononucleotide) Nicotinic acid has been shown to cause skin flushing.[4]	The form of vitamin B3 is stated on the product packaging. B3 can be written as niacinamide in the ingredients list by the company as it is often used interchangeably with nicotinamide.[17]
Administration form	Capsules, tablets, soft gels, chewable tablets, gummies, lozenges, syrups	N/A
Purity considerations	Synthetic forms are >99% pure	N/A
Patient considerations	B3 is absorbed well with or without food.	
Safety considerations	A most common side effect of B3 supplementation is skin flushing which is specific to the form of niacin[4] but high doses may also lead to diarrhea, headache, stomach discomfort, and bloating.	Though vitamin B3 is a water-soluble vitamin and large doses are excreted through urine it is advised not to exceed recommended doses as chronic megadoses have the potential to cause adverse effects.
Other considerations	Nicotinamide is contraindicated in renal patients as it has led to thrombocytopenia in hemodialysis patients.[18] High doses (gram doses) can raise blood glucose levels and thus diabetic patients are recommended to check with their doctor before taking very high B3 through supplementation.[4]	Individuals with clinical conditions and on medication are advised to seek a doctor's consultation before starting any nutritional supplementation.

INTRODUCTION

The redox pairs NADH/NAD⁺ and NADPH/NADP⁺ play an essential role in the metabolism of all organisms. They were originally discovered for their universal roles as co-enzymes to drive biosynthetic reactions.[19] The deficiency of their precursor, niacin, causes a disease called pellagra, which is characterized by symptoms affecting the skin, the digestive system, and the nervous system.[20]

DIGESTION, ABSORPTION AND STORAGE

Digestion and Absorption

Absorption of nicotinic acid and nicotinamide from the intestine is rapid. At low concentrations, it is mediated by sodium ion-dependent facilitated diffusion, while passive diffusion dominates at higher concentrations.[20]

Storage

Like all B vitamins, these are a water soluble and the body does not store it. The excess is stored in minute amounts in the liver and the rest is excreted in urine.[20]

MECHANISM OF ACTION

Nicotinamide is mainly involved in the cellular energy metabolism, DNA repair, and in regulation of transcription processes.[21]

01 | Energy Production and Photoprotection

As a precursor of NAD and NADP, niacin prevents the depletion of cellular energy. NAD is involved in the production of energy from carbohydrates, fats and proteins. NADP generally serves in biosynthetic reactions, such as in the synthesis of fatty acids and steroid hormones, cholesterol and bile. NADP is also essential for the regeneration of antioxidants and for calcium mobilization.[19]

NAD⁺ is also the substrate for the DNA repair enzyme poly (ADP ribose) polymerase 1 (PARP1). It is important in DNA unwinding to provide access to other enzymes involved in DNA repair.[22]

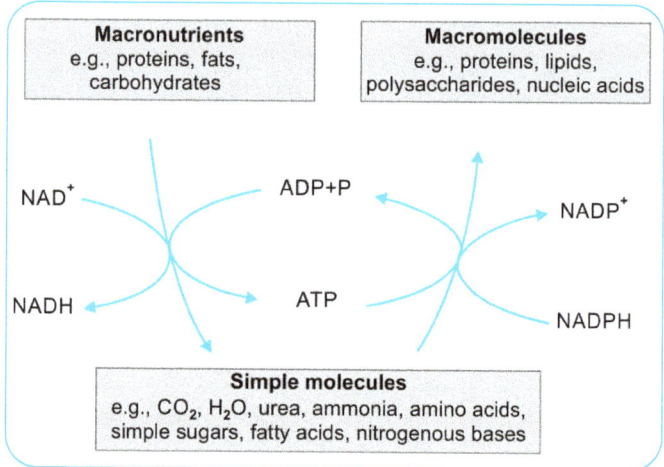

Note:
- *On the left*: In catabolic pathways, the oxidation of macronutrients is coupled with the reduction of NAD⁺; NAD⁺ accepts electrons and becomes reduced (NADH).
- *On the right*: In anabolic pathways, the oxidation of NADPH provides electrons needed for the biosynthesis of macromolecules; NADPH donates electrons and become oxidized (NADP⁺).

Figure 1: Simplified overview of NAD/NADP function in catabolic and anabolic pathways.

Thus, it makes sense that niacin deficiency can lead to severe sunlight sensitivity in exposed skin, and that niacin is used for skin cancer.[22,23] PARP1 is also one reason for the use of niacinamide for acne vulgaris.[23]

Sirtuins are a class of NAD-dependent enzymes, and their biological functions include cell differentiation, cell cycle regulation, gene silencing, and DNA damage repair. They are energy-sensing regulators involved in signaling pathways that counter the decline in cellular health that accompanies aging **(Figure 1)**.

02 | Anti-inflammatory Effect

Nicotinamide inhibits cytokines such as IL-1β, IL-6, IL-8, and TNF by controlling NF-κB (nuclear factor kappa-light-chain-enhancer of activated B cells) mediated transcription. That's why it is important in the management of acne vulgaris and autoimmune disorders like psoriasis.[23-25]

REFERENCES

1. Heidi M Rolfe. A review of nicotinamide: treatment of skin diseases and potential side effects. J Cosmet Dermatol. 2014;13(4):324-8.
2. Gehring W. Nicotinic acid/niacinamide and the skin. J Cosmet Dermatol. 2004;3(2):88-93.
3. National Institute of Nutrition Indian Council of Medical Research. Recommended Dietary Allowances and Estimated Average Requirements for Indians–2020. RDA Full Report 2020.
4. Fact Sheet for Health Professionals. Niacin [Online]. Available from: https://ods.od.nih.gov/factsheets/Niacin-HealthProfessional/
5. Overview on Tolerable Upper Intake Levels as derived by the Scientific Committee on Food (SCF) and the EFSA Panel on Dietetic Products, Nutrition and Allergies (NDA). European Food Safety Authority, 2024.
6. Igarashi Masaki, Nakagawa-Nagahama Yoshiko, Miura Masaomi, Kashiwabara Kosuke, et al. Chronic nicotinamide mononucleotide supplementation elevates blood nicotinamide adenine dinucleotide levels and alters muscle function in healthy older men. npj Aging 8, 5 (2022).
7. Gensler HL, Williams T, Huang AC, Jacobson EL. Oral niacin prevents photocarcinogenesis and photoimmunosuppression in mice. Nutr Cancer. 1999;34(1):36-41.
8. Park SM, Tricia Li WQ, Wu S, Li, Weinstock M, Qureshi AA, et al. Niacin intake and risk of skin cancer in US women and men. Int J Cancer. 2017;140(9):2023-31.
9. Chen AC, Martin AJ, Choy B, Fernández-Peñas P, et al. A Phase 3 Randomized Trial of Nicotinamide for Skin-Cancer Chemoprevention. N Engl J Med. 2015;373(17):1618-26.
10. O Tanno, Y Ota, N Kitamura, T Katsube, S Inoue. Nicotinamide increases biosynthesis of ceramides as well as other stratum corneum lipids to improve the epidermal permeability barrier. Br J Dermatol. 2000;143(3):524-31.
11. Zhou X, Du HH, Ni, Ran J, Hu J, Yu J, et al. Nicotinamide Mononucleotide Combined With *Lactobacillus fermentum* TKSN041 Reduces the Photoaging Damage in Murine Skin by Activating AMPK Signaling Pathway. Front Pharmacol. 2021:12:643089.
12. Oblong JE, Bowman A, Rovito HA, Jarrold BB, Sherrill JD, Black MR, et al. Metabolic dysfunction in human skin: Restoration of mitochondrial integrity and metabolic output by nicotinamide (niacinamide) in primary dermal fibroblasts from older aged donors. Aging Cell. 2020;19(10):e13248.
13. Hakozaki T, Minwalla L, Zhuang J, Chhoa M, Matsubara A, Miyamoto K, et al. The effect of niacinamide on reducing cutaneous pigmentation and suppression of melanosome transfer. Br J Dermatol. 2002;147(1):20-31.
14. Wessels Q, Pretorius E, Smith CM, Nel H. The potential of a niacinamide dominated cosmeceutical formulation on fibroblast activity and wound healing in vitro. Int Wound J. 2012;11(2):152-8.
15. Niren NM, Torok HM. The Nicomide Improvement in Clinical Outcomes Study (NICOS): results of an 8-week trial. Cutis. 2006;77(1 Suppl):17-28.
16. Shalita AR, Falcon R, Olansky A, Iannotta P, Akhavan A, Day D, et al. Inflammatory acne management with a novel prescription dietary supplement. J Drugs Dermatol. 2012;11(12):1428-33.
17. Huber R, Wong A. Nicotinamide: An Update and Review of Safety & Differences from Niacin. Skin Therapy Lett. 2020;25(5):7-11.
18. Lenglet A, Liabeuf S, Esper NE, Brisset S, Mansour J, Lemaire-Hurtel AS, et al. Efficacy and Safety of Nicotinamide in Haemodialysis Patients: The NICOREN Study. Nephrology Dialysis Transplantation 2017;32(5):870-9.
19. Agledal L, Niere M, Ziegler M. The phosphate makes a difference: cellular functions of NADP. Redox Rep. 2010;15(1):2-10.
20. Folate I of M (US) SC on the SE of DRI and its P on, Vitamins OB, Choline A. Niacin. In: Dietary Reference Intakes for Thiamin, Riboflavin, Niacin, Vitamin B6, Folate, Vitamin B12, Pantothenic Acid, Biotin, and Choline [Internet]. National Academies Press (US); 1998 [cited 2024 Jun 19]. Available from: https://www.ncbi.nlm.nih.gov/books/NBK114304/
21. Bains P, Kaur M, Kaur J, Sharma S. Nicotinamide: Mechanism of action and indications in dermatology. IJDVL. 2018;84:234-37.
22. Porter RM, Anstey A. Evidence and conjecture about mechanisms of cutaneous disease in photodermatology. Exp Dermatol. 2014;23(8):543-6.
23. Bj M. Seven sirtuins for seven deadly diseases of aging. Free Radic Biol Med. 2013:56:133-71.
24. Boo YC. Mechanistic Basis and Clinical Evidence for the Applications of Nicotinamide (Niacinamide) to Control Skin Aging and Pigmentation. Antioxidants (Basel). 2021;10(8):1315.
25. Damian DL. Nicotinamide for skin cancer chemoprevention. Australasian Journal of Dermatology. 2017;58(3):174-80.

04

Vitamins B6, B9, and B12

Vitamins B6, B9, and B12

Vitamins B6, B9, and B12

✎ Rohit Batra

CONTENTS

VITAMINS B6, B9, AND B12: NUTRIENT SNAPSHOT

- ▸ REQUIREMENT IN THE INDIAN CONTEXT | 33
- ▸ ACTIVE FORMS | 34
- ▸ SAFETY AND DOSAGE | 34
- ▸ CLINICAL CONDITIONS | 35
- ▸ SUPPLEMENTATION | 40

INTRODUCTION | 43

DIGESTION, ABSORPTION AND STORAGE | 43

MECHANISM OF ACTION | 43

KEY TOPICS

- ALOPECIA AREATA
- ATOPIC DERMATITIS
- COLLAGEN SYNTHESIS
- CUTANEOUS LESIONS
- HAIR FOLLICLE DEVELOPMENT
- HYPERPIGMENTATION
- PAPULOPUSTULAR ROSACEA
- PREMATURE CANITIES
- PSORIASIS
- VITILIGO
- WOUND HEALING

Nutrient Snapshot

▶ **REQUIREMENT IN THE INDIAN CONTEXT**

- B complex vitamins are water soluble vitamins that play a prominent role in the regulation of cellular metabolism. Vitamins B6 (pyridoxine), B9 (folate), and B12 (cobalamin) reduce levels of the amino acid homocysteine, a known marker of systemic inflammation.[1] They are required for the synthesis of DNA and RNA, contributing to the cell turnover process, and also contribute to the formation of red blood cells, ensuring adequate oxygen supply to the skin.

- Unrepaired DNA damage that accumulates from development throughout adulthood is correlated with and may drive the aging process. Deficiencies in these B-vitamins lead to an imbalance in DNA precursors, amongst many other cellular perturbations. Blood levels of folate have shown to decrease in the elderly.[2]

- Deficiencies of B-vitamins are rampant in India, particularly alarming for vitamin B12 and folic acid, even in apparently healthy individuals,[3] thereby adding to the burden of anemia.[4-6] Isolated vitamin B6 deficiency is not common; an inadequate status is usually associated with low levels of vitamin B12 and folate.[7]

- Vitamin B12 deficiency is still prevalent in the developing world due to a diet with more plant-derived products. This is why vegetarian and vegan diets often get insufficient vitamin B12. Furthermore, alcohol abuse and the use of gastric acid inhibitors and metformin over a period of time can cause vitamin B12 deficiency. Genetically, decreased intrinsic factor, which is required for the absorption of vitamin B12, may be another cause.[8]

▶ ACTIVE FORMS

ACTIVE FORMS	SUPPLEMENT SOURCES	SALIENT FEATURES
Vitamin B6: Pyridoxal-5-phosphate (PLP)	Synthetic	PLP is the active form of vitamin B6. Absorption of B6 from supplements is similar to that from dietary sources.[7]
Vitamin B9: 5-methyltetra-hydrofolate	Synthetic folic acid, synthetic tetrahydrofolate	Folate is the natural form of vitamin B9 in food, while folic acid is a synthetic form. Folic acid is almost entirely absorbed in the body, and is converted by the body to its biologically active form. Tetrahydrofolate may be more bioavailable than folic acid, which may be clinically relevant only in megadoses.
Vitamin B12: Methylcobalamin, adenosylcobalamin	Synthetic cyanocobalamin, synthetic methylcobalamin, natural methylcobalamin, and synthetic hydroxocobalamin	Studies suggest that methylcobalamin may be more bioavailable than cyanocobalamin. There seems to be a lot of contradictions, with some studies suggesting no difference in bioavailability. This is perhaps because bioavailability is influenced by many factors such as gastrointestinal pathologies, age, and genetics.[9,10] As per FSSAI guidelines (as of 2024), cyanocobalamin is permitted for use in food supplements. Methylcobalamin is not permitted for use in supplements.

▶ SAFETY AND DOSAGE

GENERAL REQUIREMENTS	
Indian recommendations	**RDA 2020:** B6 – RDA—Male: 1.9–3.1 mg, Female: 1.9–2.4 mg/day; TUL: 100 mg/day B9 – RDA—Male: 300 µg, Female: 220 µg/day; TUL: 1,000 µg/day B12 – RDA: 2.2 µg/day; TUL: N/A
Global recommendations and limits	**NIH RDA:** B6 – Male: 1.7 mg, Female: 1.5 mg/day; TUL: 100 mg/day B9 – 400 µg/day; TUL: 1,000 mg/day B12 – 2.4 µg/day; TUL: N/A

SAFETY AND DOSAGE (Continued)

GENERAL REQUIREMENTS	
	EFSA: B6 – Average requirements Male: 1.5 mg, Female: 1.3 mg/day; TUL: 25 mg/day[11,12] B9 – Average requirements 250 µg dietary folate equivalents (DFE)/day; TUL: 1,000 µg/day[13,14] B12 – Adequate intake-4 µg/day; TUL: N/A[15]
	B6 – NOAEL: 200 mg/day; LOAEL: 50 mg/day[12] B9 – LOAEL: 5 mg/day[16] B12 – NOAEL: 500 mg/kg of body weight/day[17]
Notes:	In the absence of clinical signs of deficiencies, the RDAs of vitamins B6, B9 and B12 should be prescribed, even though they are water-soluble. Additional dosage may either lead to imbalances between these vitamins, or increase the risk of diseases. An in vitro study demonstrated that megadoses of pyridoxine may lead to its own deficiency as an excess of this inactive form (pyridoxine) inhibits its conversion to its active form, PLP.[18] To account for differences in the absorption of naturally occurring food folate and the more bioavailable synthetic folic acid, the following formula is used: 1 µg of folic acid = 1.7 dietary equivalent folate (DFE).[19] Folic acid was found to reduce the side effects of methotrexate drug therapy given for psoriasis.[28]

CLINICAL CONDITIONS

EVIDENCE LEVEL	CONDITION OR USE CASE	DOSAGE	BENEFIT OR MECHANISM OF ACTION
+++	Collagen synthesis in the skin (vitamin B6)	Rats were fed with a different concentrations of casein diet with pyridoxine (7g/kg-control) or without pyridoxine for 4 weeks or 40 days.	Proline is an important amino acid that makes up collagen. The proline content in skin collagen fractions of the B6-deficient groups decreased compared to controls. Impaired proline production from ornithine thus leads to decreased proline content in skin collagen. This may explain the skin manifestations that are typical for B6 deficiency.[21]

▶ CLINICAL CONDITIONS (Continued)

EVIDENCE LEVEL	CONDITION OR USE CASE	DOSAGE	BENEFIT OR MECHANISM OF ACTION
+++++	Psoriasis (vitamin B9)	N/A (meta-analysis of observational studies)	According to the meta-analysis, compared with controls, patients with psoriasis had a higher serum homocysteine level, a higher prevalence of hyperhomocysteinemia and a lower serum folate level. There was no difference in serum vitamin B12 levels between patients with psoriasis and the control group.[22]
+++++	Vitiligo (vitamin B12)	N/A (meta-analysis of observational studies)	The patients with vitiligo had higher serum homocysteine levels and lower vitamin B12 levels than controls. Serum folate levels were not different between the patients and the control group.[23]
++	Vitiligo (vitamin B9)	Human epidermal melanocytes were treated with folic acid for 24 hours in vitro	Results from the experiment support the protective effects of folic acid on human melanocytes against oxidative injury via the activation of Nrf2 (master regulator of antioxidant response) and the inhibition of the proinflammatory marker HMGB1. Thus, folic acid can be used as a therapeutic agent for vitiligo.[24]

▶ CLINICAL CONDITIONS (Continued)

EVIDENCE LEVEL	CONDITION OR USE CASE	DOSAGE	BENEFIT OR MECHANISM OF ACTION
++	Premature canities (greying of hair; B-complex)	N/A (observational study)	It was observed that subjects were deficient in serum vitamin B12 and folic acid, while serum biotin levels were lower (without any obvious biotin deficiency) in premature canities cases as compared to the controls.[25]
+	Hyperpigmentation (vitamin B12)	Case study: A subject was treated with vitamin B12, intramuscular 1000 µg twice a week for a month, plus 100 µg orally daily.	Vitamin B12 dose showed an improvement in hyperpigmentation after 2 weeks and was completely resolved in the third week.[26]
++	Hyperpigmentation (vitamin B12)	Epidermal melanocytes were treated with synthesized vitamin B12 antagonist in vitro	The study showed that hypocobalaminemia disturbed melanocytes homeostasis via excess stimulation of melanogenesis (the increase of tyrosinase activity) and there was an elevation in free radicals level and imbalance. This indicates vitamin B12 deficiency plays a role in hyperpigmentation.[27]

▶ **CLINICAL CONDITIONS** (*Continued*)

EVIDENCE LEVEL	CONDITION OR USE CASE	DOSAGE	BENEFIT OR MECHANISM OF ACTION
+++	Hair follicle development (vitamin B6)	Rabbits were divided into 5 groups and fed diets supplemented with 0, 5, 10, 20, or 40 mg/kg pyridoxine. Free hair follicles were isolated from these rabbits and cultured with pyridoxine in vitro The dermal papilla cells (DPC) were isolated from the skin of these rabbits and cultured with pyridoxine in vitro	Dietary pyridoxine increased the total follicle density, secondary follicle density, and secondary-to-primary ratio. Therefore, the growth length of hair follicles cultured in the pyridoxine group was longer than that of the control group. Pyridoxine changed the DPC cycle progression, promoted cell proliferation and inhibited cell apoptosis. It affected the gene expression of components of the PI3K/Akt, Wnt and Notch signaling pathways.[28]
++	Atopic dermatitis (vitamin B6)	Human epidermal keratinocytes were treated with pyridoxine in vitro	The study reported that pyridoxine causes an increase in filaggrin production, an important protein for skin's barrier function. These results suggest that pyridoxine-induced filaggrin production may be useful in atopic dermatitis (as filaggrin levels are specifically reduced in it)[29]
++	Papulopustular Rosacea (PPR; vitamin B12 and B9)	N/A (observational study)	Serum vitamin B12 and folic acid levels were lower in PPR patients than in the healthy controls while serum homocysteine levels did not differ between PPR patients and healthy controls. PPR severity was positively correlated with serum Hcy levels.[30]

▶ CLINICAL CONDITIONS (Continued)

EVIDENCE LEVEL	CONDITION OR USE CASE	DOSAGE	BENEFIT OR MECHANISM OF ACTION
+	Alopecia areata (vitamin B9)	N/A (observational study)	The mean level of RBC folate was lower in the patient group than in controls. The level of RBC folate was lower in patients with extensive forms of the disease (alopecia totalis/alopecia universalis) in comparison with a more localized form (patchy hair loss). Patients with higher Severity of Alopecia Total (SALT) scores had lower RBC folate, as well. Serum homocysteine and blood high-sensitivity C-reactive protein levels did not show a difference.[31]
+	Cutaneous lesions (B-complex vitamins)	Patients with skin lesions were treated with intramuscular B12 injection (1000 μg) and vitamin B complex (vitamins B1, B6, and B12) tablets daily.	The skin lesions improved within 2 weeks and one month of starting treatment for both patients.[32]
+++	Wound healing in diabetes (vitamins B6, B9 and B12)	Mice were supplemented with 1 g/L B6, 1.25 mg/L B12, and 62.5 mg/L folic acid in their drinking water.	This study indicates that B vitamin supplementation may improve wound healing in diabetic mice.[33]
++	Wound healing (B-complex vitamins)	B vitamins and vitamin C were tested individually or in combination on their ability to promote the proliferation and migration of human skin fibroblasts and keratinocytes in vitro	A reduction in initial wound area was achieved by several combinations of vitamins, compared to untreated control. The expression of the cell migration marker, CXCR4 increased in fibroblasts with the vitamin combination.[34]

▶ SUPPLEMENTATION

	BASIS	WHAT TO LOOK OUT FOR
Supplementation form	B6 – Pyridoxine hydrochloride Pyridoxal 5'-phosphate B9 – n-pteroyl-l-glutamic acid (6S)-5-methyltetrahydrofolic acid glucosamine salt B12 – Cyanocobalamin Hydroxocobalamin Overall absorption of vitamin B12 is very low. Methylcobalamin, adenosylcobalamin, and hydroxycobalamin, all three forms, have superior bioavailability and safety.[10]	The form of B vitamin is stated on the ingredients list of the product packaging, except for vitamin B9, which is written as 'folic acid'.
Administration form	Capsules, tablets, gummies, soft gels, syrups, powders, chewable tablets, sublingual strips	N/A
Purity considerations	Synthetic vitamins normally have >99% purity	N/A
Patient considerations	Folic acid supplementation when taken without a meal is 100% bioavailable.[35] However, when present in a multivitamin, it can be taken with or after a meal.	N/A

▶ SUPPLEMENTATION (*Continued*)

	BASIS	WHAT TO LOOK OUT FOR
Safety considerations	B6: Adverse effects of B6 are only in case of excessive supplementation which may include nausea and other gastrointestinal symptoms, skin eruptions, and sensory neuropathies.[36] B9: Folic acid supplementation may cause hypersensitivity reactions in individuals allergic to it (this is not applicable in dietary sources as forms may differ).[37] Folic acid supplementation may mask a B12 deficiency and concerns associated with B12 deficiency could be left untreated.[9] One study also suggested that it may interfere with serum levels of other vitamins and thus high doses must be used with caution. Excess folic acid supplementation over a period of time may increase the risk of prostate cancer.[38,39] Some argue that its role is complex and the topic remains controversial.[40] B12: Vitamin B12 is generally considered to be safe because the body does not store excess amounts.	The symptoms of deficiency of B vitamins are nonspecific and overlapping thus consulting a trained practitioner is advised. While B vitamins are water-soluble vitamins and excess is excreted from the body, it is always recommended to not exceed RDA doses unless any underlying deficiency exists. Normally, vitamin B12 is prescribed to individuals when lower levels are found in blood (ELISA). Once the deficiency is treated, RDA levels can suffice.

▶ **SUPPLEMENTATION** (*Continued*)

	BASIS	WHAT TO LOOK OUT FOR
Other considerations	B6: Supplementation may be indicated in certain drug therapies for conditions such as TB, epilepsy and respiratory disorders. B9: Supplementation may be indicated in certain drug therapies or for conditions such as epilepsy and ulcerative colitis. Folic acid is used to reduce the toxicity of methotrexate, in cases of cancer and autoimmune disorders such as psoriasis (at doses is much higher than RDA).[20,35,41] B12: Certain medications such as proton pump inhibitors, or metformin may hinder the absorption of B12, thus B12 supplementation can be indicated in these conditions.	Individuals with clinical conditions and on medication are advised to seek doctor's consultation before starting any nutritional supplementation.

▶ INTRODUCTION

Among the essential nutrients, vitamin B6, vitamin B9 (folate), and vitamin B12 (cobalamin) play a fundamental role in maintaining skin vitality. Their contribution of one-carbon metabolism, makes them important for cellular homeostasis and in coordination of signaling cascades that regulate energy homeostasis and longevity.[2]

Vitamin B6 comprises a group of six related compounds. Vitamin B6 and its derivative pyridoxal 5′-phosphate (PLP) are essential to over 100 enzymes mostly involved in protein metabolism.[42]

Folate functions as a coenzyme in the metabolism of nucleic and amino acids. Folic acid, the most stable form of folate, occurs rarely in food but is the form used in vitamin supplements and in fortified food products.[42]

Vitamin B12 can be found in two form, methyl cobalamin and adenosyl cobalamin, that are active in human metabolism.[42] Although our gut bacteria are able to synthesise B12, the bacteria that produce it are located in the colon, beyond the site of B12 absorption in the terminal ileum.[43]

▶ DIGESTION, ABSORPTION AND STORAGE

Digestion and Absorption

- The human body absorbs vitamin B6 in the jejunum. Phosphorylated forms are dephosphorylated, and free vitamin B6 is absorbed by passive diffusion.[7,42]

- Folate and its derivatives are hydrolyzed in the gut, by folate conjugase, before absorption across the small intestine by a saturable transporters or passive diffusion.[44]

- The absorption of B12 begins with its release from food sources by gastric acid and pepsin in the stomach, followed by its binding to haptocorrin (HC), which is found in saliva and gastric fluid. In the duodenum, B12 is released from HC by pancreatic proteases and is then bound by intrinsic factor, which helps it get absorbed.[44]

- Vitamin C is thought to improve absorption and utilization of folic acid.[45]

- Food storage and cooking reduce the levels of B-complex vitamins in food.[46]

Storage

Like all B vitamins, these are water-soluble and the body does not store it. However, small amounts of folate and vitamin B12 are found in the liver.

▶ MECHANISM OF ACTION

One-carbon metabolism (1C; **Figure 1**) comprises a series of interlinking metabolic pathways that include the methionine and folate cycles that are central to cellular function, providing 1C units (methyl groups) for the synthesis of DNA, polyamines, amino acids, creatine, and phospholipids.[47]

Nutrients involved in 1C-folate, vitamins B6 and B12, methionine, choline, and betaine - have been inversely associated with multiple cancers,[48] and are required for normal growth and development and the maintenance of healthy skin, hair, and nails.[44] Here's how:

01 | Hair Growth

The role of folate and vitamin B12 in nucleic acid production suggests their central role in the highly proliferative hair follicle. Riboflavin, biotin, folate, and vitamin B12 deficiencies have been associated with hair loss.[49]

02 | Hair Pigmentation

Deficiencies of iron, vitamin D, folate, vitamin B12, and selenium may be involved in hair graying/whitening during childhood or early adulthood. Supplementing these micronutrients can improve premature graying.[49]

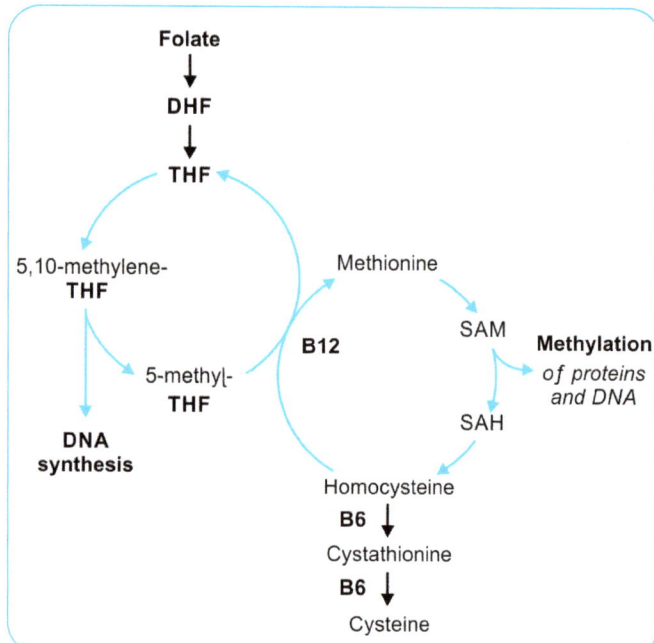

Figure 1: The role of vitamin B6, B9 and B12 in one-carbon metabolism. Vitamin B12 and folate are cofactors in one-carbon metabolism, and they facilitate Hcy remethylation. Vitamin B12 and folate shortage prevents the conversion of Hcy to methionine and leads to hyperhomocysteinemia (HHcy). Vitamin B6 shortage prevents the transfer of Hcy to cystathionine and induces HHcy, too.[44,50]

(DHF: dihydrofolate; THF: tetrahydrofolate; SAM: S-adenosylmethionine; SAH: S-adenosylhomocysteine)

03 | Regulating Immunity and Inflammation

B vitamins control DNA synthesis and methyl donor availability, which are important for the normal function of cells in the immune system.[24,30]

They influence the biosynthesis of inflammatory and anti-inflammatory long-chain polyunsaturated fatty acids (omega 6 and omega 3 fats).

Folate levels have been shown to be lower, and homocysteine levels higher, in psoriasis patients. However, the benefit of their supplementation in psoriasis has yet to be established.[21] Patients with vitiligo have also shown higher serum homocysteine levels and lower vitamin B12 levels than individuals without vitiligo, acne vulgaris, and hyperpigmentation.[43,51]

04 | Support to Antioxidant Defence Systems

These vitamins may directly or indirectly play a role in reducing oxidative stress. Cysteine synthesized by this pathway, from homocysteine, is an important contributor to synthesis of reduced glutathione.[52]

Vitamin B6 may directly react with the peroxy radicals and inhibit lipid peroxidation.[52] Vitamin B9 and B12 have also shown to have direct antioxidant properties.

05 | Sebum Production

Vitamin B6 helps regulate sebum production, and seborrheic dermatitis has been associated with low B6 levels. B-vitamins are often given to patients with acne vulgaris to help reduce sebum production.[43]

▶ REFERENCES

1. Gerhard GT, Duell PB. Homocysteine and atherosclerosis. Curr Opin Lipidol. 1999;10(5):417-28.
2. Lionaki E, Ploumi C, Tavernarakis N. One-Carbon Metabolism: Pulling the Strings behind Aging and Neurodegeneration. Cells. 2022;11(2):214.
3. Sivaprasad M, Shalini T, Reddy PY, Seshacharyulu M, Madhavi G, Kumar BN, et al. Prevalence of vitamin deficiencies in an apparently healthy urban adult population: Assessed by subclinical status and dietary intakes. Nutrition. 2019;63-64:106-13.
4. Sundarakumar JS, Shahul Hameed SK, SANSCOG Study Team, Ravindranath V. Burden of Vitamin D, Vitamin B12 and Folic Acid Deficiencies in an Aging, Rural Indian Community. Front Public Health. 2021:9:707036.
5. Kapil U, Bhadoria AS. Prevalence of Folate, Ferritin and Cobalamin Deficiencies amongst Adolescent in India. J Family Med Prim Care. 2014;3(3):247-9.
6. Chaudhary V, Saraswathy KN, Sarwal R. Dietary diversity as a sustainable approach towards micronutrient deficiencies in India. Review Indian J Med Res. 2022;156(1):31-45.
7. Fact Sheet for Health Professionals. Vitamin B6 [Online]. Available from: https://ods.od.nih.gov/factsheets/VitaminB6-HealthProfessional/
8. Singh J, Dinkar A, Gupta P, Atam V. Vitamin B12 deficiency in northern India tertiary care: Prevalence, risk factors and clinical characteristics. J Family Med Prim Care. 2022;11(6):2381-8.
9. Fact Sheet for Health Professionals. Vitamin B12 [Online]. Available from: https://ods.od.nih.gov/factsheets/Vitaminb12-HealthProfessional/
10. Paul C, Brady DM. Comparative Bioavailability and Utilization of Particular Forms of B12 Supplements With Potential to Mitigate B12-related Genetic Polymorphisms. Integr Med (Encinitas). 2017;16(1):42-9.
11. EFSA Panel on Dietetic Products, Nutrition and Allergies (NDA). Dietary Reference Values for vitamin B6. EFSA Journal. 2016;14(6):e04485.

12. EFSA Panel on Nutrition, Novel Foods and Food Allergens (NDA), Turck D, Bohn T, Castenmiller J, de Henauw S, Hirsch-Ernst KI, et al. Scientific opinion on the tolerable upper intake level for vitamin B6. EFSA Journal. 2023;21(5):e08006.
13. EFSA Panel on Dietetic Products, Nutrition and Allergies (NDA). Scientific Opinion on Dietary Reference Values for folate. EFSA Journal. 2014;12(11):3893.
14. EFSA Panel on Nutrition, Novel Foods and Food Allergens (NDA). Overview on Tolerable Upper Intake Levels as derived by the Scientific Committee on Food (SCF) and the EFSA Panel on Dietetic Products, Nutrition and Allergies (NDA). European Food Safety Authority. 2024.
15. EFSA Panel on Dietetic Products, Nutrition, and Allergies (NDA). Scientific Opinion on Dietary Reference Values for cobalamin (vitamin B12). EFSA Journal. 2015;13(7):4150.
16. Field MS, Stover PJ. Safety of folic acid. Ann N Y Acad Sci. 2018;1414(1):59-71.
17. EFSA Panel on Additives and Products or Substances used in Animal Feed (EFSA FEEDAP Panel). Safety and efficacy of vitamin B12 (in the form of cyanocobalamin) produced by Ensifer spp. as a feed additive for all animal species based on a dossier submitted by VITAC EEIG. EFSA JOURNAL. 2018;16(7):e05336.
18. Vrolijk MF, Opperhuizen A, Jansen EHJM, Hageman GJ, Bast A, Haenen GRMM. The vitamin B6 paradox: Supplementation with high concentrations of pyridoxine leads to decreased vitamin B6 function. Toxicol In Vitro. 2017 Oct;44:206-12.
19. Suitor CW, Bailey LB. Dietary folate equivalents: interpretation and application. J Am Diet Assoc. 2000;100(1):88-94.
20. Salim A, Tan E, Ilchyshyn A, Berth-Jones J. Folic acid supplementation during treatment of psoriasis with methotrexate: a randomized, double-blind, placebo-controlled trial. Br J Dermatol. 2006;154(6):1169-74.
21. Inubushi T, Takasawa T, Tuboi Y, Watanabe N, Aki K, Katunuma N. Changes of glucose metabolism and skin-collagen neogenesis in vitamin B6 deficiency. Biofactors. 2005;23(2):59-67.
22. Tsai TY, Yen H, Huang YC. Serum homocysteine, folate and vitamin B12 levels in patients with psoriasis: a systematic review and meta-analysis. Br J Dermatol. 2019;180(2):382-9.
23. Tsai TY, Kuo CY, Huang YC. Serum homocysteine, folate, and vitamin B12 levels in patients with vitiligo and their potential roles as disease activity biomarkers: A systematic review and meta-analysis. J Am Acad Dermatol. 2019;80(3):646-54.e5.
24. Du P, Zhang S, Li S, Yang Y, Kang P, Chen J, et al. Folic Acid Protects Melanocytes from Oxidative Stress via Activation of Nrf2 and Inhibition of HMGB1. Oxid Med Cell Longev. 2021;2021:1608586.
25. Daulatabad D, Singal A, Grover C, Chhillar N. Prospective Analytical Controlled Study Evaluating Serum Biotin, Vitamin B12, and Folic Acid in Patients with Premature Canities. Int J Trichology. 2017;9(1):19-24.
26. Jangda A, Voloshyna D, Ramesh K, Bseiso A, Shaik TA, Al Barznji S, et al. Hyperpigmentation as a Primary Symptom of Vitamin B12 Deficiency: A Case Report. Cureus. 2022;14(9):e29008.
27. Rzepka Z, Respondek M, Rok J, Beberok A, ó Proinsias K, Gryko D, et al. Vitamin B12 Deficiency Induces Imbalance in Melanocytes Homeostasis—A Cellular Basis of Hypocobalaminemia Pigmentary Manifestations. Int J Mol Sci. 2018;19(9):2845.
28. Liu G, Cheng G, Zhang Y, Gao S, Sun H, Bai L, et al. Pyridoxine regulates hair follicle development via the PI3K/Akt, Wnt and Notch signalling pathways in rex rabbits. Anim Nutr. 2021;7(4):1162-72.
29. Fujishiro M, Yahagi S, Takemi S, Nakahara M, Sakai T, Sakata I. Pyridoxine stimulates filaggrin production in human epidermal keratinocytes. Mol Biol Rep. 2021;48(7):5513-8.
30. Chung BY, Kim HO, Park CW, Yang NG, Kim JY, Eun YS, et al. Relationships of Serum Homocysteine, Vitamin B12, and Folic Acid Levels with Papulopustular Rosacea Severity: A Case-Control Study. Biomed Res Int. 2022;2022:5479626.
31. Yousefi M, Namazi MR, Rahimi H, Younespour S, Ehsani AH, Shakoei S. Evaluation of Serum Homocysteine, High-Sensitivity CRP, and RBC Folate in Patients with Alopecia Areata. Indian J Dermatol. 2014;59(6):630.
32. Kannan R, Ng MJM. Cutaneous lesions and vitamin B12 deficiency. Can Fam Physician. 2008;54(4):529-32.
33. Mochizuki S, Takano M, Sugano N, Ohtsu M, Tsunoda K, Koshi R, et al. The effect of B vitamin supplementation on wound healing in type 2 diabetic mice. J Clin Biochem Nutr. 2016;58(1):64-8.
34. Rembe JD, Fromm-Dornieden C, Stuermer EK. Effects of Vitamin B Complex and Vitamin C on Human Skin Cells: Is the Perceived Effect Measurable?
35. Fact Sheet for Health Professionals. Folate [Online]. Available from: https://ods.od.nih.gov/factsheets/Folate-HealthProfessional/
36. Elgharably N, Al Abadie M, Al Abadie M, Ball PA, Morrissey H. Vitamin B group levels and supplementations in dermatology. Dermatol Reports. 2022;15(1):9511.
37. Nucera E, Aruanno A, Mezzacappa S, Pascolini L, Buonomo A, Schiavino D. Hypersensitivity reactions to folic acid: Three case reports and a review of the literature. Int J Immunopathol Pharmacol. 2018;32: 2058738418817704.
38. Wien TN, Pike E, Wisløff T, Staff A, Smeland S, Klemp M. Cancer risk with folic acid supplements: a systematic review and meta-analysis. BMJ Open. 2012;2(1):e000653.
39. Circulating Folate and Vitamin B12 and Risk of Prostate Cancer: A Collaborative Analysis of Individual Participant Data from Six Cohorts Including 6875 Cases and 8104 Controls. European Urology. 2016;70(6):941-51.
40. Maitin-Shepard M, O'Tierney-Ginn P, Kraneveld AD, Lyall K, Fallin D, Arora M, et al. Food, nutrition, and autism: from soil to fork. The American Journal of Clinical Nutrition [Internet]. 2024 Apr 25 [cited 2024 Jun 20];0(0) [Online]. Available from: https://ajcn.nutrition.org/article/S0002-9165(24)00443-X/fulltext
41. Czarnecka-Operacz M, Sadowska-Przytocka A. The possibilities and principles of methotrexate treatment of psoriasis – the updated knowledge. Postepy Dermatol Alergol. 2014;31(6):392-400.
42. Institute of Medicine (US) Standing Committee on the Scientific Evaluation of Dietary Reference Intakes and its Panel on Folate, Other B Vitamins, and Choline. Dietary Reference Intakes for Thiamin, Riboflavin, Niacin, Vitamin B6, Folate, Vitamin B12, Pantothenic Acid, Biotin, and Choline. National Academies Press (US). 1998. doi:10.17226/6015.
43. Elgharably N, Al Abadie M, Al Abadie M, Ball PA, Morrissey H. Vitamin B group levels and supplementations in dermatology. Dermatol Reports. 2022;15(1):9511.
44. Lyon P, Strippoli V, Fang B, Cimmino L. B Vitamins and One-Carbon Metabolism: Implications in Human Health and Disease. Nutrients. 2020;12(9):2867.

45. Sahin K, Onderci M, Sahin N, Gursu MF, Kucuk O. Dietary Vitamin C and Folic Acid Supplementation Ameliorates the Detrimental Effects of Heat Stress in Japanese Quail. J Nutr. 2003;133(6):1882-6.
46. Bureau S, Mouhoubi S, Touloumet L, Garcia C, Moreau F, Bédouet V, el al. Are folates, carotenoids and vitamin C affected by cooking? Four domestic procedures are compared on a large diversity of frozen vegetables. LWT - Food Science and Technology. 2015;64(2):735-41.
47. Clare CE, Brassington AH, Kwong WY, Sinclair KD. One-Carbon Metabolism: Linking Nutritional Biochemistry to Epigenetic Programming of Long-Term Development. Annu Rev Anim Biosci. 2019;7:263-87.
48. Dhana A, Yen H, Li T, Holmes MD, Qureshi AA, Cho E. Intake of folate and other nutrients related to one-carbon metabolism and risk of cutaneous melanoma among US women and men. Cancer Epidemiol. 2018;55:176-83.
49. Almohanna HM, Ahmed AA, Tsatalis JP, Tosti A. The Role of Vitamins and Minerals in Hair Loss: A Review. Dermatol Ther (Heidelb). 2018;9(1):51-70.
50. Ueno A, Hamano T, Enomoto S, Shirafuji N, Nagata M, Kimura H, et al. Influences of Vitamin B12 Supplementation on Cognition and Homocysteine in Patients with Vitamin B12 Deficiency and Cognitive Impairment. Nutrients. 2022;14(7):1494.
51. Tsai TY, Kuo CY, Huang YC. Serum homocysteine, folate, and vitamin B12 levels in patients with vitiligo and their potential roles as disease activity biomarkers: A systematic review and meta-analysis. J Am Acad Dermatol. 2019;80(3):646-54.e5.
52. Hsu CC, Cheng CH, Hsu CL, Lee WJ, Huang SC, Huang YC. Role of vitamin B6 status on antioxidant defenses, glutathione, and related enzyme activities in mice with homocysteine-induced oxidative stress. Food Nutr Res. 2015;59:10.3402/fnr.v59.25702.

05

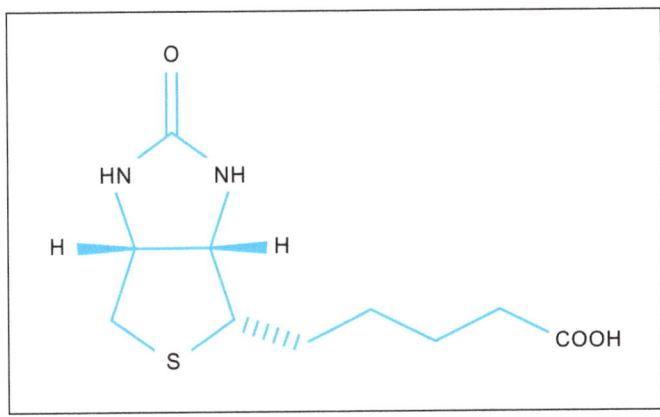

Biotin

Biotin (Vitamin B7)

✍ Abhishek De

CONTENTS

BIOTIN (VITAMIN B7): NUTRIENT SNAPSHOT

- ▶ REQUIREMENT IN THE INDIAN CONTEXT | 48
- ▶ ACTIVE FORMS | 49
- ▶ SAFETY AND DOSAGE | 49
- ▶ CLINICAL CONDITIONS | 49
- ▶ SUPPLEMENTATION | 51

INTRODUCTION | 52

DIGESTION, ABSORPTION AND STORAGE | 52

MECHANISM OF ACTION | 52

KEY TOPICS

- HAIR ISSUES RELATED TO ACNE VULGARIS
- HAIR LOSS
- HAIR LOSS RELATED TO BIOTINIDASE DEFICIENCY
- PREMATURE CANITIES
- UNCOMBABLE HAIR SYNDROME IN CHILDREN

Nutrient Snapshot

▶ **REQUIREMENT IN THE INDIAN CONTEXT**

- Biotin, also known as vitamin B7 or vitamin H, is a water-soluble vitamin that functions as a cofactor to four carboxylases involved in fatty acid synthesis, gluconeogenesis, and amino acid metabolism.[1]

- Biotin is widely found in food, and good dietary sources include egg yolk, liver, cereals, and some vegetables. Intestinal bacteria are thought to produce biotin more than the body's daily requirements.[2] Hence, a biotin deficiency is very rare. There isn't enough evidence to suggest a daily requirement, and so guidelines by authorities often provide an intake for adequacy.[3] With recommendations in microgram quantities, oral supplementation with as much as 5–30 mg of biotin are available in many hair and nail supplements. Research suggests that most of the ingested biotin in a single dose (upwards of 600 µg to 2 mg) is simply excreted.[4-6]

- Pharmacological doses of biotin are beneficial in the case of hereditary biotin metabolism defects and in the treatment of multiple sclerosis.[7] Furthermore, high doses would provide a benefit in alopecia only if deficiency is the cause.[2]

- Despite inconclusive evidence to support its therapeutic benefit, biotin has been glamorized in the media to improve hair and nails, which has been further encouraged by supplement companies.[7] Unfortunately, this belittles the importance of many other nutrients for hair health, like vitamin D, iron and zinc, in the mind of consumers. Additionally, unprecedented effects of pharmacological doses may also occur. For example, it may interfere with certain biochemical tests[8,9] and even some cellular functions.[10]

- Nutritional biotin deficiency is rare, but the consumption of raw eggs on a regular basis, a practise followed by bodybuilders, may cause biotin deficiency. This is due to avidin, a protein present in raw eggs, which denatures upon cooking. Avidin strongly binds to biotin, thus making it unavailable for intestinal absorption in a syndrome, called "egg white injury".[2,5]

- While the role of biotin in dermatology is irreplaceable and verified, its current pharmacological dosage must be reconsidered, i.e., to be based on evidence rather than current perspectives and anecdotal observations. Aiming for adequacy via recommended doses may suffice.[8]

▶ ACTIVE FORMS

ACTIVE FORMS	SUPPLEMENT SOURCES	SALIENT FEATURES
Biotin	Synthetic: Natural source from *Sesbania grandiflora*	The purity of synthetic biotin is 100% and is completely absorbed.[11,12] The purity of natural sources of biotin is not standardized.

▶ SAFETY AND DOSAGE

GENERAL REQUIREMENTS	
Indian recommendations	ICMR-NIN Adequate intake (AI): 25 µg/day
Global recommendations and limits	NIH adequate intake: 30 µg/day
	EFSA adequate intake (AI): 40 µg/day[13]
	NOAEL: 39 g biotin/day for a 70 kg human[14]
Notes:	Despite no evidence in hair growth, large doses of biotin are being used. Biotin has shown benefits on hair only when the cause of hair loss is a biotin deficiency. A large dose of biotin may interfere with other biochemical tests.

▶ CLINICAL CONDITIONS

EVIDENCE LEVEL	CONDITION OR USE CASE	DOSAGE	BENEFIT OR MECHANISM OF ACTION
+	Uncombable hair syndrome in children	2 young patients (siblings: girl and boy) were started with oral biotin 5 mg/day for 3 months.	There was an improvement in hair and nails observed after 3 months period. At 6 months, when the boy's hair was thicker and more combable, scanning electron microscopy (SEM) showed the hair unchanged. Stopping biotin supplementation reversed improvements.[15]

▶ **CLINICAL CONDITIONS** (*Continued*)

EVIDENCE LEVEL	CONDITION OR USE CASE	DOSAGE	BENEFIT OR MECHANISM OF ACTION
+++	Hair loss	N/A (Observational study)	Biotin deficiency was found in 38% of women complaining of hair loss. Of those, 24% showed diffuse telogen effluvium in trichograms, and 35% had evidence of associated seborrheic-like dermatitis.[2]
+++++	Hair issues related to acne vulgaris	Groups A and B received 0.5 mg/kg/day isotretinoin, and a 10 mg/day biotin supplement was added to Group B for 4 months.	In group B, the anagen hair ratio increased and the telogen hair ratio decreased significantly. Skin sebum and skin retraction values decreased in both groups. Skin hydration decreased in group A, but it was maintained in group B. The study suggests that biotin can prevent the mucocutaneous adverse effects of isotretinoin treatment.[16]
+	Hair loss related to biotinidase deficiency	Case study 1: A 3-year-old girl was treated with oral biotin 10 mg twice a day for 6 months. Case study 2: A 3-year old boy was supplemented daily with 30 mg biotin for 6 months.	Case study 1: Air grew back in 6 months of treatment.[17] Case study 2: After 6 weeks, there was a dramatic improvement with a thick crop of black hair replacing the diffusely alopecic scalp.[18]
++	Premature canities (greying of hair)	N/A (observational study)	Subjects were deficient in serum vitamin B12 and folic acid, while serum biotin levels were lower (without any obvious biotin deficiency) in premature canities cases as compared to the controls.[19]

▶ SUPPLEMENTATION

	BASIS	**WHAT TO LOOK OUT FOR**
Supplementation form	D-biotin *Sesbania grandiflora* extracts	The form of biotin is given in the ingredients list. Many brands add extracts to provide high doses of biotin but the concentration of biotin in extracts may not be standardized.
Administration form	Capsules, gummies, tablets, chewable tablets, soft gels	N/A
Purity considerations	Pharmaceutical grade or synthetic biotin normally has > 99% purity. Purity of natural extracts may vary.	N/A
Patient considerations	Biotin is present in most multivitamins or can be available as a stand-alone product so it is recommended to be taken with or after a meal.	Though biotin is present in most of the nail and hair supplements, the research on efficacy is limited and it should be used mindfully.[7] A dose higher than the RDA is needed only in case of a deficiency under the guidance of a doctor. The dose per serving is stated on the nutritional label of the product packaging.
Safety considerations	The tolerability of biotin is excellent and there is no risk of hypervitaminosis even in the case of high doses.	N/A
Other considerations	High doses of biotin falsely alter the biochemical test results of hormonal tests, and cardiac health so it is suggested to wait for at least 8 hours before doing the tests in case the individuals are on heavy doses of biotin.[20,21] Individuals on anticonvulsant treatments may have lower serum levels of biotin and thus may need supplementation.[11]	Most hair and skin supplements contain biotin in them. A dose exceeding the RDA may interfere with the laboratory tests of the individuals and hence should be informed accordingly.

▶ INTRODUCTION

Biotin is required as a cofactor for four carboxylases found in mammalian species. Of these, three are mitochondrial [pyruvate carboxylase, methylcrotonyl-coenzyme A (CoA) carboxylase, and propionyl-CoA carboxylase], whereas the fourth (acetyl-CoA carboxylase) is found in both the mitochondria and the cytosol.[1]

▶ DIGESTION, ABSORPTION AND STORAGE

Digestion and Absorption

- Biotin in food is largely protein bound. It is released to its free form during digestion via gastrointestinal proteases and peptidases that produce biotin-l-lysine (biocytin) and biotin-oligopeptides which are then converted into free biotin by biotinidase.

- Absorption of free biotin in the small and large intestine involves a saturable sodium-dependent process by a transporter known as human sodium-dependent multivitamin transporter (hSMVT), which is shared with pantothenic and α-lipoic acid.[5]

- Large doses of pantothenic acid (vitamin B5) have the potential to compete with biotin for intestinal and cellular uptake by the hSMVT.[5]

- Biotin is 100% bioavailable, and that the elimination half-life time from plasma of a single oral biotin dose (of 600 μg) is about 110 minutes.[6]

- Avidin, a protein found in appreciable amounts in raw egg white, has been shown to bind biotin in the small intestine and prevent its absorption.[1]

Storage

Like all B vitamins, biotin is water soluble and the body does not store it. However, some biotin may be stored in the liver and the bacteria in the intestine can make biotin.[1,22] That's why, even in diets designed to lack biotin, the body is able to cover its biotin needs for about one month.[5]

▶ MECHANISM OF ACTION

Symptoms of biotin deficiency include dermatitis, conjunctivitis, alopecia, and central nervous system abnormalities.[1,23,24]

Biotin functions as a covalently bound cofactor required for the biological activity of the four known mammalian biotin-dependent carboxylases, which are essential for metabolic reactions for:[24]

01 | Energy Production

Biotin-dependent carboxylases are required in the mitochondria for regulating fatty acid oxidation and for gluconeogenesis, the formation of glucose from sources other than carbohydrates, such as pyruvate, lactate, glycerol, and amino acids.[23]

Carboxylases also allow for the catabolism of branched-chain amino acids (leucine, isoleucine, and valine), methionine and threonine.

02 | Gene Expression and Protein Synthesis

'Biotinylation' refers to the covalent addition of biotin to any molecule. Biotinylation of histone proteins in nuclear chromatin is a post-translational modification that plays a role in chromatin stability and gene expression. Approximately 2,000 genes have been identified so far that are biotin-dependent. Biotin levels also affect transcriptional factors, such as nuclear factor kappa B (NF-κB).[23]

Biotin, is therefore, required for production of skin's matrix components like collagen, keratin, elastin, etc.

03 | Immune Function

Finally, biotin also regulates immunological and inflammatory functions - in the maturation and responsiveness of immune cells, and in the function of natural killer (NK) lymphocytes. Evidence shows increasing interleukin-1 beta (IL-1β) and proinflammatory cytokines TNF-α in biotin deficiency.[23]

These functions are important for skin repair and turnover, and for the rapidly growing cells in the hair follicle, eventually leading to healthier skin, hair and nails.[23]

▶ REFERENCES

1. The National Academies, Panel on Folate, Other B Vitamins, And Choline. In: Dietary Reference Intakes for Thiamin, Riboflavin, Niacin, Vitamin B6, Folate, Vitamin B12, Pantothenic Acid, Biotin, and Choline. Chapter 11: Biotin. National Academies Press (US); 1998.
2. Trüeb RM. Serum Biotin Levels in Women Complaining of Hair Loss. Int J Trichology. 2016;8(2):73-7.
3. National Institute of Nutrition Indian Council of Medical Research. Recommended Dietary Allowances and Estimated Average Requirements for Indians – 2020. RDA Full Report 2020.
4. Zempleni J, Mock DM. Bioavailability of biotin given orally to humans in pharmacologic doses. Am J Clin Nutr. 1999;69(3):504-8.
5. ScienceDirect Topics. Biotin - an overview. https://www.sciencedirect.com/topics/neuroscience/biotin
6. Bitsch R, Salz I, Hötzel D. Studies on bioavailability of oral biotin doses for humans. Int J Vitam Nutr Res. 1989;59(1):65-71.
7. Patel DP, Swink SM, Castelo-Soccio L. A Review of the Use of Biotin for Hair Loss. Skin Appendage Disord. 2017;3(3):166-9.
8. Thompson KG, Kim N. Dietary supplements in dermatology: A review of the evidence for zinc, biotin, vitamin D, nicotinamide, and Polypodium. J Am Acad Dermatol. 2021;84(4):1042-50.
9. Deleterious side effects of nutritional supplements. Clinics in Dermatology. 2021;39(5):745-56.
10. In Vivo Biotin Supplementation at a Pharmacologic Dose Decreases Proliferation Rates of Human Peripheral Blood Mononuclear Cells and Cytokine Release. The Journal of Nutrition. 2001;131(5):1479-84.
11. Fact Sheet for Health Professionals. Biotin [Online]. Available from: https://ods.od.nih.gov/factsheets/Biotin-HealthProfessional/
12. Zempleni J, Mock DM. Bioavailability of biotin given orally to humans in pharmacologic doses. Am J Clin Nutr. 1999;69(3):504-8.
13. EFSA Panel on Dietetic Products, Nutrition and Allergies (NDA). Scientific Opinion on Dietary Reference Values for biotin. EFSA Journal. 2014;12(2):3580.
14. Blum JL, Ellis M, Chen JX, Mendes O, Sylla S, Ojalvo SP, et al. Toxicologic evaluation of a novel, highly soluble biotin salt, magnesium biotinate. Food Chem Toxicol. 2021;153:112267.
15. Boccaletti V, Zendri E, Giordano G, Gnetti L, De Panfilis G. Familial Uncombable Hair Syndrome: Ultrastructural Hair Study and Response to Biotin. Pediatr Dermatol. 2007;24(3):E14-6.
16. Aksac SE, Bilgili SG, Yavuz GO, Yavuz IH, Aksac M, Karadag AS. Evaluation of biophysical skin parameters and hair changes in patients with acne vulgaris treated with isotretinoin, and the effect of biotin use on these parameters. Int J Dermatol. 2021;60(8):980-5.
17. A girl with spastic tetraparesis associated with biotinidase deficiency. European Journal of Paediatric Neurology. 2011;15(6):551-3.
18. Mukhopadhyay D, Das MK, Dhar S, Mukhopadhyay M. Multiple Carboxylase Deficiency (Late Onset) Due to Deficiency of Biotinidase. Indian J Dermatol. 2014;59(5):502-4.
19. Daulatabad D, Singal A, Grover C, Chhillar N. Prospective Analytical Controlled Study Evaluating Serum Biotin, Vitamin B12, and Folic Acid in Patients with Premature Canities. Int J Trichology. 2017;9(1):19-24.
20. Samarasinghe S, Meah F, Singh V, Basit A, Emanuele N, Emanuele MA, et al. Biotin Interference with Routine Clinical Immunoassays: Understand The Causes and Mitigate The Risks. Endocr Pract. 2017;23(8):989-98.
21. Rigopoulos D, Elewski B, Tosti A. Is Biotin Safe for Dermatology Patients? Skin Appendage Disord. 2018;4(4):201.
22. Balamurugan K, Ortiz A, Said HM. Biotin uptake by human intestinal and liver epithelial cells: role of the SMVT system. American Journal of Physiology-Gastrointestinal and Liver Physiology. 2003;285(1):G73–7.
23. Saleem F, Soos MP. Biotin Deficiency. In: StatPearls. Treasure Island (FL): StatPearls Publishing; 2024.
24. Bistas KG, Tadi P. Biotin. In: StatPearls. Treasure Island (FL): StatPearls Publishing; 2024.

06

Ascorbic Acid (Vitamin C)

Vitamin C

✍ Sachin Varma

CONTENTS

VITAMIN C: NUTRIENT SNAPSHOT

- ▶ REQUIREMENT IN THE INDIAN CONTEXT | 55
- ▶ ACTIVE FORMS | 56
- ▶ SAFETY AND DOSAGE | 56
- ▶ CLINICAL CONDITIONS | 56
- ▶ SUPPLEMENTATION | 59

INTRODUCTION | 61

DIGESTION, ABSORPTION AND STORAGE | 61

MECHANISM OF ACTION | 62

KEY TOPICS

- ATOPIC DERMATITIS
- CERAMIDE PRODUCTION
- GENITAL WARTS
- OXIDATIVE STRESS IN THE SKIN
- PIGMENTED PURPURIC DERMATOSIS
- PSORIASIS
- SKIN BARRIER FUNCTION
- UVB INDUCED SUNBURN (DNA DAMAGE)
- UVA MEDIATED MELANOGENESIS
- WRINKLES

Nutrient Snapshot

▶ **REQUIREMENT IN THE INDIAN CONTEXT**

- Vitamin C, also known as ascorbic acid, is a water-soluble vitamin. Humans do not have the ability to synthesize it and must obtain it from our diet. Ingestion of L-ascorbic acid or its reversibly oxidized form, dehydroascorbic acid (DHAA), raises the plasma concentration of ascorbate, the anion of ascorbic acid, and the predominant form at physiological pH.[1] With a half-life of a few minutes, DHAA is normally reduced back to ascorbate. This process, and the recycling of vitamin C, are efficient in healthy individuals, but may be compromised in disease states or in smokers.[2]

- Vitamin C is ubiquitous in our food, particularly in fruits and vegetables.[2] The Indian diet is skewed toward cereal intake, with daily consumption of fruit and vegetables making up only 2.3–3.5 servings on average, compared to the recommended minimum of 5 servings/day (80 g/serving).[3,4]

- Vitamin C deficiency is more prevalent in men, with increasing age, users of tobacco and biomass fuels, and in those with anthropometric indicators of poor nutrition.[5] Tobacco use is common in India with a third of adults smoking or chewing tobacco.[5] In diabetes, which is also extremely prevalent in India,[6] reduced levels of plasma vitamin C have been reported.[2]

- In addition to low dietary intake, low plasma levels of vitamin C in India may be due to the haptoglobin (Hp) allele status (Hp1 or Hp2). When the antioxidant function of Hp is insufficient, vitamin C acts in its place, subsequently depleting serum ascorbic acid. The Hp2/Hp2 genotype is substantially higher in India (around 70–80%) compared to those of European ancestry (30–40%).[5] The capacity of Hp2 to inhibit oxidation is less than that of Hp1, and therefore causes a higher depletion in vitamin C.[7] Other genetic modifiers of vitamin C levels are yet to be investigated.[5]

- Topical application of vitamin C may be a challenge due to its instability and aqueous solubility. While it has been stabilized and successfully used in many topical concoctions, its dietary intake helps deliver it to all layers of the skin effectively by the body's transport mechanisms.

- In dermatology, vitamin C is used for limiting UV damage, signs of aging, and for the treatment of hair fall, acne, allergies, dermatitis, psoriasis, progressive purpura and many more. It is normally seen as an adjuvant for use in combination with other drugs, nutrients or therapies.[8]

▶ ACTIVE FORMS

ACTIVE FORMS	SUPPLEMENT SOURCES	SALIENT FEATURES
L-ascorbic acid	Synthetic	The steady state comparative bioavailability studies in humans have shown no differences between synthetic and natural vitamin C. Some pharmacokinetic human studies show transient differences which are likely to have little physiological impact.[9,10]
	Natural form from *amla*, acerola cherry extract	

▶ SAFETY AND DOSAGE

GENERAL REQUIREMENTS	
Indian recommendations	RDA 2020: 80 mg/day
	TUL: 2,000 mg/day, LOAEL: 3,000 mg/day
Global recommendations and limits	NIH-RDA: Male—90 mg, Female—75 mg/day
	TUL: 2,000 mg/day
	EFSA:
	Average requirement: Men—90 mg, Women—80 mg/day[11]
	LOAEL: 3,000 mg/day
	NOAEL: N/A
Notes:	Absorption decreases to about 50% or less with single doses above 1 g.[12]
	About 100–200 mg of vitamin C per day is an adequate amount to saturate plasma concentrations in healthy individuals and covers general requirements for the reduction of chronic disease risk.[12,13]

▶ CLINICAL CONDITIONS

EVIDENCE LEVEL	CONDITION OR USE CASE	DOSAGE	BENEFIT OR MECHANISM OF ACTION
+++	Oxidative stress in the skin	Subjects ingested either 100 mg or 180 mg of vitamin C per day or a placebo daily for 12 weeks.	The intake of 100 mg resulted in an increase in the radical-scavenging activity by 22% after 4 weeks while the intake of 180 mg resulted in an increase of 37%. The placebo group did not show any changes.[14]

▶ **CLINICAL CONDITIONS** (*Continued*)

EVIDENCE LEVEL	CONDITION OR USE CASE	DOSAGE	BENEFIT OR MECHANISM OF ACTION
+	Psoriasis and atopic dermatitis (AD)	Ex vivo observation	The study demonstrated higher iron concentration in the AD dermis compared to healthy controls and a lower concentration of vitamin C in the AD dermis than in the dermis of healthy controls.[15,16]
++	Atopic dermatitis	Ex vivo observation	Atopic dermatitis patients had high levels of malondialdehyde and low levels of glutathione, vitamin A, C, and E as compared to healthy controls.[17]
+++	UVB induced sunburn (DNA damage)	Subjects took 1 g of ascorbic acid and 500 IU of D-α-tocopherol (vitamin E) twice daily for 3 months.	After 3 months, the median minimal erythema dose (MED) rose demonstrating that oral vitamins E plus C decreases the skin's susceptibility to sunburn. After antioxidant treatment, the number of thymine-dimer-positive cells (produced by UV radiation, a potential factor to cause skin cancer) reduced showing the protective effect against UV-inflicted DNA damage.[18]
++++	Wrinkles	N/A (observational study)	Higher vitamin C intakes were associated with a lower likelihood of a wrinkled appearance.[19]
++	UVA mediated melanogenesis	Human melanoma cells were treated with L-ascorbic acid for 30 minutes before exposing to UVA radiation in vitro.	Ascorbic acid protects against UVA-dependent melanogenesis possibly through the improvement of antioxidant defence capacity and inhibition of nitric oxide production.[20]

▶ **CLINICAL CONDITIONS** (*Continued*)

EVIDENCE LEVEL	CONDITION OR USE CASE	DOSAGE	BENEFIT OR MECHANISM OF ACTION
++	Skin barrier function	Rat epidermal keratinocytes were treated with vitamin C supplementation in vitro.	Vitamin C enhanced the normal wavy pattern of the stratum corneum, the number of keratohyalin granules present (cross-linking of keratin filaments), and the quantity and organization of intercellular lipid lamellae in the interstices of the stratum corneum. Vitamin C correlated with improved epidermal barrier function. Filaggrin was increased by vitamin C.[21]
++	Ceramide production	Human keratinocytes were grown in 1.2 mM calcium with or without vitamin C (50 μg/mL) for 11 days.	The ceramide content increased with terminal differentiation of keratinocytes as compared to controls. The sphingosine-1-phosphate (S1P) hydrolysis was stimulated by vitamin C supplementation, contributing to enhanced ceramide production.[22]
+++	Genital warts	Subjects were divided into two groups. Group A1 received laser vaporization treatment while A2 received additional treatment with pidotimod (two sachets daily) + vitamin C (1,000 mg daily) for 15 days, and reduced doses for two more months: Pidotimod (one sachet daily) + vitamin C (500 mg daily).	The additional treatment with pidotimod and vitamin C shortened the time of warts remission and marginally decreased the rate of warts' recurrence (81% vs. 67%): Nonsignificant difference.[23]

▶ CLINICAL CONDITIONS (Continued)

EVIDENCE LEVEL	CONDITION OR USE CASE	DOSAGE	BENEFIT OR MECHANISM OF ACTION
+++	Pigmented purpuric dermatosis	Subjects were treated with 50 mg of rutoside twice a day and 1,000 mg of vitamin C daily for 6 years.	71.4% of the participants experienced complete clearance of symptoms and 20% showed more than 50% improvement in symptoms and quality of life. For patients who had relapsed, supplementation was re-initiated and all responded again. Participants with shorter disease duration showed better therapeutic success, shorter time to response and lower risk of recurrence.[24]

Note: There are many studies showing improvements in skin, hair, and nail health with multiple ingredients that include vitamin C, which have not been included herein.

▶ SUPPLEMENTATION

	BASIS	WHAT TO LOOK OUT FOR
Supplementation form	L- ascorbic acid: Most of the vitamin C and/ or multivitamin supplements available in the Indian market have this form. Some supplements have the mineral salts of vitamin C like sodium L-ascorbate. One of the studies comparing ascorbic acid versus a product containing calcium ascorbate and dehydroascorbate showed the same bioavailability in humans.	Vitamin C form is stated on the nutrition table or in the ingredients section of the product packaging.
Administration form	Tablets, effervescent tablets, chewable capsules, powders, liquids, lozenges, strips, and gummies	N/A

▶ SUPPLEMENTATION (Continued)

	BASIS	WHAT TO LOOK OUT FOR
Purity considerations	Synthetic vitamin C normally has >99% purity. Vitamin C purity from a natural source is not known and varies according to the extract used (typically, 4% of *amla*, 25% for acerola cherry fruit). Purity is not standardized by the FSSAI.	Purity of natural sources should be inquired from the manufacturer.
Patient considerations	At lower concentrations, most vitamin C is absorbed and reabsorbed in the body.[25]	
Safety considerations	Large doses of vitamin C may lead to gastrointestinal issues such as diarrhea, nausea, abdominal cramps, and other gastrointestinal disturbances due to the osmotic effect of unabsorbed vitamin C in the gastrointestinal tract[26]	Dose per serving is stated on the nutrition table.
Other considerations	Chewable tablets or gummies with high doses of vitamin C may lead to erosion of teeth.	
	Individuals at risk of kidney stones should avoid consuming high doses of vitamin C in supplements. High doses are also contraindicated in blood disorders like thalassemia, G6PD deficiency, sickle cell disease, and hemochromatosis.[27]	Individuals with any medical conditions should consult their doctors before consuming any nutritional supplement.

INTRODUCTION

Vitamin C is essential for the body as a water-soluble vitamin. As an antioxidant, vitamin C has both oxidized (DHAA) and reduced forms in the body (ascorbic acid).[2] Severe vitamin C deficiency causes scurvy, which is characterized by symptoms related to connective tissue defects.[12]

Ascorbic acid acts as an electron donor for eight enzymes-responsible for the hydroxylation of collagen and the biosynthesis of carnitine, catecholamines, and bile acids. It functions as a reducing agent for oxidases in the microsomal drug-metabolizing system that inactivates a variety of endogenous hormones or xenobiotics. The activity of both, the microsomal drug-metabolizing enzymes and cytochrome P450 enzymes, is lowered by vitamin C deficiency.[13]

In contrast to vitamin C synthesizing species, adaptational processes exist, wherein our ability to prevent vitamin C deficiency has been improved by various measures, including more efficient absorption, recycling, and its renal reuptake.[2] However, a diet that supplies 100–200 mg of vitamin C per day, provides an adequate amount to saturate plasma concentrations in healthy individuals and covers general requirements for the reduction of chronic disease risk.[12,13]

DIGESTION, ABSORPTION AND STORAGE

Digestion and Absorption

- Both forms of vitamin C are absorbed from the lumen of the intestine (by enterocytes) and reabsorbed in renal tubules (by renal epithelial cells).[1]

- Three modes of membrane transport exist: Passive diffusion, facilitated diffusion (via carrier proteins), and active transport (via transporters). The majority of intestinal uptake, tissue distribution, and renal reuptake is handled by the sodium-dependent vitamin C transporter (SVCT) family of proteins, which cotransports sodium ions and ascorbate.[1]

- Vitamin C circulates in the blood and enters all of the cells. Specific mechanisms of transport concentrate vitamin C intracellularly to enhance its function as an enzyme cofactor and antioxidant.[1]

- Dose-dependent absorption and renal regulation of ascorbate allows its conservation during low intakes and limits plasma levels at high intakes. Little unmetabolized ascorbate is excreted with dietary intakes up to about 80 mg/day, which is the current RDA, and its renal excretion increases proportionately with higher intakes.

- With large intakes of vitamin C, unabsorbed ascorbate is degraded in the intestine, which may account for the intestinal discomfort and diarrhea sometimes reported.[12]

- DHAA competes with glucose for uptake through the mammalian facilitative glucose transporters GLUT1, GLUT3, and GLUT4.[1]

Storage

- As a water-soluble vitamin, vitamin C is readily excreted in urine; not much is stored in the body.[28] Only a negligible amount is found in the blood and saliva of healthy individuals,[2] while high levels are maintained in leukocytes, the pituitary and adrenal glands, eye tissues and the brain.[12]

- Most cell types efficiently recycle DHAA to ascorbic acid, so their combined pool is considered as the total available vitamin C capacity.[2]

- Catabolic turnover varies widely. A total body pool of < 300 mg is associated with scurvy symptoms, while maximum body pools are limited to about 2 g.[12]

- There is a large difference in the content of vitamin C within the layers of the skin. The content of ascorbic acid in the epidermis is 425% higher than that in the dermis.[8]

▶ MECHANISM OF ACTION

01 | Antioxidant Activity and Photoprotection

As an electron donor, vitamin C neutralizes free radicals and takes part in numerous physiological reactions.[8] Although Vitamin C has no UV absorption spectra in the UVA (320 to 400 nm) or UVB (290 to 320 nm) range, topical ascorbic acid is able to exert photoprotection against UV radiation due to its antioxidant and anti-inflammatory properties.[29]

Vitamin C is particularly effective at reducing oxidative damage to the skin when used in conjunction with vitamin E. It can regenerate oxidized vitamin E, thereby effectively recycling this lipid-soluble antioxidant and limiting oxidative damage to cell membranes **Figure 1**.[28]

02 | Collagen Synthesis

Enzymatic hydroxylation is a post-translation modification of proline (by prolyl hydroxylase) and lysine (by lysyl hydroxylase), to make hydroxyproline and hydroxylysine, respectively. This step, which requires vitamin C as a cofactor, is critical for the stabilization of the triple helix conformation of collagen during its synthesis.

This makes vitamin C fundamental for skin turnover and in wound healing. When ascorbic acid is deficient, fibroblasts produce unstable collagen.[30]

03 | Boosting Cell Metabolism

Carnitine is essential for the transport of long-chain fatty acids into the mitochondria and plays an important role in energy production of cells. Vitamin C is an essential cofactor for enzymatic reactions required for the synthesis of carnitine. Carnitine may also favor hair growth by increasing energy supply to the proliferating cells in the hair follicle,[31,32] metabolic decline of which is implicated in hair loss.[33,34]

Vitamin C promotes late keratinocyte differentiation, which is an important prerequisite for the integrity of the skin barrier. Perturbation of the skin barrier can lead to water loss as well as skin disorders.[8] Studies have also shown that vitamin C promotes synthesis and organization of barrier lipids and increased cornified envelope formation during differentiation, the mechanism of which is not yet elucidated.[28]

Vitamin C appears to have a role in the utilization and perhaps absorption of folic acid, which is a major player in cellular metabolism.[35]

04 | Reducing Pigmentation

Tyrosinase is the main enzyme responsible for converting tyrosine into melanin. Ascorbic acid plays a role as an anti-pigmentary agent. It interacts with copper ions at the active site of the tyrosinase enzyme thereby inhibiting its action.[29,36]

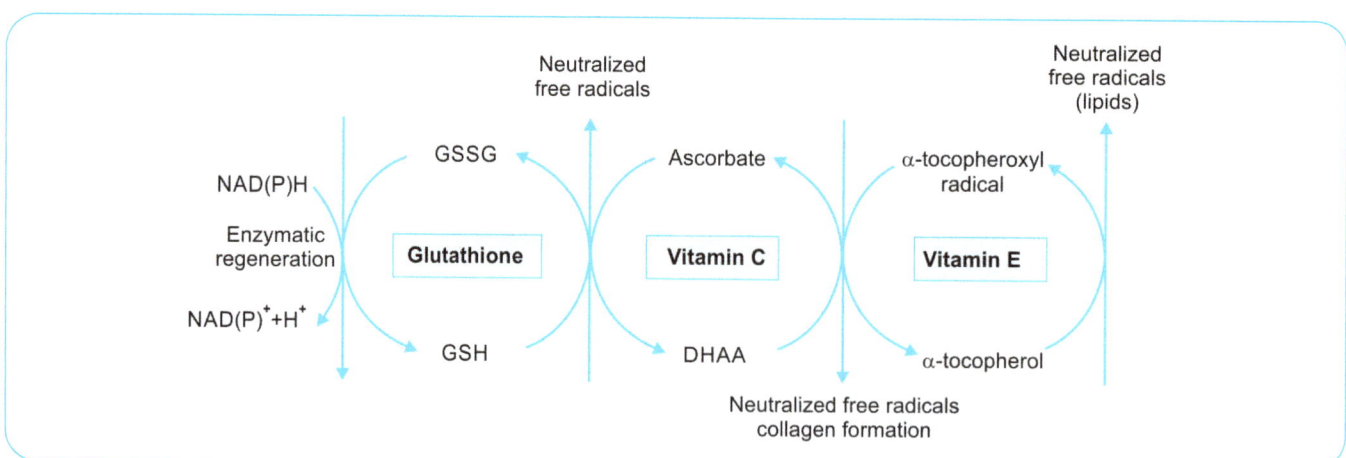

Figure 1: Vitamin C and other antioxidants in the skin scavenge free radicals and regenerate other reduced antioxidants. Vitamin E is in the lipid fraction of the cell, whereas vitamin C and glutathione (GSSG; GSH) are water-soluble and present in the cytosol. (DHAA: dehydroascorbic acid) *Source: Adapted from Pullar (2017).*[28]

Just like UV protection, vitamin C's combination with vitamin E inhibits melanocyte production more significantly than vitamin C alone.[8]

05 | Immunoregulation

Vitamin C stimulates both the production and function of leucocytes, especially neutrophils, lymphocytes, and phagocytes, by improving cellular motility, chemotaxis, and phagocytosis. Vitamin C accumulates in leucocytes and protects them from the reactive oxygen species they produce to kill pathogens, and supports neutrophil clearance by macrophages. Vitamin C also helps increase the absorption of non-heme iron, which plays a significant role in skin health and its immune response.[9,10]

06 | Epigenetic Regulation

Vitamin C influences the methylation status of DNA and histones in mammalian cells, thereby safeguarding genome integrity. By functioning as a co-factor for the ten-eleven translocation (TET) family of enzymes, vitamin C can prevent UV-induced apoptosis and melanoma progression. Vitamin C therefore, plays a role in health and disease beyond what was previously understood.[28]

▶ REFERENCES

1. Wilson John X. Regulation of Vitamin C transport. Annual Review of Nutrition. 2005;25:105-25.
2. Lykkesfeldt J, Tveden-Nyborg P. The Pharmacokinetics of Vitamin C. Nutrients. 2019;11(10):2412.
3. Mukherjee A, Dutta S, Goyal TM. India's Phytonutrient Report: A Snapshot of Fruits and Vegetables Consumption, Availability and Implications for Phytonutrient Intake --Think Tank, Indian Council for Research on International Economic Relations (ICRIER) 2016.
4. Choudhury S, Shankar B, Aleksandrowicz L, Tak M, Green R, Harris F, et al. What underlies inadequate and unequal fruit and vegetable consumption in India? An exploratory analysis. Global Food Security. 2020;24:100332.
5. Ravindran RD, Vashist P, Gupta SK, Young IS, Maraini G, Camparini M, et al. Prevalence and Risk Factors for Vitamin C Deficiency in North and South India: A Two Centre Population Based Study in People Aged 60 Years and Over. PLoS One. 2011;6(12):e28588.
6. Pradeepa R, Viswanathan M. Epidemiology of type 2 diabetes in India. Indian J Ophthalmol. 2021;69(11):2932-8.
7. Imamura F. On the gene-nutrient analyses of Cahill et al. Am J Clin Nutr. 2010;91(4):1070-1.
8. Wang K, Hui J, Li Wenshuang, Mingyue Q, Dong T, Hongbin Li. Role of Vitamin C in Skin Diseases. Front Physiol. 2018;9:819.
9. Carr AC, Silvia M. Vitamin C and Immune Function. Nutrients. 2017;9(11):1211.
10. Carr AC, Margreet CMV. Synthetic or Food-Derived Vitamin C --Are They Equally Bioavailable? Nutrients. 2013;5(11):4284-304.
11. EFSA Panel on Dietetic Products, Nutrition and Allergies (NDA). Scientific Opinion on Dietary Reference Values for vitamin C. EFSA Journal 2013;11(11):3418, 68.
12. Institute of Medicine (US) Panel on Dietary Antioxidants and Related Compounds. Dietary Reference Intakes for Vitamin C, Vitamin E, Selenium, and Carotenoids. National Academies Press (US), 2000.
13. National Institute of Nutrition Indian Council of Medical Research. Recommended Dietary Allowances and Estimated Average Requirements for Indians - 2020. RDA Full Report 2020.
14. Lauer AC, Groth N, Haag SF, Darvin ME, Lademann J, Meinke MC. Dose-dependent vitamin C uptake and radical scavenging activity in human skin measured with in vivo electron paramagnetic resonance spectroscopy. Skin Pharmacol Physiol. 2013;26(3):147-54.
15. Leveque N, Robin S, Muret P, Mac-Mary S, Makki S, Berthelot A, et al. In vivo assessment of iron and ascorbic acid in psoriatic dermis. Acta Derm Venereol. 2004;84(1):2-5.
16. Leveque N, Robin S, Muret P, Mac-Mary S, Humbert P. High iron and low ascorbic acid concentrations in the dermis of atopic dermatitis patients. Dermatology. 2003;207(3):261-4.
17. Sivaranjani N, Rao S Venkata, Rajeev G. Role of Reactive Oxygen Species and Antioxidants in Atopic Dermatitis. J Clin Diagn Res. 2013;7(12):2683-5.
18. Placzek M, Gaube S, Kerkmann U, Gilbertz KP, Herzinger T, Haen E, et al. Ultraviolet B-Induced DNA Damage in Human Epidermis Is Modified by the Antioxidants Ascorbic Acid and D-α-Tocopherol. Clinical Trial J Invest Dermatol. 2005;124(2):304-7.
19. Cosgrove MC, Franco OH, Granger SP, Murray PG, Mayes AE. Dietary nutrient intakes and skin-aging appearance among middle-aged American women. Am J Clin Nutr. 2007;86(4):1225-31.
20. Panich U, Tangsupa-a-nan V, Onkoksoong T, Kongtaphan K, Kasetsinsombat K, Akarasereenont P, et al. Inhibition of UVA-mediated melanogenesis by ascorbic acid through modulation of antioxidant defense and nitric oxide system. Arch Pharm Res. 2011;34(5):811-20.
21. Pasonen-Seppänen S, Suhonen TM, Kirjavainen M, Suihko E, Urtti A, Miettinen M, et al. Vitamin C enhances differentiation of a continuous keratinocyte cell line (REK) into epidermis with normal stratum corneum ultrastructure and functional permeability barrier. Histochem Cell Biol. 2001;116(4):287-97.
22. Kun PK, Shin KO, Park K, Yun HJ, Mann S, Lee MY, et al. Vitamin C Stimulates Epidermal Ceramide Production by Regulating Its Metabolic Enzymes. Biomol Ther (Seoul). 2015;23(6):525-30.
23. Zervoudis S, Iatrakis G, Peitsidou A, Papandonopolos L, Nikolopoulou MK, Papadopoulos L, et al. Complementary treatment with oral Pidotimod plus vitamin C after laser vaporization for female genital warts: a prospective study. J Med Life. 2010;3(3):286-8.
24. Schober SM, Peitsch WK, Gisela B, Metze D, Thomas K, Goerge T, et al. Early treatment with rutoside and ascorbic acid is highly effective for progressive pigmented purpuric dermatosis. J Dtsch Dermatol Ges. 2014;12(12):1112-9.

25. Nelson EW, Lane H, Fabri PJ, Scott B. Demonstration of saturation kinetics in the intestinal absorption of vitamin C in man and the guinea pig. J Clin Pharmacol. 1978;18(7):325-35.
26. Jacob RA, Sotoudeh G. Vitamin C function and status in chronic disease. Nutr Clin Care. 2002;5(2):66-74.
27. Abdullah M, Jamil RT, Attia FN. Vitamin C (Ascorbic Acid). In: StatPearls. Treasure Island (FL): StatPearls Publishing; 2024.
28. Pullar JM, Carr AC, and Vissers MCM. The Roles of Vitamin C in Skin Health. Nutrients 2017;9(8):866.
29. Ravetti S, Clemente C, Brignone S, Hergert L, Allemandi D, Palma S. Ascorbic Acid in Skin Health. Cosmetics 2019;6(4):58.
30. Yamauchi M, Sricholpech M. Lysine post-translational modifications of collagen. Essays Biochem. 2012;52:113-33.
31. Foitzik K, Hoting E, Förster T, Pertile P, Paus R. L-Carnitine -L-tartrate promotes human hair growth in vitro. Exp Dermatol. 2007;16(11):936-45.
32. Foitzik K, Hoting E, Heinrich U, Tronnier H, Paus R. Indications that topical L-carnitin-L-tartrate promotes human hair growth in vivo. J Dermatol Sci. 2007;48(2):141-4.
33. Badolati N, Sommella E, Riccio G, Salviati E, Heintz D, Bottone S, et al. Annurca Apple Polyphenols Ignite Keratin Production in Hair Follicles by Inhibiting the Pentose Phosphate Pathway and Amino Acid Oxidation. Nutrients. 2018;10(10):1406.
34. Piccini I, Sousa M, Altendorf S, Jimenez F, Rossi A, Funk W, et al. Intermediate Hair Follicles from Patients with Female Pattern Hair Loss Are Associated with Nutrient Insufficiency and a Quiescent Metabolic Phenotype. Nutrients. 2022;14(16):3357.
35. Shin J, Kim YJ, Kwon O, Kim NI, and ChoY. Associations among plasma vitamin C, epidermal ceramide and clinical severity of atopic dermatitis. Nutr Res Pract. 2016;10(4):398-403.
36. Ando H, Kondoh H, Ichihashi M, Hearing VJ. Approaches to identify inhibitors of melanin biosynthesis via the quality control of tyrosinase. J Invest Dermatol. 2007;127(4):751-61.

Nutrition in Dermatology

Cholecalciferol (D3)

Vitamin D

✍ Sachin Varma

CONTENTS

VITAMIN D: NUTRIENT SNAPSHOT

- ▶ REQUIREMENT IN THE INDIAN CONTEXT | 66
- ▶ ACTIVE FORMS | 67
- ▶ SAFETY AND DOSAGE | 67
- ▶ CLINICAL CONDITIONS | 67
- ▶ SUPPLEMENTATION | 70

INTRODUCTION | 71

DIGESTION, ABSORPTION AND STORAGE | 71

MECHANISM OF ACTION | 71

KEY TOPICS

- ATOPIC DERMATITIS
- PSORIASIS
- *STAPHYLOCOCCUS AUREUS* COLONIZATION
- SUNBURN
- TELOGEN EFFLUVIUM
- URTICARIA
- VITILIGO

Nutrient Snapshot

▶ **REQUIREMENT IN THE INDIAN CONTEXT**

- Vitamin D, the sunshine vitamin, is a fat soluble vitamin that is essential for skin and hair health. While foods can provide some vitamin D, synthesis in skin exposed to UVB radiation is its main source. Ergocalciferol (vitamin D2) is sourced from the UV irradiation of ergosterol, which is a steroid found in some plants but largely in fungi. Cholecalciferol (vitamin D3) is synthesized via the UV irradiation of 7-dehydrocholesterol to previtamin D3 in the skin of animals exposed to UVB rays.[1]

- Exposing your arms and legs to midday sun (between 11 AM and 2 PM) for just 15 to 30 minutes (twice a week) can be sufficient to meet vitamin D requirements. However, season, latitude, and skin pigmentation all affect cutaneous synthesis of vitamin D.[2]

- In India, Vitamin D deficiency is widespread. Various factors such as an indoor and sedentary lifestyle, clothing, air pollution and skin complexion are some of the reasons for it. Furthermore, there is a decline in vitamin D synthesis with age.[3-5] Measurement of serum levels of vitamin D should be considered upon suspicion of deficiency or excess.

Nutrition in Dermatology

▶ ACTIVE FORMS

ACTIVE FORMS	SUPPLEMENT SOURCES	SALIENT FEATURES
Vitamin D3	Lanolin (wool source)	Research indicates that vitamin D3 is more efficacious at raising serum 25(OH)D concentrations than is vitamin D2.[1]
	Lichen (vegan source)	Lichen is the only source of vegan vitamin D3.
Vitamin D2	Mushroom or yeast	Since vitamin D2 is cheaper to produce, it's the most common form in fortified foods.

▶ SAFETY AND DOSAGE

GENERAL REQUIREMENTS	
Indian recommendations	ICMR-NIN RDA: 600 IU, EAR: 400 IU, TUL: 4,000 IU
Global recommendations and limits	NIH (USA) RDA: 600 IU, TUL: 4,000 IU
	EFSA: NOAEL—10,000 IU
Notes:	1 µg of vitamin D is equal to 40 IU.
	Vitamin D needs to be taken after a meal as it is fat soluble.
	Caution must be exercised when providing high doses of vitamin D. Magnesium supplementation should be given for doses >RDA, as large doses of vitamin D can lead to Mg depletion.

▶ CLINICAL CONDITIONS

EVIDENCE LEVEL	CONDITION OR USE CASE	DOSAGE	BENEFIT OR MECHANISM OF ACTION
+++	Telogen effluvium	6 doses of 2,00,000 IU were given fortnightly and assessments were done after 15 days of last dose.	The use of oral vitamin D3 (200,000 IU, fortnightly) for 3 months resulted in improvement in hair regrowth in the patient of TE.[6]
+++	Psoriasis and vitiligo	Patients with psoriasis and vitiligo received 35,000 IU daily for 6 months along with a low-calcium diet (avoiding dairy products and calcium-enriched foods like oat, rice or soya "milk") and hydration (minimum 2.5 L daily).	The Psoriasis Area and Severity Index (PASI) score improved in all patients with psoriasis. Patients with vitiligo had 25–75% repigmentation.[7]

▶ **CLINICAL CONDITIONS** (*Continued*)

EVIDENCE LEVEL	CONDITION OR USE CASE	DOSAGE	BENEFIT OR MECHANISM OF ACTION
+++++	Atopic dermatitis (AD)	One group of patients received 1,600 IU of vitamin D3 and other the group received placebo for 2 months	Scoring Atopic Dermatitis (SCORAD) and Three Item Severity (TIS) score value index in the vitamin D group showed improvement in patients with mild, moderate and severe AD and in patients with placebo, no improvement was seen.[8]
+++	Atopic dermatitis and *Staphylococcus aureus* colonization	Patients either received oral 2,000 IU/ day of vitamin D supplement or placebo for 4 weeks	*Staphylococcus aureus* colonization in the skin of AD patients reduces cathelicidin, which plays a crucial role in innate and adaptive immunity. With Vitamin D supplementation, there was reduction in *S. aureus* skin colonization, SCORAD score (of AD severity) and erythema index.[10]
++	Atopic dermatitis	Patients received 2,000 IU daily of vitamin D3 for 3 months	After supplementation, both mean objective SCORAD and SCORAD index were lowered significantly.[11]
+++	Urticaria	Patients were treated with vitamin D 50,000 IU weekly followed by daily supplementation (dose not given) for 8–12 weeks duration.	With vitamin D treatment, 70% of subjects had complete resolution of symptoms. Symptom recurrence was seen in subsequent months only if vitamin D insufficiency recurred.[12]

▶ CLINICAL CONDITIONS (Continued)

EVIDENCE LEVEL	CONDITION OR USE CASE	DOSAGE	BENEFIT OR MECHANISM OF ACTION
+++	Urticaria	Subjects with chronic urticaria either received high (4,000 IU/day) or low (600 IU/day) vitamin D3 supplementation for 12 weeks along with a standardized triple-drug therapy (cetirizine, ranitidine, and montelukast)	Triple-drug therapy decreased total Urticaria Symptom Severity (USS) scores in the first week with further decrease in total USS scores in the high, but not low, vitamin D3 treatment group by week 12. Compared with low treatment, the high treatment group demonstrated a trend toward lower total USS scores at week 12, driven by significant decreases in body distribution and number of days with hives. Beneficial trends for sleep quality and pruritus scores were observed with high vitamin D3. There was no correlation between 25-hydroxyvitamin D levels and USS scores.[13]
++++	Sunburn	200,000 IU 1 hour after induced UV radiation	Compared to placebo, participants receiving vitamin D3 demonstrated reduced expression of pro-inflammatory mediators tumor necrosis factor-alpha (TNF-α) and inducible nitric oxide synthase (iNOS) in skin biopsy specimens 48 hours after experimental sunburn. Global gene expression profiles revealed that participants with higher serum vitamin D3 levels after treatment demonstrated increased skin expression of the anti-inflammatory mediator arginase-1, and a sustained reduction in skin redness, correlating with expression of genes related to skin barrier repair.

▶ SUPPLEMENTATION

	BASIS	WHAT TO LOOK OUT FOR
Supplementation form	Vitamin D3 is superior to D2 in raising and maintaining serum concentrations of vitamin D and also produces 2–3 times more storage than D2.[15,16]	The vitamin D source should be mentioned in the ingredients section on the label.
Administration form	Capsules, tablets, soft gels, flavored lozenges, flavored syrups	Either form is suitable. Vitamin D needs to be taken after a meal as it is fat soluble.
Purity considerations	Vitamin D normally has >99% purity.	N/A
Patient considerations	Vitamin D2 is obtained from a veg source but vitamin D3 is more potent than D2. Lichen is the only vegan source of vitamin D3.	The vitamin D source should be mentioned in the ingredients section on the label. Normally, vitamin D3 in supplements is non-vegan, unless stated otherwise.
Safety considerations	Mega doses of vitamin D are indicated in case of deficiency and should be given only for specific periods and frequency varies from once in a week, once in fortnight to once in a month. Magnesium supplementation should be given when vitamin D in doses >RDA are given. A dose above 10,000 IU for a longer period of time can lead to toxicity and thus frequency and duration of supplementation need to be confirmed by the doctor. Vitamin D3 doses above RDA (600 IU) should not be taken without a doctor's recommendation.	Measurement of serum levels of $1,25(OH)_2D$ should be considered when providing mega doses.
Other considerations	Vitamin D2 is more sensitive to humidity and fluctuations in temperature. For this reason, vitamin D2 supplements may be more likely to degrade over time and have a shorter shelf-life.[17]	The vitamin D type should be mentioned in the ingredients section on the label. Storage conditions should be considered for vitamin D2.

▶ INTRODUCTION

Vitamin D is more like a hormone than a vitamin. The vitamin D receptor (VDR) is found in nearly all, if not all, cells in the body. The enzyme that produces the active hormone of vitamin D, 1,25-dihydroxyvitamin D3 (calcitriol; 1,25(OH)$_2$D), namely CYP27B1, likewise is widely expressed in many cells of the body. These observations indicate that the role of vitamin D is not limited to regulation of bone and mineral homeostasis.

Evidence suggests vitamin D has anti-inflammatory and immunoregulatory properties. It has a major role to play in the regulation of keratinocytes, the balance of the cutaneous immune system, and the process of apoptosis. It also helps to regulate the synthesis of glycosylceramides needed for barrier function and permeability in the stratum corneum.[18]

▶ DIGESTION, ABSORPTION AND STORAGE

Digestion and Absorption

- Vitamin D absorption occurs by passive diffusion or may be carrier-mediated, especially cholesterol transporters.[19]

- Fat consumed concomitantly with vitamin D improves vitamin D absorption. Phytosterols and long-chain fatty acids reduce the absorption of vitamin D.[19]

- Factors that could interfere with vitamin D uptake include uremia, gastrectomy and malabsorptive and inflammatory conditions. Intestinal absorption of vitamin D might be greater in states of vitamin D deficiency.[19]

- Vitamin D3 enters the circulation and is transported to the liver, where it is hydroxylated to form 25-hydroxyvitamin D3 (calcidiol; the major circulating form of vitamin D). In the kidneys, the 25-hydroxyvitamin D3-1-hydroxylase enzyme catalyzes a second hydroxylation, resulting in the formation of 1,25-dihydroxyvitamin D3 (calcitriol).

- Keratinocytes of the epidermis also possess the enzymes needed to convert vitamin D to 1,25(OH)$_2$D.

Storage

As a fat soluble vitamin, vitamin D is stored mainly in adipose tissue.

▶ MECHANISM OF ACTION

Vitamin D signaling may involve nongenomic as well as genomic mechanisms of action.

01 | Keratinocyte Regulation and Photoprotection

1,25(OH)$_2$D functions as a steroid hormone. Upon entering the nucleus, it associates with the VDR, which heterodimerizes with the retinoic acid X receptor (RXR). This complex binds sequences of DNA known as vitamin D response elements (VDREs); this initiates a cascade of molecular interactions that modulate the transcription of certain genes. In this manner, vitamin D inhibits the expression of genes responsible for keratinocyte proliferation and induces the expression of genes responsible for keratinocyte differentiation.

In addition to its steroid hormone actions, vitamin D regulates biochemical steps that result in a cellular influx of calcium, which is important in cell differentiation and apoptosis. Because uncontrolled proliferation of cells with certain mutations may lead to cancer, vitamin D and VDR are known to be protective against carcinogenesis.

1,25(OH)$_2$D has shown to prevent UV-induced apoptosis and DNA damage in human skin cells.[20,21] UV protective benefits occur through its ability to reduce nitric oxide metabolites (that otherwise cause DNA damage), upregulate p53 (tumor surpressor) and promote inherent antioxidant systems.[21]

02 | Hair Growth

Vitamin D's role in cell division and keratinocyte regulation, and therefore hair growth, is undisputed. Furthermore, VDR is essential for β-catenin induction of stem cell proliferation and differentiation required for anagen entry. Whether regulation of hair follicle cycling is an independent action of VDR or whether it requires vitamin D or another ligand is currently unclear.[22]

03 | Barrier Function

Vitamin D mediates its effect on the epidermal barrier by enhanced synthesis of structural proteins of the cornified envelope. Additionally, 1,25(OH)$_2$D regulates the processing of the long-chain glycosylceramides essential for lipid barrier formation.[23]

04 | Immunomodulation and Wound Healing

The processes of epidermal proliferation and differentiation are essential for wound healing as well. Moreover, 1,25(OH)$_2$D regulates the expression of cathelicidin, an antimicrobial protein that appears to modulates inflammation, induces angiogenesis, and improves reepithelialization.[24-26]

The influence of 1,25(OH)$_2$D on the immune system is one of its most important roles. VDR is present in most immune cell types, particularly in monocytes, macrophages and dendritic cells. Together with cathelicidin, 1,25(OH)$_2$D also expresses beta defensins which attack pathogens. In general, the innate immune system is enhanced and the adaptive immune system is inhibited by 1,25(OH)$_2$D. Thus, vitamin D performs a balancing act on the inflammatory system.[27]

In cutaneous adaptive immunity, T helper (Th) cells appear to be the principal target for 1,25(OH)$_2$D, which can suppress Th cell proliferation as well as modulate cytokines production by these cells. Another group of T cells known to be potently induced by 1,25(OH)$_2$D are regulatory T cells (Tregs). Although part of the Th cell family, Tregs act to suppress immune responses by other T cells as part of the machinery to prevent over-exuberant or autoimmune responses.[28] This is thought to be the reason that vitamin D treatment shows improvement in conditions like psoriasis and atopic dermatitis, where immune dysregulation occurs.[23]

▶ REFERENCES

1. Tripkovic L, Lambert H, Hart K, Smith CP, Bucca G, Penson S, et al. Comparison of vitamin D2 and vitamin D3 supplementation in raising serum 25-hydroxyvitamin D status: a systematic review and meta-analysis. Am J Clin Nutr. 2012;95(6):1357-64.
2. Harinarayan CV, Holick MF, Prasad UV, Vani PS, Himabindu G. Vitamin D status and sun exposure in India. Dermatoendocrinol. 2013;5(1):130-41.
3. Aparna P, Muthathal S, Nongkynrih B, Gupta SK. Vitamin D deficiency in India. J Family Med Prim Care. 2018;7(2):324-30.
4. National Institute of Nutrition Indian Council of Medical Research. Recommended Dietary Allowances and Estimated Average Requirements for Indians - 2020. RDA Full Report 2020.
5. MacLaughlin J, Holick MF. Aging decreases the capacity of human skin to produce vitamin D3. J Clin Invest. 1985;76(4):1536-8.
6. Sattar F, Almas U, Ibrahim NA, Akhtar A, Shazad MK, Akram S, et al. Efficacy of Oral Vitamin D3 Therapy in Patients Suffering from Diffuse Hair Loss (Telogen Effluvium). J Nutr Sci Vitaminol (Tokyo). 2021;67(1):68-71.
7. Finamor DC, Sinigaglia-Coimbra R, Neves Luiz CM, Gutierrez M, Silva JJ, Torres LD, et al. A pilot study assessing the effect of prolonged administration of high daily doses of vitamin D on the clinical course of vitiligo and psoriasis. Dermatoendocrinol. 2013;5(1):222-34.
8. Amestejani M, Salehi BS, Vasigh M, Sobhkhiz A, Karami M, Alinia H, et al. Vitamin D supplementation in the treatment of atopic dermatitis: a clinical trial study. J Drugs Dermatol. 2012;11(3):327-30.
9. Javanbakht MH, Keshavarz SA, Djalali M, Siassi F, Eshraghian MR, Firooz A, et al. Randomized controlled trial using vitamins E and D supplementation in atopic dermatitis. J Dermatolog Treat. 2011;22(3):144-50.
10. Udompataikul M, Huajai S, Chalermchai T, Taweechotipatr M, Kamanamool N. The Effects of Oral Vitamin D Supplement on Atopic Dermatitis: A Clinical Trial with Staphylococcus aureus Colonization Determination. J Med Assoc Thai. 2015;98(Suppl 9):S23-30.
11. Samochocki Z, Bogaczewicz J, Jeziorkowska R, Sysa-Jędrzejowska A, et al. Vitamin D effects in atopic dermatitis. Journal of the American Academy of Dermatology. 2013;69(2):238-44.
12. Goetz DW. Idiopathic itch, rash, and urticaria/angioedema merit serum vitamin D evaluation: a descriptive case series. W V Med J. 2011;107(1):14-20.
13. Rorie A, Goldner WS, Lyden E, Poole JA. Beneficial role for supplemental vitamin D3 treatment in chronic urticaria: a randomized study. Ann Allergy Asthma Immunol. 2014;112(4):376-82.
14. Scott JF, Das LM, Ahsanuddin S, Qiu Y, Binko AM, Traylor ZP, et al. Oral vitamin D rapidly attenuates inflammation from sunburn: an interventional study. J Invest Dermatol. 2017;137(10):2078-86.
15. Heaney RP, Recker RR, Grote J, Horst RL, Armas Laura AG. Vitamin D(3) is more potent than vitamin D(2) in humans. J Clin Endocrinol Metab. 2011;96(3):E447-52.

16. Balachandar R, Pullakhandam R, Kulkarni B, Sachdev HS. Relative Efficacy of Vitamin D2 and Vitamin D3 in Improving Vitamin D Status: Systematic Review and Meta-Analysis. Nutrients. 2021;13(10):3328.
17. Houghton LA, Vieth R. The case against ergocalciferol (vitamin D2) as a vitamin supplement. Am J Clin Nutr. 2006;84(4):694-7.
18. Barrea L, Savanelli MC, Di Somma C, Napolitano M, Megna M, Colao A, et al. Vitamin D and its role in psoriasis: An overview of the dermatologist and nutritionist. Rev Endocr Metab Disord. 2017;18(2):195-205.
19. Silva MC, Furlanetto TW. Intestinal absorption of vitamin D: a systematic review. Nutrition Reviews. 2018;76(1):60-76.
20. De Haes P, Garmyn M, Degreef H, Vantieghem K, Bouillon R, Segaert S. 1,25-Dihydroxyvitamin D3 inhibits ultraviolet B-induced apoptosis, Jun kinase activation, and interleukin-6 production in primary human keratinocytes. J Cell Biochem. 2003;89(4):663-73.
21. Dixon KM, Tongkao-On W, Sequeira VB, Carter SE, Song EJ, Rybchyn MS, et al. Vitamin D and Death by Sunshine. Int J Mol Sci. 2013;14(1):1964-77.
22. Pálmer HG, Anjos-Afonso F, Carmeliet G, Takeda H, Watt FM. The Vitamin D Receptor Is a Wnt Effector that Controls Hair Follicle Differentiation and Specifies Tumor Type in Adult Epidermis. PLoS One. 2008;3(1):e1483.
23. Umar M, Sastry KS, Al Ali F, Al-Khulaifi M, Wang E, Chouchane AI. Vitamin D and the Pathophysiology of Inflammatory Skin Diseases. Skin Pharmacology and Physiology. 2018;31(2):74-86.
24. Heilborn JD, Nilsson MF, Kratz G, Weber G, Sørensen O, Borregaard N, et al. The cathelicidin anti-microbial peptide LL-37 is involved in re-epithelialization of human skin wounds and is lacking in chronic ulcer epithelium. J Invest Dermatol. 2003;120(3):379-89.
25. Wang TT, Nestel FP, Bourdeau V, Nagai Y, Wang Q, Liao J, et al. Cutting edge: 1,25-dihydroxyvitamin D3 is a direct inducer of antimicrobial peptide gene expression. J Immunol. 2004;173(5):2909-12.
26. Frohm M, Agerberth B, Ahangari G, Ståhle-Bäckdahl M, Lidén S, Wigzell H, et al. The expression of the gene coding for the antibacterial peptide LL-37 is induced in human keratinocytes during inflammatory disorders. J Biol Chem. 1997;272(24):15258-63.
27. Mangin M, Sinha R, Fincher K. Inflammation and vitamin D: the infection connection. Inflamm Res. 2014;63(10):803-19.
28. Mostafa WZ, Hegazy RA. Vitamin D and the skin: Focus on a complex relationship: A review. J Adv Res. 2015;6(6):793-804.

08

Tocopherols and Tocotrienols

Vitamin E

✍ Sachin Varma

CONTENTS

VITAMIN E: NUTRIENT SNAPSHOT

- ▶ REQUIREMENT IN THE INDIAN CONTEXT | **75**
- ▶ ACTIVE FORMS | **76**
- ▶ SAFETY AND DOSAGE | **76**
- ▶ CLINICAL CONDITIONS | **77**
- ▶ SUPPLEMENTATION | **82**

INTRODUCTION | **83**

DIGESTION, ABSORPTION AND STORAGE | **83**

MECHANISM OF ACTION | **84**

KEY TOPICS

- ACNE VULGARIS
- AUTOANTIBODY PRODUCTION IN LUPUS ERYTHEMATOUS
- CHLOASMA AND PIGMENTED CONTACT DERMATITIS
- HAIR LOSS
- LEPROSY
- PHOTOPROTECTION
- PSORIASIS
- THERMAL STRESS
- VITILIGO

Nutrient Snapshot

▶ **REQUIREMENT IN THE INDIAN CONTEXT**

- Vitamin E is a collective term for tocopherols and tocotrienols.[1] It is a fat soluble vitamin that is essential for skin and hair health. Vitamin E can prevent lipid peroxidation of the cell membrane and the sebum, which otherwise results in cell damage, barrier issues, aging and induces various skin pathologies.[2] That's why vitamin E is the most prominent antioxidant in the lipophilic phase, while vitamin C and glutathione (GSH) have the highest abundance in the cytosol, together forming the bulk of the cellular redox system.

- Vitamin E deficiency is seldom found in adult humans.[3] Vegetable oil and unseen fats from cereal, nuts and vegetables contribute to adequate tocopherol content in Indian diets. While limited, the available information suggests that α-tocopherol levels in blood are of 0.5 mg/kg/mL, which is considered satisfactory.[4] However, low carbohydrate diets like the ketogenic diet (that are high in fat) are often low in vitamin E.[5]

- Vitamin E is of prime importance in dermatology. Alopecia patients generally exhibit lower levels of antioxidants in their scalp and a higher lipid peroxidation index.[6] It is also imperative for photoprotection. Irradiation of skin with UV at doses below those that cause a mild redness can deplete α-tocopherol by almost 50% in the stratum corneum.[7] That perhaps causes the characteristic vitamin E gradient in the stratum corneum, with lower levels toward the outer layers.[8]

- Although many cosmeceuticals contain vitamins C and E, the benefit of using oral administration is to deliver them in their active form to deeper layers; they do not have issues of crossing the skin layers. Topical products may be degraded by light and air.[9]

- Supplemental vitamin E is useful for general dermatological purposes. It is particularly useful for skin conditions like alopecia and atopic dermatitis, where lipid peroxidation, leading to damage of epidermal keratinocytes and inflammation, is a key concern.[1,6]

▶ ACTIVE FORMS

ACTIVE FORMS	SUPPLEMENT SOURCES	SALIENT FEATURES
Tocopherol	Palm oil, sunflower oil or synthetic	α-tocopherol is most commonly used in supplements. Other naturally occurring forms of vitamin E (β-, γ-, and δ-tocopherols and the tocotrienols) do not contribute toward meeting the vitamin E requirement because (although absorbed) they are not converted to α-tocopherol by humans and are recognized poorly by the α-tocopherol transfer protein (α-TTP) in the liver. While other forms of vitamin E do get transported to extrahepatic tissue, the significance of TTP in their transport is unclear at present.[10]
Tocotrienol	Tocotrienol-rich extract of palm oil, rice bran oil, synthetic	Tocotrienols display greater antioxidant potential than tocopherols due to their unsaturated and isoprenoid side chain.[1] Studies found that tocotrienols exhibit biological activities not shared by tocopherols, including neuroprotective, radioprotective, anticancer, anti-inflammatory and lipid lowering properties[11]

▶ SAFETY AND DOSAGE

GENERAL REQUIREMENTS	
Indian recommendations	ICMR-NIN RDA: 7.5–10 mg α-tocopherol TUL: N/A
Global recommendations and limits	NIH (USA) RDA: 15 mg, TUL: 1,000 mg (2,325 μmol)/day of any form of supplemental α-tocopherol based on the adverse effect of increased tendency to hemorrhage.[10] EFSA: AI for α-tocopherol is 13 mg/day for Male and 11 mg/day for Female[12] NOAEL: 540 mg α-tocopherol equivalent (TE)/day[12] UL: 300 mg α-TE/day
Notes:	1 mg of vitamin E is equal to 1.5 IU d-α-tocopherol (natural) or 1.1 IU dL-α-tocopherol (synthetic). Vitamin E needs to be taken after a meal as it is a fat soluble vitamin.

▶ CLINICAL CONDITIONS

EVIDENCE LEVEL	CONDITION OR USE CASE	DOSAGE	BENEFIT OR MECHANISM OF ACTION
++++	Psoriasis, atopic dermatitis, acne and vitiligo	N/A (meta-analysis of observational studies)	This meta-analysis showed that levels of serum vitamin E were lower in individuals suffering from psoriasis, atopic dermatitis, vitiligo, and acne.[13]
++++	Atopic dermatitis (AD)	Subjects were divided into 4 groups. Group P received vitamins D and E placebos; group D ingested 1600 IU vitamin D3 + vitamin E placebo; group E ingested 600 IU α-tocopherol + vitamin D placebo; and group DE 1600 IU vitamin D3 + 600 IU α-tocopherol for 60 days.	There was reduction in SCORing Atopic Dermatitis (SCORAD) after 60 days in groups D, E and DE. Objective SCORAD also showed improvements. There was a positive correlation between SCORAD and intensity, objective, subjective and extent and negative association between plasma α-tocopherol and SCORAD, intensity, objective and extent.[15]
+++++	Atopic dermatitis (AD)	Patients received either 400 IU vitamin E or placebo daily for 4 months	There was an improvement in all symptoms such as itching, extent of lesion, and SCORAD index in the group receiving vitamin E, compared to placebo.[14]
+++++	Atopic dermatitis (AD)	Subjects ingested 400 IU (268 mg) of vitamin E or placebo for 8 months	Females showed less progression of AD than males in both groups and a higher percentage of almost complete remission. Subjects with great improvement and near remission of AD in the vitamin E group demonstrated a decrease in serum IgE. In the placebo group, the difference was half of that seen in the vitamin E group. There was remarkable improvement in facial erythema, lichenification, and the presence of apparently normal skin was reported. Eczematous lesions healed mostly as a result of decreased pruritus.[16]

▶ **CLINICAL CONDITIONS** *(Continued)*

EVIDENCE LEVEL	CONDITION OR USE CASE	DOSAGE	BENEFIT OR MECHANISM OF ACTION
+++	UV induced erythema	Subjects received a carotenoid supplement (25 mg) daily with or without a vitamin E supplement (500 IU or 335 mg) for 12 weeks.	Serum β-carotene and α-tocopherol concentrations increased with supplementation. Erythema on dorsal skin (back) was diminished after week 8, and erythema suppression was greater with the combination of carotenoids and vitamin E than with carotenoids alone.[17]
++++	UV induced skin inflammation	Subjects were divided in 4 groups Group 1: α-tocopherol (α-Toc)- 2 g/day, Group 2: Ascorbic acid (Asc) 3 g/day Group 3: α-Toc 2 g/day combined with Asc 3 g/day Group 4: Placebo, for 50 days.	After 50 days of supplementation, α-Toc keratinocyte levels were increased in groups 1 and 3, Asc concentrations were elevated in groups 2 and 3, and the α/γ-Toc ratio increased in groups 1 and 3. The minimal erythema dose (MED) increased after supplementation in group 3, when both vitamins were combined.[18]
++	Sunburn	Subjects received either 2 g of vitamin C plus 1000 IU (approximately 667 mg) vitamin E or placebo for 8 days	The median minimal erythema dose (MED) of those taking vitamins increased, whereas it declined in the placebo group.[19]
+++	Photoprotection	Subjects were divided into 3 groups. Group 1 received d-α- tocopherol 1,200 IU (approximately 800 mg); Group 2 received ascorbic acid 2 g and Group 3 received ascorbic acid 2 g + d-α-tocopherol 1,200 IU (approximately 800 mg) daily for 1 week	The results showed that the median minimal erythema dose (MED) increased in group 1 and in group 3 (both groups with supplemental vitamin E). No modifications were observed in group 2 (the group given only ascorbic acid).[20]

▶ CLINICAL CONDITIONS (Continued)

EVIDENCE LEVEL	CONDITION OR USE CASE	DOSAGE	BENEFIT OR MECHANISM OF ACTION
+++	Psoriasis	Severe erythrodermic (EP) and arthropathic (PsA) forms of psoriasis patients received either coenzyme Q10 (50 mg), vitamin E (50 mg), and selenium (48 mg) or placebo for 30–35 day.	Plasma levels of oxidative stress markers were greater than normal in psoriatic patients. Supplementation resulted in an improvement of clinical conditions, which corresponded to the faster normalization of the oxidative stress markers compared to placebo.[21]
+++	Vitiligo	Subjects were divided into 2 groups: Group A treated with narrowband ultraviolet B (NB-UVB) + oral supplement of α-tocopherol 400 IU daily for 6 months (started 2 weeks before NB-UVB) Group B included 12 patients treated with NB-UVB as monotherapy for 6 months.	There was improvement recorded in the extent of repigmentation in the existing lesions. Number of patients with repigmentation was higher in group A than in group B. After treatment, there was a reduction in plasma malondialdehyde (MDA; product of lipid peroxidation) in group A than in group B, but the increase in plasma GSH was not significant.[22]

▶ **CLINICAL CONDITIONS** *(Continued)*

EVIDENCE LEVEL	CONDITION OR USE CASE	DOSAGE	BENEFIT OR MECHANISM OF ACTION
+++	Chloasma and pigmented contact dermatitis (PCD)	Subjects received either a combination of vitamin C and E or a single preparation for vitamin C and E. Dose and duration not available	The objective data from color difference measurements and color photographs revealed better results with combination treatment in chloasma than vitamin C alone and, in PCD, than vitamin E or C alone. Differences in skin luminosity between hyperpigmented and normal areas decreased in all three groups, with the combination group producing the most change. The total serum lipoperoxide level declined in the combination group, and decreased significantly in the vitamin E group. The sebum lipoperoxide level decreased significantly only in the combination group.[23]
+++	Hair loss	Each subject received a capsule containing 50 mg of mixed tocotrienols (30.8% α-tocotrienol, 56.4% γ-tocotrienol and 12.8% δ-tocotrienol) as well as 23 IU of α-tocopherol twice daily for 8 months	The number of hairs of the subjects in the supplementation group increased as compared to the placebo. The cumulative weight of 20 strands of hair clippings did not differ much from the baseline for both groups.[6]

▶ CLINICAL CONDITIONS (Continued)

EVIDENCE LEVEL	CONDITION OR USE CASE	DOSAGE	BENEFIT OR MECHANISM OF ACTION
++	Thermal stress	Human epidermal keratinocytes were treated with 100 µM vitamin E for 24 hours followed by thermal stress at 51°C for 10 minutes in vitro	Vitamin E preconditioning resulted in improved cell morphology, enhanced viability and reduced lactate dehydrogenase release. Vitamin E preconditioned cells exposed to thermal stress showed down-regulated expression of BAX (proapoptotic protein) and up-regulated expression of PCNA (component of replication and repair), BCL-XL (antiapoptotic protein), vascular endothelial growth factor (VEGF), involucrin, transglutaminase 1 (TGM1) and filaggrin (FLG) escorted by increased paracrine release of VEGF, basic fibroblast growth factor (bFGF) and epidermal growth factor (EGF).[24]
++	Leprosy	Leprosy patients received multiple drug therapy (MDT) with or without 400 IU of vitamin E supplementation for 12 months	Coadministration of vitamin E along with MDT decreased oxidative stress and improved antioxidant status.[25]
++	Autoantibody production in lupus erythematous	Patients received vitamin E (150 to 300 mg/day) together with prednisolone (PSL) versus a prednisolone only group	Urinary 8-hydroxydeoxyguanosine (8-OHdG), an indicator of oxidative DNA damage, and the anti-double-stranded DNA (anti-ds DNA) antibody, a predictor of disease activity, were assayed. The anti-ds DNA antibody titer in the PSL with vitamin E group was significantly lower than that in the PSL without vitamin E group.[26]

Note: There are many studies showing improvements in skin, hair and nail health with multiple ingredients that include vitamin E, which have not been included herein.

▶ SUPPLEMENTATION

	BASIS	WHAT TO LOOK OUT FOR?
Supplementation form	d-α-tocopherol is a natural form dL-α-tocopherol is a synthetic form α-tocotrienol is a natural form	The form is mentioned in the ingredients list of the product packaging. If it is not stated, the manufacturer can provide the information.
Administration form	Softgels, capsules, syrups	N/A
Purity considerations	Synthetic vitamin E has >99% purity. Purity of natural forms may vary.	N/A
Patient considerations	Vitamin E being a fat soluble vitamin should be taken after meals for better absorption.	N/A
Safety considerations	Acute doses of mixed tocotrienols ranging from 200 to 1011 mg were considerably safe for human consumption and no adverse events was reported.[11] Most people do not experience any side effects when taking the recommended daily doses. High doses can cause nausea, diarrhea, stomach cramps, fatigue, weakness, headache, blurred vision, rash, bruising, and bleeding.[9] Patients taking anticoagulants should be monitored for increased bleeding tendencies.[9]	The best indicator of the vitamin E level is serum α-tocopherol. However, this test may be unnecessary, unless an excess is suspected.[27] Patients with chronic disorders should consult their doctors before starting any nutritional supplement.
Other considerations	Combining vitamin E with vitamin C or coenzyme Q10, and some carotenoids and polyphenols, can promote its antioxidant benefits as they act synergistically.[9,28,29]	

INTRODUCTION

Cellular redox homeostasis ensures the balance between reducing and oxidizing reactions and regulates a plethora of biological events. Vitamin E is part of this system, alongside other cellular antioxidants like vitamin C and glutathione. Synergistically they maintain the concentration of vitamin E and keep its radical concentrations low.[3] Since this system is coupled with the energy status of the organism, prolonged energy deficit, or deficiencies of niacin (component of NADP or NADPH) or riboflavin (cofactor for glutathione reductase) can compromise the system.[4]

Of the eight naturally occurring forms of vitamin E (four tocopherols and four tocotrienols), the main forms in the diet are α- and γ-tocopherol, due to the highest content in food products. However, only the α-tocopherol form is maintained in human plasma and has the highest tissue concentration. This is because it has the highest affinity for α-tocopherol transfer protein (α-TTP) in the human liver. The α- forms of both tocopherols and tocotrienols are considered as the most metabolically active.[30]

As mentioned earlier, the main function of vitamin E in humans is that of a fat-soluble antioxidant. Fats are an integral part of every cell membrane, and are vulnerable to damage through lipid peroxidation by free radicals, which is especially true for unsaturated fats.[4] It therefore helps maintain cell membrane fluidity and stability.[27]

By virtue of a shorter hydrocarbon tail, tocotrienols are considered stronger free radical quenchers than tocopherols, about 40- to 60-fold more potent,[6] due to their greater flexibility and agility **(Figure 1)**.[31] The unsaturated side chain of tocotrienol allows for more efficient penetration into tissue as well.[32]

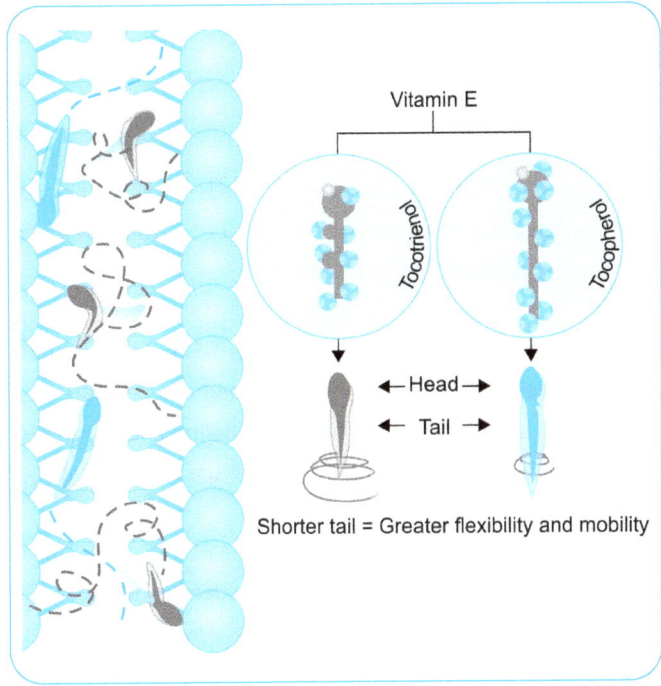

Figure 1: The vitamin E molecule looks like a tadpole with a head and a tail. Tocotrienols have a shorter tail than tocopherols, giving them greater flexibility and agility within cellular membranes.

DIGESTION, ABSORPTION AND STORAGE

Digestion and Absorption

- Fat-soluble vitamins are absorbed in the small intestine into newly forming micelles. This process is dependent on bile and pancreatic enzymes secretion.[27]

- After absorption into enterocytes, α-tocotrienol is taken up by small HDL particles whilst α-tocopherol is taken up by chylomicrons, that are secreted into the lymphatic system before entering the bloodstream.[11,27]

- Chylomicrons are metabolized by lipoprotein lipase, which release vitamin E into tissue for use and storage.[27]

- α-tocopherol is targeted into lipoproteins in the liver by a α-tocopherol transfer protein (TTP),[27] while α-tocotrienol may be absorbed via an α-TTP independent pathway.[11,30]

- The absorption of tocopherols and tocotrienols in the intestine is 20–80%.[30]

Storage

- As a fat-soluble vitamin, vitamin E is stored mainly in adipose tissue. They also accumulate in many tissue including the liver and adrenal glands.[27,30]

- Plasma and body tissue are 90% saturated with α-tocopherol while other forms of are believed to be degraded and excreted. However, their hepatically-formed metabolites show promise in the prevention of diseases driven by acute inflammatory and oxidative processes.[33]

- Accumulated tocotrienols are difficult to detect and largely unknown; however, their supplementation in animals has shown an increase in adipose tissue.[30]

▶ MECHANISM OF ACTION

01 | Antioxidant Activity

Vitamin E is a peroxyl radical scavenger and especially protects PUFAs within cell membrane phospholipids and in plasma lipoproteins.[34] Peroxyl radicals react with vitamin E a thousand times more rapidly than they do with PUFA.[10] The phenolic hydroxyl group of tocopherol reacts with an organic peroxyl radical to form the corresponding organic hydroperoxide and the tocopheroxyl radical, which can undergo several possible fates.[10,34]

- It can be reduced by other antioxidants (like vitamin C) to tocopherol

- It can react with another tocopheroxyl radical to form non-reactive products such as tocopherol dimers

- It can undergo further oxidation to tocopheryl quinone

- It can act as a prooxidant and oxidize other lipids (which is why vitamin E radicals are maintained at low levels)[3]

The antioxidant activity of vitamin E benefits skin structure and promotes hair growth.[6] In terms of androgenic alopecia, androgen-inducible transforming growth factor beta 1 (TGF-B1), is mediated by free radicals and could be prevented by antioxidants in hair follicle dermal papilla cells.[6]

02 | Barrier Function

A series of studies have demonstrated that vitamin E is the predominant physiological barrier antioxidant in human skin. Vitamin E accumulates in the sebum, which is then delivered to the skin surface.[35] On the surface and within the skin, vitamin E acts like an antioxidant, preventing lipid peroxidation.

Vitamin E also increases ceramide synthesis[36] and upregulates gene expression of keratinocyte differentiation markers (transglutaminase 1, cytokeratin 10, involucrin and loricrin), and intracellular Ca^{2+} concentrations.[1,36]

03 | Immunoregulation and Photoprotection

Apart from its antioxidant activity, vitamin E prevents DNA damage caused by UV radiation and is able to suppress inflammation.[37] Vitamin E has an inhibitory effect on pro-inflammatory cytokine expression by inhibiting the activation of nuclear transcription factor kappa B (NF-κB).[38,39]

Some isoforms of vitamin E are also able to suppress cyclooxygenase-2 (COX-2) expression in cells.[40,41] COX-2 is induced in response to ROS and UV radiation leading to an increased production of PGE2, a major contributor to UV-induced inflammation and immunosuppression. Vitamin E can therefore reduce photodamage.[42] It has also shown to delay the growth of the melanoma by promoting apoptosis of tumor cells and inhibiting VEGF-mediated angiogenesis.[43]

Vitamin E modulates T cell function by impacting cell membrane integrity, cell division and signal transduction, and also indirectly by affecting inflammatory mediators.[44] It also inhibits IgE responses to allergic stimuli, making it useful for managing dermatoses.[45] It's long-term immunomodulatory role may also involve its ability to reduce the abundance of certain gut microbes, like *Bacteroidetes*, and decreased the ratio of Bacteroidetes/Firmicutes.[46]

04 | Depigmentation

Vitamin E derivatives have shown to limit melanogenesis in vitro via inhibition of tyrosinase, an important enzyme for melanin synthesis.[47,48] The increase in intracellular glutathione content is another explanation for its depigmenting effect.[49]

05 | Microcirculation

Microcirculation surrounding the hair follicle is essential for hair maintenance and nutrient delivery. By virtue of reducing oxidative stress and regulation of nitric oxide synthase, vitamin E can improve endothelial function and promote the growth of hair.[50] This is especially true in combination with vitamin C.[51,52]

▶ REFERENCES

1. Teo CWL, Tay SHY, Tey HL, Ung YW, Yap WN. Vitamin E in Atopic Dermatitis: From Preclinical to Clinical Studies. Dermatology. 2020;237(4):553-64.
2. Niki E. Lipid oxidation in the skin. Free Radic Res. 2015;49(7):827-34.
3. Packer L. Interactions among Antioxidants in Health and Disease: Vitamin E and Its Redox Cycle. Proc Soc Exp Biol Med. 1992;200(2):271-6.
4. National Institute of Nutrition Indian Council of Medical Research. Recommended Dietary Allowances and Estimated Average Requirements for Indians – 2020. RDA Full Report 2020.
5. Crosby L, Davis B, Joshi S, Jardine M, Paul J, Neola M, et al. Ketogenic Diets and Chronic Disease: Weighing the Benefits Against the Risks. Front Nutr. 2021;8:702802.
6. Beoy Lim Ai, Woei Wong Jia, Hay Yuen Kah. Effects of Tocotrienol Supplementation on Hair Growth in Human Volunteers. Trop Life Sci Res. 2010;21(2):91-9.
7. Thiele JJ, Traber MG, Packer L. Depletion of human stratum corneum vitamin E: an early and sensitive in vivo marker of UV induced photo-oxidation. J Invest Dermatol. 1998;110(5):756-61.
8. Packer L, Valacchi G. Antioxidants and the response of skin to oxidative stress: vitamin E as a key indicator. Skin Pharmacol Appl Skin Physiol. 2002;15(5):282-90.
9. Keen Mohammad Abid, Hassan Iffat. Vitamin E in dermatology. Indian Dermatol Online J. 2016;7(4):311-5.
10. Institute of Medicine (US) Panel on Dietary Antioxidants and Related Compounds. Dietary Reference Intakes for Vitamin C, Vitamin E, Selenium, and Carotenoids. Chapter 6: Vitamin E. National Academies Press (US); 2000.
11. Fu J-Y, Che H-L, Tan DM-Y, Teng K-T. Bioavailability of tocotrienols: evidence in human studies. Nutr Metab (Lond). 2014;11(1):5.
12. EFSA Panel on Dietetic Products, Nutrition, and Allergies (NDA). Scientific Opinion on Dietary Reference Values for vitamin E as α-tocopherol. EFSA Journal. 2015;13(7):4149.
13. Liu X, Yang G, Luo M, Lan Q, Shi X, Deng H, et al. Serum vitamin E levels and chronic inflammatory skin diseases: A systematic review and meta-analysis. PLoS One. 2021;16(12):e0261259.
14. Jaffary F, Faghihi G, Mokhtarian A, Hosseini SM. Effects of oral vitamin E on treatment of atopic dermatitis: A randomized controlled trial. J Res Med Sci. 2015;20(11):1053-7.
15. Javanbakht MH, Keshavarz SA, Djalali M, Siassi F, Eshraghian MR, Firooz A, et al. Randomized controlled trial using vitamins E and D supplementation in atopic dermatitis. J Dermatolog Treat. 2011;22(3):144-50.
16. Tsoureli-Nikita E, Hercogova J, Lotti T, Menchini G. Evaluation of dietary intake of vitamin E in the treatment of atopic dermatitis: a study of the clinical course and evaluation of the immunoglobulin E serum levels. Int J Dermatol. 200;41(3):146-50.
17. Stahl W, Heinrich U, Jungmann H, Sies H, Tronnier H. Carotenoids and carotenoids plus vitamin E protect against ultraviolet light-induced erythema in humans. Am J Clin Nutr. 2000;71(3):795-8.
18. Modulation of UV-light-induced skin inflammation by D-alpha-tocopherol and L-ascorbic acid: a clinical study using solar simulated radiation. Free Radical Biology and Medicine. 1998;25(9):1006-12.
19. Eberlein-König B, Placzek M, Przybilla B. Protective effect against sunburn of combined systemic ascorbic acid (vitamin C) and D-alpha-tocopherol (vitamin E). J Am Acad Dermatol. 1998;38(1):45-8.
20. Mireles-Rocha H, Galindo I, Huerta M, Trujillo-Hernández B, Elizalde A, Cortés-Franco R. UVB photoprotection with antioxidants: effects of oral therapy with D-alpha-tocopherol and ascorbic acid on the minimal erythema dose. Acta Derm Venereol. 2002;82(1):21-4.
21. Kharaeva Z, Gostova E, De Luca C, Raskovic D, Korkina L. Clinical and biochemical effects of coenzyme Q(10), vitamin E, and selenium supplementation to psoriasis patients. Nutrition. 2009;25(3):295-302.
22. Elgoweini M, Nour El Din N. Response of vitiligo to narrowband ultraviolet B and oral antioxidants. J Clin Pharmacol. 2009;49(7):852-5.
23. Hayakawa R, Ueda H, Nozaki T, Izawa Y, Yokotake J, Yazaki K, et al. Effects of combination treatment with vitamins E and C on chloasma and pigmented contact dermatitis. A double blind controlled clinical trial. Acta Vitaminol Enzymol. 1981;3(1):31-8.
24. Butt H, Mehmood A, Ali M, Tasneem S, Tarar MN, Riazuddin S. Vitamin E preconditioning alleviates in vitro thermal stress in cultured human epidermal keratinocytes. Life Sci. 2019;239:116972.
25. Vijayaraghavan R, Suribabu CS, Sekar B, Oommen PK, Kavithalakshmi SN, Madhusudhanan N, et al. Protective role of vitamin E on the oxidative stress in Hansen's disease (Leprosy) patients. Eur J Clin Nutr. 2005;59(10):1121-8.
26. Maeshima E, Liang XM, Goda M, Otani H, Mune M. The efficacy of vitamin E against oxidative damage and autoantibody production in systemic lupus erythematosus: a preliminary study. Clin Rheumatol. 2007;26(3):401-4.
27. Reddy P, Jialal I. Biochemistry, Fat Soluble Vitamins. In: StatPearls. Treasure Island (FL): StatPearls Publishing; 2024.
28. Kagan VE, Fabisiak JP, Quinn PJ. Coenzyme Q and vitamin E need each other as antioxidants. Protoplasma. 2000;214(1):11-8.
29. Scheidegger S. Infantile Herzhypertrophie. Schweizerische Zeitschrift für allgemeine Pathologie und Bakteriologie. 2008;8(5):295-7.
30. Szewczyk K, Chojnacka A, Górnicka M. Tocopherols and Tocotrienols—Bioactive Dietary Compounds; What Is Certain, What Is Doubt? Int J Mol Sci. 2021;22(12):6222.

31. Watson RR, Preedy VR. Tocotrienols: Vitamin E Beyond Tocopherols. CRC Press; 2008. 424 p.
32. Sen CK, Khanna S, Roy S. Tocotrienols: Vitamin E Beyond Tocopherols. Life Sci. 2006;78(18):2088-98.
33. Ziegler M, Wallert M, Lorkowski S, Peter K. Cardiovascular and Metabolic Protection by Vitamin E: A Matter of Treatment Strategy? Antioxidants (Basel). 2020;9(10):935.
34. Burton GW, Joyce A, Ingold KU. Is vitamin E the only lipid-soluble, chain-breaking antioxidant in human blood plasma and erythrocyte membranes? Arch Biochem Biophys. 1983;221(1):281-90.
35. Thiele JJ, Weber SU, Packer L. Sebaceous gland secretion is a major physiologic route of vitamin E delivery to skin. J Invest Dermatol. 1999;113(6):1006-10.
36. Kato E, Takahashi N. Improvement by sodium dl-α-tocopheryl-6-O-phosphate treatment of moisture-retaining ability in stratum corneum through increased ceramide levels. Bioorg Med Chem. 2012;20(12):3837-42.
37. Placzek M, Gaube S, Kerkmann U, Gilbertz KP, Herzinger T, Haen E, et al. Ultraviolet B-induced DNA damage in human epidermis is modified by the antioxidants ascorbic acid and D-alpha-tocopherol. J Invest Dermatol. 2005;124(2):304-7.
38. Asbaghi O, Sadeghian M, Nazarian B, Sarreshtedari M, Mozaffari-Khosravi H, Maleki V, et al. The effect of vitamin E supplementation on selected inflammatory biomarkers in adults: a systematic review and meta-analysis of randomized clinical trials. Sci Rep. 2020;10(1):17234.
39. Qureshi AA, Tan X, Reis JC, Badr MZ, Papasian CJ, Morrison DC, et al. Inhibition of nitric oxide in LPS-stimulated macrophages of young and senescent mice by δ-tocotrienol and quercetin. Lipids Health Dis. 2011;10:239.
40. Yam ML, Abdul Hafid SR, Cheng HM, Nesaretnam K. Tocotrienols suppress proinflammatory markers and cyclooxygenase-2 expression in RAW264.7 macrophages. Lipids. 2009;44(9):787-97.
41. Jiang Q, Yin X, Lill MA, Danielson ML, Freiser H, Huang J. Long-chain carboxychromanols, metabolites of vitamin E, are potent inhibitors of cyclooxygenases. Proc Natl Acad Sci U S A. 2008;105(51):20464-9.
42. Kato E, Sasaki Y, Takahashi N. Sodium DL-α-tocopheryl-6-O-phosphate inhibits PGE_2 production in keratinocytes induced by UVB, IL-1β and peroxidants. Bioorg Med Chem. 2011;19(21):6348-55.
43. Pinto CAS de O, Martins TEA, Martinez RM, Freire TB, Velasco MVR, Baby AR, et al. Vitamin E in Human Skin: Functionality and Topical Products. In: Vitamin E in Health and Disease - Interactions, Diseases and Health Aspects [Internet]. IntechOpen; 2021 [cited 2024 Jun 20]. Available from: https://www.intechopen.com/chapters/77087
44. Lewis ED, Meydani SN, Wu D. Regulatory role of vitamin E in the immune system and inflammation. IUBMB Life. 2019;71(4):487-94.
45. Fogarty A, Lewis S, Weiss S, Britton J. Dietary vitamin E, IgE concentrations, and atopy. The Lancet. 2000;356(9241):1573-4.
46. Kim DJ, Yoon S, Ji SC, Yang J, Kim Y-K, Lee SH, et al. Ursodeoxycholic acid improves liver function via phenylalanine/tyrosine pathway and microbiome remodelling in patients with liver dysfunction. 2018;8(1):11874.
47. Ichihashi M, Funasaka Y, Ohashi A, Chacraborty A, Ahmed NU, Ueda M, et al. The inhibitory effect of DL-alpha-tocopheryl ferulate in lecithin on melanogenesis. Anticancer Res. 1999;19(5A):3769-74.
48. Kamei Y, Otsuka Y, Abe K. Comparison of the inhibitory effects of vitamin E analogues on melanogenesis in mouse B16 melanoma cells. Cytotechnology. 2009;59(3):183-90.
49. del Marmol V, Solano F, Sels A, Huez G, Libert A, Lejeune F, et al. Glutathione depletion increases tyrosinase activity in human melanoma cells. J Invest Dermatol. 1993;101(6):871-4.
50. Boa BCS, Barros CMMR, Souza M das GC, Castiglione RC, Cyrino FZGA, Bouskela E. α-Tocopherol Improves Microcirculatory Dysfunction on Fructose Fed Hamsters. PLOS ONE. 2015;10(8):e0134740.
51. Ülker S, McKeown PP, Bayraktutan U. Vitamins Reverse Endothelial Dysfunction Through Regulation of eNOS and NAD(P)H Oxidase Activities. Hypertension. 2003;41(3):534-9.
52. Engler MM, Engler MB, Malloy MJ, Chiu EY, Schloetter MC, Paul SM, et al. Antioxidant Vitamins C and E Improve Endothelial Function in Children With Hyperlipidemia. Circulation. 2003;108(9):1059-63.

Nutrition in Dermatology

09

Phylloquinone, Menaquinones

Vitamin K

✍ Sachin Varma

CONTENTS

VITAMIN K: NUTRIENT SNAPSHOT

▸ REQUIREMENT IN THE INDIAN CONTEXT | 88

▸ ACTIVE FORMS | 89

▸ SAFETY AND DOSAGE | 89

▸ CLINICAL CONDITIONS | 90

▸ SUPPLEMENTATION | 91

INTRODUCTION | 93

DIGESTION, ABSORPTION AND STORAGE | 93

MECHANISM OF ACTION | 94

KEY TOPICS

- AGING- RELATED PRO-INFLAMMATORY FACTORS
- COLLAGEN METABOLISM
- OXIDATIVE STRESS
- PEDIATRIC ATOPIC DERMATITIS
- PSEUDOXANTHOMA ELASTICUM (PXE)
- WOUND HEALING

Nutrient Snapshot

▶ **REQUIREMENT IN THE INDIAN CONTEXT**

- Vitamin K is a fat-soluble, "multitasking" vitamin that was originally identified for its role in the activation of vitamin K-dependent coagulation factors.[1] Naturally, vitamin K appears as two variants—vitamin K1 is known as phylloquinone and vitamin K2 refers to a family of molecules called menaquinones (MKs).[2] Other than coagulation, vitamin K-dependent proteins are involved in tissue renewal and cell growth control. Other functions of vitamin K are mainly ascribed to vitamin K2 including the support of bone mineralization, calcium homeostasis and endothelial integrity, and inhibiting vessel wall calcification.[2,3]

- A deficiency of vitamin K is uncommon in healthy adults, due to its homeostatic control and it is widespread in food.[1] Vitamin K1 is found in green leafy vegetables and some plant oils, which is why it is more abundant in our diet. However, it is less bioactive than vitamin K2, especially compared to MK-7.

- Vitamin K2 forms are usually found in cheese, animal products, and certain fermented foods,[2] and tend to be lower in the Indian diet.[4] Although vitamin K2 is produced by the microbiota of the large intestine, our diet is its principal source, as it is absorbed in the small intestine.[5-7]

- Our body prioritizes the use of vitamin K for essential, life-sustaining, vitamin K-dependent proteins (e.g., the activation of blood coagulation proteins). The remaining vitamin K1 is converted to vitamin K2. However, vitamin K2 is thought to be insufficient for a number of other vitamin K-dependent proteins, nonessential for survival, that promote immune, cardiovascular, skeletal, and neuromuscular health.[4]

- From a dermatological perspective, vitamin K is not given much importance. It's topical application shows beneficial effects, such as suppression of pigmentation and alleviation of bruising, and promoting wound healing. It is also used prophylactically to limit the acneiform side effects in patients receiving the monoclonal antibody cetuximab. However, its photodegradation and phototoxicity limit its topical use.[8]

- From a supplement perspective, a case can be made for vitamin K2 insufficiency. Its ability to promote vascular health may benefit aging factors with a vascular component, including the appearance of undereye dark circles, hair loss, varicose veins, and bruising.

▶ ACTIVE FORMS

ACTIVE FORMS	SUPPLEMENT SOURCES	SALIENT FEATURES
Vitamin K1 (phylloquinone)	Plant based extraction or synthetic[9]	Vitamin K1 is well absorbed but has a shorter shelf-life.[10,11]
Vitamin K2 (menaquinones; MKs)	Bacterial fermentation synthetic	Menaquinone is analogous to ubiquinone in function as ubiquinone is used as an electron carrier in electron transport chain by bacteria.[12] K2-MK7 has a longer half life and thus is stable in serum.[10]
Vitamin K3 (menadione)	Synthetic	Vitamin K3 is not allowed for human consumption as per the FSSAI, and is usually used in animal feeds.

▶ SAFETY AND DOSAGE

GENERAL REQUIREMENTS	
Indian recommendations	RDA 2020: 55 μg/day, TUL: N/A
Global recommendations and limits	Adequate intake, NIH: Male—120 μg, Females—90 μg/day TUL: Not established.[13]
	EFSA AI: 70 μg/day for phylloquinone[14] NOAEL: Not established.
Notes:	Because of the lack of data to estimate an average requirement, an adequate intake (AI) is given. Vitamin K needs to be taken after a meal as it is a fat soluble vitamin.

▶ **CLINICAL CONDITIONS**

EVIDENCE LEVEL	CONDITION OR USE CASE	DOSAGE	BENEFIT OR MECHANISM OF ACTION
+++	Collagen metabolism	Rats were injected with Vikasol solution (converts to vitamin K2) for 10 days or pelentan (anticoagulant) by mouth for 15–20 days, or both preparations together for 20 days. Rats getting pelentan suffered from avitaminosis; they were started with Vikasol for 8 days.	In avitaminosis-K rats, the total collagen content in the skin was reduced. There was a parallel increase in the rate of its hydrolysis and in the level of free hydroxyproline, suggesting an increase in catabolism of collagen.[15]
+++++	Wound healing	N/A (meta-analysis)	According to various studies, vitamin K has shown to increase the rate of wound healing in animal models.[16]
+	Pseudoxanthoma elasticum (PXE)—calcium accumulation in elastin fibers	N/A (observational study)	The serum levels of vitamin K in patients with PXE were lower than the controls.[17]
++	Oxidative stress	Human embryonic kidney cells were treated with vitamin K (in vitro).	Cell viability under conditions of no induced oxidative stress was increased by the presence of vitamins K1 and K2 but not ubinquinone-10 and was specifically dependent on VKORC1L1 expression. Intracellular oxidative damage to membrane intrinsic proteins was inversely dependent on VKORC1L1 expression and the presence of vitamin K1.[18]

▶ CLINICAL CONDITIONS (Continued)

EVIDENCE LEVEL	CONDITION OR USE CASE	DOSAGE	BENEFIT OR MECHANISM OF ACTION
++	Aging-related proinflammatory factors	Vitamin K2-MK7 was added in cell culture human monocyte derived macrophages (hMDMs) for 30 hours (in vitro).	MK-7 was able to modulate immune and inflammatory reactions by a dose-dependent inhibition of TNF-α, IL-1α, and IL-1β gene expression and protein production in healthy hMDMs.[19]
+++	Pediatric atopic dermatitis	Peripheral blood mononuclear cells of children with and without atopic dermatitis were collected and treated with vitamin K2.	Vitamin K2 attenuated activated T-cell immunity in atopic dermatitis patients through the inhibition of mitogen activated protein kinase (Mek1), extracellular signal-regulated kinases (ERK 1/2), and stress activated protein kinase (SAPK) or c-Jun N-terminal kinase (JNK) signaling pathway.[20]

▶ SUPPLEMENTATION

	BASIS	WHAT TO LOOK OUT FOR
Supplementation form	Vitamin K1 (phylloquinones) Vitamin K2-MK7 (menaquinones) Both K1 and K2-MK7 are well absorbed but K2-MK7 has a longer half life.[10,11] Vitamin K2 can be supplemented, as vitamin K1 is plenty in the Indian diet.	The form of vitamin K is stated on the nutritional table or in ingredients of the product packaging.
Administration form	Capsules, tablets, softgels, powders, gummies	N/A
Purity considerations	Vitamin K normally has >99% purity.	N/A
Patient considerations	Vitamin K is a fat soluble vitamin, and thus should be taken after meals.	
Safety considerations	There are no severe side effects from vitamin K supplementation.[13,21]	N/A

▶ **SUPPLEMENTATION** (*Continued*)

	BASIS	**WHAT TO LOOK OUT FOR**
Other considerations	Individuals on warfarin and other blood thinners should be careful while taking vitamin K supplements as it acts as an antagonist and might reduced the effect of warfarin.[21]	Most of the multivitamin formulations will have vitamin K.
	Prolonged use of antibiotics accompanied with low vitamin K intake may require vitamin K supplementation. A multivitamin formulation with vitamin K can be given.[13]	

INTRODUCTION

Carboxylation is a post-translational modification of proteins that converts specific glutamate residues (Glu) to γ-carboxyglutamate residues (Gla). It is catalyzed by γ-glutamyl carboxylase (GGCX), which utilizes the reduced form of vitamin K as a cofactor. Both vitamin K1 and K2 can function as cofactors for blood coagulation proteins. With the discovery of new vitamin K-dependent proteins, we now know that vitamin K2 is involved in bone metabolism and other important physiological processes.[22]

The body stores very small amounts of vitamin K, which is probably why the body recycles it through a process called the vitamin K-epoxide cycle. Briefly, vitamin K hydroquinone (reduced form; KH_2) is oxidized to vitamin K epoxide (oxidized form; KO). An enzyme called vitamin K-oxidoreductase (VKOR) converts KO to vitamin K and back to KH_2. The anticoagulant drug warfarin acts as a vitamin K antagonist by inhibiting this enzyme and preventing vitamin K recycling **(Figure 1)**.[23]

DIGESTION, ABSORPTION AND STORAGE

Digestion and Absorption

- Vitamin K1 is absorbed in the intestine via active transport in the jejunum, whilst vitamin K2 is absorbed in the small intestine by diffusion. Bile salts and products of pancreatic lipase are required for optimal absorption.[6]

- Vitamin K1 is metabolized and more than half the amount is excreted by the organism, while vitamin K2 is transported by LDL to extrahepatic tissue.[23]

- Bioavailability and pharmacokinetics vary widely amongst the different forms. Some of them have very short half-life, like vitamin K1, are found in the circulation from 4-10 hours after ingestion, whilst others, like vitamin K2 MK-7, are present for more than 96 hours.[6] Typically, longer chain MKs, such as MK-7, MK-8 and MK-9, have a longer half-life in circulation in comparison to K1. However, MK-9, being even more lipophilic, has a very long half-life, but is poorly absorbed. That's why MK-7, providing high bioavailability and a long half-life, is frequently used in supplements.[3]

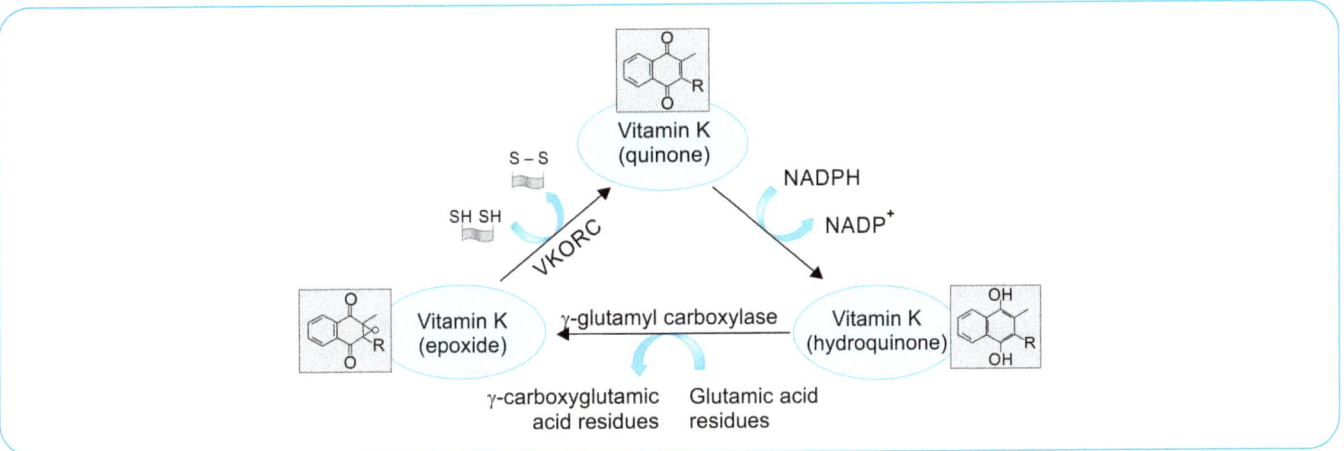

Figure 1: Metabolic redox-cycle of vitamin K.
(VKORC: vitamin K-dependent epoxide reductase complex)
Source: Adapted from Ivanova.

Storage

- As a fat-soluble vitamin, vitamin K is stored mainly in adipose tissue. Vitamin K1 is stored in the liver and vitamin K2 accumulates in many tissue.[3]

- With limited vitamin K storage capacity, the body reuses it by recycling it in the vitamin K oxidation-reduction cycle.

▶ MECHANISM OF ACTION

01 | Antioxidant Activity

Vitamin K's reduced form, KH_2, has been recognized as a potent biological antioxidant, nearly 10- to 100-fold higher than any other known antioxidants, such as α-tocopherol and coenzyme Q10.[3,24]

Both vitamin K1 and K2 have shown to increase survival of oxidatively stressed cells caused by depleted glutathione levels. They have been recognized to be important for limiting oxidative damage to membrane proteins.[18,25]

02 | Regulation of Cellular Function

Vitamin K-dependent signaling pathways in osteogenic cells have been long established. Due to its ability to bind to the intranuclear receptor SXR (steroid and xenobiotic receptor), which activates several genes, vitamin K2 is being called a hormone.[26]

Similar to coenzyme Q10, vitamin K2 has been reported to facilitate ATP production and rescue mitochondrial dysfunction.[27] Decline of mitochondrial activity is a result of cellular aging, and has been implicated in conditions such as female pattern hair loss.[28]

Vitamin K has been shown to be cytotoxic to cancer cells via redox mechanisms involving cell growth arrest and suppression of proliferation. This has been exploited for cancer suppression and preventing bacterial growth during wound healing.[16,23]

03 | Immunoregulation

Vitamin K has shown to reduce the expression of pro-inflammatory markers, TNF-α, IL-6, IL-1α and IL-1β, via the inactivation of the NF-κB signaling pathway.[19,29] This is one of the reasons for its use in managing type 2 diabetes.[29]

Other than blood clotting, in wound healing, vitamin K is thought to promote the expression of transforming growth factor beta (TGF-β) and platelet-derived growth factor (PDGF), but the exact mechanism is still unclear.[16]

Vitamin K2 can also modulate T-cell function. This has been shown in vitro, where it suppressed the proliferation of T-cell mitogen-activated peripheral blood mononuclear cells acquired from atopic dermatitis patients.[20,30]

▶ REFERENCES

1. Institute of Medicine (US) Panel on Micronutrients. Dietary Reference Intakes for Vitamin A, Vitamin K, Arsenic, Boron, Chromium, Copper, Iodine, Iron, Manganese, Molybdenum, Nickel, Silicon, Vanadium, and Zinc. Chapter 5: Vitamin K. National Academies Press (US); 2001
2. Gröber U, Reichrath J, Holick MF, Kisters K. Vitamin K: an old vitamin in a new perspective. Dermatoendocrinol. 2015;6(1):e968490.
3. Halder M, Petsophonsakul P, Akbulut AC, Pavlic A, et al. Vitamin K: Double Bonds beyond Coagulation Insights into Differences between Vitamin K1 and K2 in Health and Disease. Int J Mol Sci. 2019;20(4):896.
4. Vaidya R, Vaidya ADB, Sheth J, Jadhav S, Mahale U, Mehta D, et al. Vitamin K Insufficiency in the Indian Population: Pilot Observational Epidemiology Study. JMIR Public Health Surveill. 2022;8(2):e31941.
5. Lai Y, Masatoshi H, Ma Y, Guo Y, Zhang B. Role of Vitamin K in Intestinal Health. Front Immunol. 2022;12.
6. Alonso N, Meinitzer A, Fritz-Petrin E, Enko D, Herrmann M. Role of Vitamin K in Bone and Muscle Metabolism. Calcif Tissue Int. 2023;112(2):178-96.
7. Walther B, Karl JP, Booth SL, Boyaval P. Menaquinones, Bacteria, and the Food Supply: The Relevance of Dairy and Fermented Food Products to Vitamin K Requirements. Adv Nutr. 2013;4(4):463-73.
8. Goto S, Setoguchi S, Matsunaga K, Takata J. Overcoming the Photochemical Problem of Vitamin K in Topical Application. In: Vitamin K - Recent Topics on the Biology and Chemistry. IntechOpen. 2021.
9. Kang M-J, Baek K-R, Lee Y-R, Kim G-H, Seo S-O. Production of Vitamin K by Wild-Type and Engineered Microorganisms. Microorganisms. 2022;10(3):554.
10. Schurgers LJ, Teunissen KJF, Hamulyák K, Knapen MHJ, Vik H, Vermeer C. Vitamin K -containing dietary supplements: comparison of synthetic vitamin K1 and natto-derived menaquinone-7. Blood. 2006;109(8):3279-83.

11. Simes DC, Viegas CSB, Araújo N, Marreiros C. Vitamin K as a Diet Supplement with Impact in Human Health: Current Evidence in Age-Related Diseases. Nutrients. 2020;12(1):138.
12. Marles RJ, Roe AL, Oketch-Rabah HA. US Pharmacopeial Convention safety evaluation of menaquinone-7, a form of vitamin K. Nutr Rev. 2017;75(7):553-78.
13. Fact Sheet for Health Professionals. Vitamin K [Online]. Available from: https://ods.od.nih.gov/factsheets/vitaminK-HealthProfessional/
14. EFSA Panel on Dietetic Products, Nutrition and Allergies (NDA). Dietary reference values for vitamin K. 2017.
15. Sharaev PN, Bogdanov NG, Yamaldinov RN. Effect of body vitamin K level on collagen metabolism in the skin. Bull Exp Biol Med. 1976;81(6):822-3.
16. Tang S, Ruan Z, Ma A, Wang D, Kou J. Effect of vitamin K on wound healing: A systematic review and meta-analysis based on preclinical studies. Front Pharmacol. 2022;13:1063349.
17. Vanakker OM, Martin L, Schurgers LJ, Quaglino D, Costrop L, Vermeer C, et al. Low serum vitamin K in PXE results in defective carboxylation of mineralization inhibitors similar to the GGCX mutations in the PXE-like syndrome. Lab Invest. 2010;90(6):895-905.
18. Westhofen P, Watzka M, Marinova M, Hass M, Kirfel G, Müller J, et al. Human Vitamin K 2,3-Epoxide Reductase Complex Subunit 1-like 1 (VKORC1L1) Mediates Vitamin K-dependent Intracellular Antioxidant Function. J Biol Chem. 2011;286(17):15085-94.
19. Pan M-H, Maresz K, Lee P-S, Wu J-C, Ho C-T, Popko J, et al. Inhibition of TNF-α, IL-1α, and IL-1β by Pretreatment of Human Monocyte-Derived Macrophages with Menaquinone-7 and Cell Activation with TLR Agonists In Vitro. J Med Food. 2016;19(7):663-9.
20. Zhang M, Miura T, Suzuki S, Chiyotanda M, Tanaka S, Sugiyama K, et al. Vitamin K2 Suppresses Proliferation and Inflammatory Cytokine Production in Mitogen-Activated Lymphocytes of Atopic Dermatitis Patients through the Inhibition of Mitogen-Activated Protein Kinases. Biol Pharm Bull. 2021;44(1):7-17.
21. Jadhav N, Ajgaonkar S, Saha P, Gurav P, Pandey A, Basudkar V, et al. Molecular Pathways and Roles for Vitamin K2-7 as a Health-Beneficial Nutraceutical: Challenges and Opportunities. Front Pharmacol. 2022;13:896920.
22. Hao Z, Jin DY, Stafford DW, Tie JK. Vitamin K-dependent carboxylation of coagulation factors: insights from a cell-based functional study. Haematologica. 2020;105(8):2164-73.
23. Ivanova D, Zhelev Z, Getsov P, Nikolova B, Aoki I, Higashi T, et al. Vitamin K: Redox-modulation, prevention of mitochondrial dysfunction and anticancer effect. Redox Biology. 2018;16:352-8.
24. Mukai K, Morimoto H, Kikuchi S, Nagaoka S. Kinetic study of free-radical-scavenging action of biological hydroquinones (reduced forms of ubiquinone, vitamin K and tocopherol quinone) in solution. Biochim Biophys Acta. 1993;1157(3):313-7.
25. Li J, Lin JC, Wang H, Peterson JW, Furie BC, Furie B, et al. Novel Role of Vitamin K in Preventing Oxidative Injury to Developing Oligodendrocytes and Neurons. J Neurosci. 2003;23(13):5816-26.
26. Gordeladze Jan Oxholm. Vitamin K2: A Vitamin that Works like a Hormone, Impinging on Gene Expression. In: Cell Signalling - Thermodynamics and Molecular Control. IntechOpen, 2019.
27. Vos M, Esposito G, Edirisinghe JN, Vilain S, Haddad DM, Slabbaert JR, et al. Vitamin K2 is a mitochondrial electron carrier that rescues pink1 deficiency. Science. 2012;336(6086):1306-10.
28. Piccini I, Sousa M, Altendorf S, Jimenez F, Rossi A, Funk W, et al. Intermediate Hair Follicles from Patients with Female Pattern Hair Loss Are Associated with Nutrient.
29. Li Y, Chen JP, Duan L, Li S. Effect of vitamin K2 on type 2 diabetes mellitus: A review. Diabetes Res Clin Pract. 2018;136:39-51.
30. Meng K, Xu W, Miura T, Suzuki S, Chiyotanda M, Tanaka S, et al. The effects of vitamin K1 and vitamin K2 on the proliferation, cytokine production and regulatory T-cell frequency in peripheral blood mononuclear cells of paediatric atopic dermatitis patients. Exp Dermatol. 2018;27(9):1058-60

SECTION 02

Minerals

10.	Iron	*Rasya Dixit*
11.	Zinc	*Rasya Dixit*
12.	Magnesium	*Abhishek De*
13.	Calcium	*Abhishek De*
14.	Selenium	*Abhishek De*
15.	Copper	*Rasya Dixit*
16.	Iodine	*Abhishek De*

10

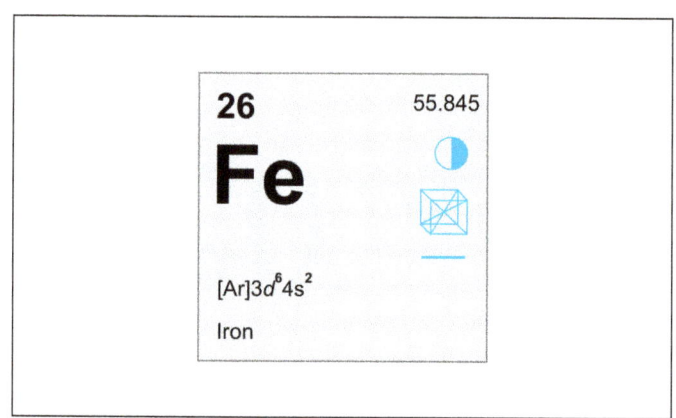

Iron

Iron

✎ Rasya Dixit

CONTENTS

IRON: NUTRIENT SNAPSHOT

- ▶ REQUIREMENT IN THE INDIAN CONTEXT | **99**
- ▶ ACTIVE FORMS | **100**
- ▶ SAFETY AND DOSAGE | **100**
- ▶ CLINICAL CONDITIONS | **100**
- ▶ SUPPLEMENTATION | **101**

INTRODUCTION | **103**

DIGESTION, ABSORPTION AND STORAGE | **103**

MECHANISM OF ACTION | **103**

KEY TOPICS

- CHRONIC TELOGEN EFFLUVIUM
- EXCESSIVE HAIR LOSS
- FEMALE PATTERN HAIR LOSS

Nutrient Snapshot

▶ **REQUIREMENT IN THE INDIAN CONTEXT**

- Iron is an essential trace mineral that exists in two biologically relevant oxidation states: The ferrous form (Fe^{2+}) and the ferric form (Fe^{3+}). Iron is an essential component of hundreds of proteins and enzymes supporting essential biological functions, such as oxygen transport, energy production, DNA synthesis, and cell growth and replication. Iron is a double-edged sword, especially in the skin. In addition to its role in development, maintenance and function of skin, iron is also required for oxidative stress processes.[1]

- Iron deficiency is the most common micronutrient deficiency globally, especially in India. Women of childbearing age are particularly vulnerable to iron deficiency because of their greater requirements of iron for menstruation and pregnancy.[2]

- Lower iron absorption could be a major mechanism by which iron deficiency affects populations. Plant-based diets, commonly consumed in India, contain an abundance of phytates and polyphenols that inhibit the absorption of dietary non-heme iron, which constitutes 91% of the total iron present in the Indian diet.[2] Suboptimal intake of protein, and specifically the essential amino acid, L-lysine, is also thought to be a contributing factor, putting vegetarians at a higher risk of iron deficiency.[3] Due to these reasons, iron is often added to hair supplements.

▶ ACTIVE FORMS

ACTIVE FORMS	SUPPLEMENT SOURCES	SALIENT FEATURES
Ferrous state (Fe^{2+})	Inorganic ferrous salts, chelated ferrous form, ferrous polymaltose complex	The ferrous form has better bioavailability as compared to the ferric form.[4] Most of the iron supplements available in the market are in the ferrous form.
Ferric state (Fe^{3+})	Inorganic ferric salts, ferric polymaltose complex	Ferric state has less solubility over ferrous and thus is 3–4 times less bioavailable. The iron in the ferric form has to be converted to the ferrous form to get absorbed.[4]

▶ SAFETY AND DOSAGE

GENERAL REQUIREMENTS	
Indian recommendations	ICMR-NIN (RDA 2020): Male—19 mg/day, Female—29 mg/day
	EAR: Male—11 mg/day, Female—15 mg/day[5]
	TUL: 45 mg/day[5,6]
Global recommendations and limits	IOM's Food and Nutrition Board: Male—8 mg/day, Female—18 mg/day
	TUL: 45 mg/day.[7]
	EFSA: Male—11 mg, Female—16 mg (premenopausal).[8]
	Upper limit: 45 mg/day
	LOAEL: 70 mg/day
Notes:	The risk of exceeding the TUL of iron remains low when receiving supplementation of 10 mg/day, but is much higher if consumed in greater amounts.[5] That's why long-term use can be limited to 10 mg in the absence of a deficiency.
	Iron and zinc may interfere with each others absorption. However, when taken with food, this issue may not persist. As a rule of thumb, Iron:Zinc ratio should be 1:1 or maximum 2:1.

▶ CLINICAL CONDITIONS

EVIDENCE LEVEL	CONDITION OR USE CASE	DOSAGE	BENEFIT OR MECHANISM OF ACTION
++	Excessive hair loss (unknown cause)	N/A (Observational study)	Among the women affected by excessive hair loss, a larger proportion of women (59%) had low iron stores (< 40 μg/L) compared to the remainder of the population (48%).[9]

▶ CLINICAL CONDITIONS (Continued)

EVIDENCE LEVEL	CONDITION OR USE CASE	DOSAGE	BENEFIT OR MECHANISM OF ACTION
++	Female pattern hair loss (FPHL)	N/A (Observational study)	Premenopausal FPHL patients showed significantly lower serum ferritin than age/sex-matched controls.[10]
+++	Chronic telogen effluvium	20 mg iron alongside other nutrients including L-lysine, for 6 months.	There was a reduction in the amount of hair being shed, along with an increase in the mean serum ferritin level.[3]

Note: There are a number of clinical studies on a variety of hair supplements containing iron alongside other vitamins, minerals and antioxidants that have shown benefits in hair growth and quality parameters.

▶ SUPPLEMENTATION

	BASIS	WHAT TO LOOK OUT FOR
Supplementation form	Ferrous sulphate (20% elemental iron) Ferrous gluconate (12% elemental iron) Ferrous fumarate (33% elemental iron)[11] Ferrous ascorbate (16% elemental iron)[12] Ferrous salts normally have a higher purity than chelates, but have lower bioavailability. Among the salt forms, ferrous fumarate is the most preferred form as it is inexpensive.[4] Ferrous ascorbate has a lower incidence of GI distress, followed by ferrous sulphate.[13]	Stated in the ingredients section of the packaging.
	Ferrous bisglycinate: This chelated iron is considered the best form of iron as it has high bioavailability and negligible effects on the gastrointestinal tract (GI).[14] The amount of elemental iron in chelated forms varies as per manufacturer.	
	Iron polymaltose complex (IPC)—ferrous or ferric iron is coupled with a sugar. Ferrous sulphate and IPC preparations are generally available in the market. According to studies, IPC has poorer bioavailability and efficacy (in terms of anemia) than ferrous ascorbate and ferrous bisglycinate.[15-18]	

▶ SUPPLEMENTATION (Continued)

	BASIS	WHAT TO LOOK OUT FOR
	Liposomal iron Inorganic form of iron is encapsulated in a liposomes. Manufacturers claim it has the highest bioavailability and lower GI distress.	Clinical studies can be referred to.
Administration form	Capsules, tablets, syrups, gummies, and lozenges	N/A
Purity considerations	The elemental form of iron varies as per its form.	The elemental iron is often mentioned on the product packaging. If not, this information can be provided by the manufacturer.
Patient considerations	20 mg of iron (and less) can give gastric distress. Ferrous ascorbate has the lowest GI distress among salts while ferrous bisglycinate has the highest bioavailability and low incidence of GI distress.	The dose per serving is mentioned on the nutritional table, while the form of iron is given in the ingredients list.
Safety considerations	Acute iron toxicity can occur with supplementation in the range 20–60 mg/kg body weight per day causing symptoms such as constipation, nausea, abdominal pain and vomiting.[19]	Recommending mega doses of iron should be based on biochemical reports of the patients (i.e., incase of deficiency).
Other considerations	High intake of iron can also affect zinc absorption.[19] The presence of calcium decreases iron absorption from both non-heme and heme sources.[7] Vitamin A deficiency often coexists with iron deficiency and may exacerbate iron deficiency.[20]	If prescribing iron and calcium, both can be recommended separately in different times of the day.[7]

INTRODUCTION

Iron is a vital co-factor for proteins and enzymes involved in energy metabolism, respiration, DNA synthesis, cell cycle arrest and apoptosis. Over the past 10 years, major advances have been made in understanding the genetics of iron metabolism. Historically, it has long been known that iron is essential for healthy skin, mucous membranes, hair and nails.[1] For example, iron-containing proteins have specific functions, such as the metabolism of collagen by procollagen-proline dioxygenase.[1]

Clinical features of iron deficiency include skin pallor, pruritus, and predisposition to skin infection (impetigo, boils and candidiasis), angular cheilitis, swollen tongue, fragile nails, koilonychia, and dry brittle hair.[1]

DIGESTION, ABSORPTION AND STORAGE

Digestion and Absorption

- The absorption of most dietary iron occurs in the duodenum and proximal jejunum. At physiological pH, iron exists in the oxidized, ferric (Fe^{3+}) state, which must be converted to the ferrous (Fe^{2+}) state and can also be bound by a protein such as heme to be absorbed. The low pH of gastric acid in the duodenum allows an enzyme on the brush border of the enterocytes to convert ferric (Fe^{3+}) to absorbable ferrous (Fe^{2+}) ions.[21]

- Gastric acid production plays a key role in plasma iron homeostasis. When proton-pump inhibiting drugs such as omeprazole are used, iron absorption is greatly reduced. Once ferric iron is reduced to ferrous iron in the intestinal lumen, iron is transported into the enterocytes.[21]

- Heme iron, derived from animal food sources (meat, seafood, poultry) is the most easily absorbable form (15–35%) and contributes 10% or more of our total absorbed iron. Non-heme iron is derived from plants and iron-fortified foods and is absorbed less.[21]

- Ascorbic acid (vitamin C) helps with iron absorption by forming a chelate with ferric (Fe^{3+}) iron in the low pH of the stomach, which persists and remains soluble in the alkaline environment of the duodenum.[21-23]

- Protein intake improves iron status as amino acids (like lysine) increase iron absorption.

Storage

- The human body contains 3–5 g of iron, of which up to 75% may be bound in hemoglobin, with lesser amounts in storage compounds (ferritin and hemosiderin) and in muscle cells as myoglobin. Iron is also found bound to proteins (hemoprotein) and non-heme enzymes involved in oxidation-reduction reactions and the transfer of electrons (cytochromes and catalase). Additionally, approximately 2.2% of total body iron is found in the so-called labile pool, a poorly defined and reactive pool of iron that forms reactive oxygen species (ROS) via the Fenton reaction.[21,24]

- Iron is not actively excreted from the body, however the skin is a key organ in iron homeostasis as iron is lost through the skin by desquamation.[1]

MECHANISM OF ACTION

The most widely cited nutritional causes of hair loss include iron, one of the key micronutrients in metabolism of our body.[25] Iron is a critical factor in regulating keratin expression in epidermal tissues, as well as in hair follicle growth and maturation.[26] Studies have demonstrated that the mean ferritin level in patients with androgenic alopecia and alopecia areata is significantly lower than that in normal individuals without hair loss.[27]

Under normal conditions, low levels of ROS actively participate in redox reactions and act as second messengers for regulatory functions. Iron plays a key role in oxidative stress processes, as it is a transition metal, which exists in two stable states, Fe^{2+} (electron donor) and Fe^{3+} (electron acceptor). Catalase and some peroxidases are heme-containing enzymes that protect cells against the accumulation of ROS. Iron also catalyses the formation of ROS as part of the immune response. This defensive role, may, however, become one of attack when production of ROS overwhelms cellular scavenging systems. The iron-catalyzed ROS can severely damage cell constituents, as observed e.g., after UVA irradiation in skin cells.[28,29]

In addition, in the thyroid gland, heme-containing thyroid peroxidase catalyzes the iodination of thyroglobulin for the production of thyroid hormones such that thyroid metabolism can be impaired in iron deficiency anemia. Thyroid hormones are important regulators of epidermal homeostasis[30] as well as hair follicle cycling and pigmentation.[31]

► REFERENCES

1. Wright JA, Richards T, Srai SKS. The role of iron in the skin and cutaneous wound healing. Front Pharmacol. 2014;5:156.
2. Thankachan P, Walczyk T, Muthayya S, Kurpad AV, Hurrell RF. Iron absorption in young Indian women: The interaction of iron status with the influence of tea and ascorbic acid1-3. Am J Clin Nutr. 2008;87(4):881-6.
3. Rushton DH, Norris MJ, Dove R, Busuttil N. Causes of hair loss and the developments in hair rejuvenation. Int J Cosmet Sci. 2002;24:17-23.
4. Santiago, P. Ferrous versus Ferric Oral Iron Formulations for the Treatment of Iron Deficiency: A Clinical Overview. ScientificWorldJournal. 2012:2012:846824.
5. Ghosh S, Sinha S, Thomas T, Sachdev HS, Kurpad AV. Revisiting Dietary Iron Requirement and Deficiency in Indian Women: Implications for Food Iron Fortification and Supplementation. J Nutr. 2019;149:366.
6. National Institute of Nutrition Indian Council of Medical Research. Recommended Dietary Allowances and Estimated Average Requirements for Indians – 2020. RDA Full Report 2020.
7. Iron - Health Professional Fact Sheet. [Online] Available from https://ods.od.nih.gov/factsheets/Iron- HealthProfessional/
8. Bresson JL. Scientific Opinion on Dietary Reference Values for iron. EFSA Journal. 2015.
9. Deloche C, Bastien P, Chadoutaud S, Galan P, Bertrais S, Hercberg S, et al. Low iron stores: a risk factor for excessive hair loss in non-menopausal women. Eur J Dermatol. 2007;17(6):507-12.
10. Park SY, Na SY, Kim JH, Cho S, Lee JH. Iron Plays a Certain Role in Patterned Hair Loss. J Korean Med Sci. 2013;28(6):934-8.
11. Nguyen M, Tadi P. Iron Supplementation. StatPearls (2023).
12. Ferrous Ascorbate Formulation with 16:84 Iron: Ascorbic Acid Ratio Might Have Better Gastrointestinal Tolerability than Conventional Formulations | CiplaMed. https://ciplamed-library.com/content/ferrous-ascorbate-formulation-with-1684-iron-ascorbic-acid-ratio-might-have-better.
13. Chavan S, Rana P, Tripathi R, Tekur U. Comparison of efficacy & safety of iron polymaltose complex & ferrous ascorbate with ferrous sulphate in pregnant women with iron-deficiency anaemia. Indian J Med Res. 2021;154:78.
14. Abdel Moety GAF, Ali AM, Fouad R, Ramadan W, Belal DS, Haggag HM. Amino acid chelated iron versus an iron salt in the treatment of iron deficiency anemia with pregnancy: A randomized controlled study. Eur J Obstet Gynecol Reprod Biol. 2017:210:242-6.
15. Pisani A, Riccio E, Sabbatini M, Andreucci M, Rio AD, Visciano B. Effect of oral liposomal iron versus intravenous iron for treatment of iron deficiency anaemia in CKD patients: a randomized trial. Nephrol Dial Transplant. 2015;30(4):645-52.
16. Fanzaga M, Bollati C, Ranaldi G, Sucato S, Fustinoni S, Roda G, et al. Bioavailability Assessment of an Iron Formulation Using Differentiated Human Intestinal Caco-2 Cells. Foods. 2023;12(16):3016.
17. Patil P, Geevarghese P, Khaire P, Joshi T, Suryawanshi A, Mundada S, et al. Comparison of Therapeutic Efficacy of Ferrous Ascorbate and Iron Polymaltose Complex in Iron Deficiency Anemia in Children: A Randomized Controlled Trial. Indian J Pediatr. 2019;86(12):1112-7.
18. Name JJ, Vasconcelos AR, Maluf MCVR. Iron Bisglycinate Chelate and Polymaltose Iron for the Treatment of Iron Deficiency Anemia: A Pilot Randomized Trial. Curr Pediatr Rev. 2018;14(4):261-8.
19. National Institute of Nutrition (India). Expert Group. & Indian Council of Medical Research. Nutrient requirements for Indians: recommended dietary allowances and estimated average requirement-2020. 321.
20. Piskin E, Cianciosi D, Gulec S, Tomas M, Capanoglu E. Iron Absorption: Factors, Limitations, and Improvement Methods. ACS Omega. 2022;7(24):20441-56.
21. Li Y, Jiang H, Huang G. Protein Hydrolysates as Promoters of Non-Haem Iron Absorption. Nutrients. 2017;9(6):609.
22. Jiang S, Wang C-xu, Lan L, Zhao D. Vitamin A deficiency aggravates iron deficiency by upregulating the expression of iron regulatory protein-2. Nutrition. 2012;28(3):281-7.
23. Ems T, Lucia KS, Huecker MR. Biochemistry, Iron Absorption. StatPearls (2023).
24. Hirobe T. Iron and skin health: iron stimulates skin function. 2012;196–214.
25. Park SY, Na SY, Kim JH, Cho S, Lee JH. Iron Plays a Certain Role in Patterned Hair Loss. J Korean Med Sci. 2013;28:934.
26. Miniaci MC, Irace C, Capuozzo A, Piccolo M, Pascale AD, Russo A, et al. Cysteine Prevents the Reduction in Keratin Synthesis Induced by Iron Deficiency in Human Keratinocytes. J Cell Biochem. 2016;117:402-12.
27. Kantor J, Kessler LJ, Brook DG, Cotsarelis G. Decreased Serum Ferritin is Associated With Alopecia in Women. J Invest Dermatol. 2003;121(5):985-8.
28. Pourzand C, Albieri-Borges A, Raczek NN. Shedding a New Light on Skin Aging, Iron- and Redox-Homeostasis and Emerging Natural Antioxidants. Antioxidants (Basel). 2022;11(3):471.
29. Cabantchik ZI. Labile iron in cells and body fluids: Physiology, pathology, and pharmacology. Front Pharmacol. 2014:5:45.
30. Safer JD. Thyroid hormone action on skin. Dermatoendocrinol. 2011;3(3):211-5.
31. Van Beek N, Bodó E, Kromminga A, Gáspár E, Meyer K, Zmijewski MA, et al. Thyroid hormones directly alter human hair follicle functions: anagen prolongation and stimulation of both hair matrix keratinocyte proliferation and hair pigmentation. J Clin Endocrinol Metab. 2008;93(11):4381-8.

11

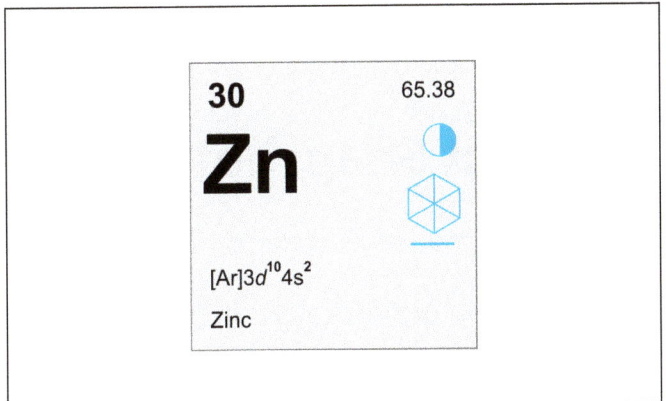

Zinc

Zinc

✍ Rasya Dixit

CONTENTS

ZINC: NUTRIENT SNAPSHOT
- ▸ REQUIREMENT IN THE INDIAN CONTEXT | 106
- ▸ ACTIVE FORMS | 107
- ▸ SAFETY AND DOSAGE | 107
- ▸ CLINICAL CONDITIONS | 108
- ▸ SUPPLEMENTATION | 111

INTRODUCTION | 113
DIGESTION, ABSORPTION AND STORAGE | 113
MECHANISM OF ACTION | 113

KEY TOPICS

- ACNE VULGARIS
- ALOPECIA AREATA
- ANDROGENIC ALOPECIA
- BEHCET'S DISEASE
- CUTANEOUS LEISHMANIASIS
- ERYTHROMYCIN-RESISTANT ACNE VULGARIS
- HIDRADENITIS SUPPURATIVA
- PSORIASIS
- ROSACEA
- SEBORRHEIC DERMATITIS
- VIRAL WARTS
- VITILIGO
- WOUND HEALING

Nutrient Snapshot

▶ **REQUIREMENT IN THE INDIAN CONTEXT**

- Zinc, a divalent cation, is an essential micronutrient for humans. It is an essential component of more than 1,000 enzymatic reactions and over 2,000 transcription factors that are needed for regulation of lipid, protein and nucleic acid metabolism, and gene transcription.[1]

- Half of the global population is predictably at the risk of low intakes of zinc. Reliable national-level data are scant to clearly demonstrate the extent of the prevalence of zinc deficiency. The lack of a suitable biomarker for physiological zinc status is a major obstacle.[2] However, numerous small studies indicate persistently worsening trends for zinc deficiency.[3,4] The cereal-rich Indian diet, which is high in phytate (that blocks zinc absorption), and lacks foods from animal origin drive zinc deficiency.

- Inadequacy of zinc can be connected to insufficient food supply, but mostly results from poor bioavailability from the diet. Zinc excess, on the other hand, is mainly associated with disturbed copper homeostasis.[2] Zinc is often prescribed as part of hair supplements or daily multivitamins within RDA limits. Higher doses of zinc must be balanced with copper intake.

ACTIVE FORMS

ACTIVE FORMS	SUPPLEMENT SOURCES	SALIENT FEATURES
Zinc	Inorganic zinc	Inorganic salts have higher purity but poor bioavailability.
	Chelated zinc	Chelated form of zinc has a higher bioavailability as compared to inorganic salts.

SAFETY AND DOSAGE

GENERAL REQUIREMENTS		
Indian recommendations	ICMR-NIN: Male—17 mg/day, Female—13.2 mg/day[45]	
	TUL (RDA 2020): 40 mg/day	
Global recommendations and limits	IOM: Males—11 mg/day and Female—8 mg/day	
	Upper limit: 25 mg/day or 40 mg/day (IOM)	
	NOAEL: 50 mg/day or 40 mg/day	
	No established LOAEL	
Notes:	High doses of iron supplementation can inhibit zinc absorption when given together. This is not applicable for iron from the dietary sources. As a rule of thumb, Iron: Zinc ratio should be 1:1 or maximum 2:1.	
	Calcium may also interfere with zinc absorption due to the formation of calcium zinc complexes.	
	High doses of zinc can interfere with copper absorption as zinc acts as an antagonist. Thus, copper supplementation is necessary in case of zinc supplementation to take care of copper requirements. As a general rule of thumb, for every 8–15 mg zinc, 1 mg of copper can help prevent zinc-induced copper deficiency.[6]	
	Protein intake has a beneficial effect on zinc absorption.	

▶ **CLINICAL CONDITIONS**

EVIDENCE LEVEL	CONDITION OR USE CASE	DOSAGE	BENEFIT OR MECHANISM OF ACTION
+++	Alopecia areata (zinc deficiency-related telogen effluvium)	150 mg zinc zinc chelate of L-carnosine (34 mg elemental zinc) for 6 months (in zinc deficient individuals)	Zinc is an essential cofactor for multiple enzymes and it is involved with important functional activities in the hair follicle. However, it may be used alongside other micronutrients as the rapidly growing cells in the hair follicle require all micronutrients.[7]
+++	Psoriasis	Oral zinc sulfate 50–200 mg three times per day + 5 mg copper sulfate for 3–4 months	Lesions in most cases revealed a moderate degree of improvement, while itching and scaling markedly reduced.[8]
++	Wound healing	N/A (review papers)	Zinc is involved in regulating every phase of the wound healing process; from membrane repair, oxidative stress, coagulation, inflammation and immune defence, tissue re-epithelialization, angiogenesis, to fibrosis/scar formation.[9] Zinc deficiency and high-dose zinc supplementation delay wound healing as a result of altered inflammatory responses.[10]
+++++	Acne vulgaris	N/A (Meta-analysis)	Zinc supplementation showed reduction in inflammatory papule count.[11]

▶ CLINICAL CONDITIONS *(Continued)*

EVIDENCE LEVEL	CONDITION OR USE CASE	DOSAGE	BENEFIT OR MECHANISM OF ACTION
+++	Acne vulgaris	Participants with acne and healthy controls received 220 mg of zinc sulphate heptahydrate capsules, 3 times daily, 1 hour before meals, for a period of 1 month.	Further to its anti-inflammatory action, zinc can inhibit the lipases of follicular bacterial species. It can also increase the serum level of retinol binding protein. The role of zinc in essential fatty acid metabolism, deficiency of which induces hyperkeratosis in animal models, may be a possible mechanism.[12]
+++	Erythromycin-resistant acne vulgaris	30 mg zinc gluconate for 60 days	There was a reduction in inflammatory lesions (papules and pustules) after 30 and 60 days of zinc supplementation.[13]
++++	Rosacea	The patients randomly received either zinc sulfate 100 mg or placebo capsules 3 time a day. The patients crossed over after 3 months.	The mean severity score of zinc group decreased after the first month of therapy to a lower level. After shifting to placebo treatment, the mean started to rise gradually in the fifth month but remained lower than the levels before therapy. In the group started on placebo, the mean severity score remained high in the first 3 months of therapy while the patients were on placebo. After shifting to zinc sulfate, the mean started to decrease after the fourth month to significantly low levels.[14]
++	Seborrheic dermatitis	N/A (observational study)	Patients who had seborrheic dermatitis had lower levels of serum zinc levels than healthy subjects.[15]
+++	Viral warts	10 mg/kg/day (maximum dose of 600 mg/day) oral zinc sulfate for 2 months	40–50% of patients showed complete resolution of warts.[16,17]

▶ **CLINICAL CONDITIONS** (*Continued*)

EVIDENCE LEVEL	CONDITION OR USE CASE	DOSAGE	BENEFIT OR MECHANISM OF ACTION
++++	Cutaneous leishmaniasis	Oral zinc sulfate in doses of 2.5, 5, and 10 mg/kg/day for 45 days	Results showed that the cure rate for the 2.5 mg/kg group was 83.9%, for the 5 mg/kg treatment group it was 93.1% and for the 10 mg/kg treatment group it was 96.9%. No lesions in the control group showed any sign of healing during the follow-up period.[18]
+++	Hidradenitis suppurativa	Zinc gluconate 90 mg/day (15 mg elemental zinc)	There was a clinical improvement, with 8 complete remissions and 14 partial remissions.[19]
+	Vitiligo	N/A (observational study)	Serum zinc levels are low in patients with generalized vitiligo.[20]
+++	Behcet's disease	Patients in group A received 100 mg zinc sulfate while those in group B received identical placebo tablet three times daily. After 3 months of starting treatment, patients were crossed over.	In group A, the mean clinical manifestations index (CMI) started to decline directly after the first month of therapy. After shifting to placebo treatment, the mean of CMI started to rise again gradually but remained lower than levels before therapy. In group B (started with placebo), the mean of CMI remained high for the first 3 months. After crossing over, the mean of CMI started to decrease after the fourth month. An inverse correlation between CMI and serum zinc level was found.[21]

Note: There are a number of clinical studies on a variety of hair supplements containing zinc alongside other vitamins, minerals and antioxidants that have shown benefits in hair growth and quality parameters.

▶ SUPPLEMENTATION

	BASIS	**WHAT TO LOOK OUT FOR**
Supplementation form	**Inorganic zinc salts:** Zinc acetate (30% zinc) Zinc oxide (80% zinc) Zinc sulfate (23% zinc) Zinc citrate (31% zinc) Zinc gluconate (14% zinc) Absorption of zinc gluconate and citrate has been estimated to be 60–61%, while that of zinc oxide was 50%.[22]	The form is mentioned in the ingredients section of the product packaging.
	Chelated form: Zinc methionine (or monomethionine) Zinc glycine In vitro and in vivo (animal) studies reveal that amino acid chelated zinc supplementation had higher absorption (particularly zinc methionine) as compared to zinc sulfate.[6,23] Chelated zinc, i.e., zinc methionine has higher bioavailability than sources of zinc.[24]	
Administration form	Multinutrient or multimineral formula designed in the tablets, capsules, powders, syrups, dispersible tablets format.	The administration form is mentioned on the product packaging
Purity considerations	Different forms of zinc contain different amounts of elemental zinc, which refers to the weight of the zinc molecule by itself.	The form and elemental zinc must be mentioned on the product packaging.

Nutrition in Dermatology

▶ **SUPPLEMENTATION** (*Continued*)

	BASIS	WHAT TO LOOK OUT FOR
Patient considerations	Zinc has a metallic aftertaste and astringency. Zinc chelates like zinc monomethionine have a strong odor. Chronic supplementation of zinc above TUL can result in gastrointestinal symptoms such as vomiting, nausea, abdominal pain and diarrhea.[25]	Capsules/tablets of zinc rather than a drink may be better for avoiding the aftertaste. Gummies may have lower amounts of zinc due to taste considerations. Supplementation above RDA should be based on biochemical test reports of the patient (i.e., in case of known deficiency)
Safety considerations	Zinc is fat-soluble, so caution must be exercised when providing more than RDA levels.	The amount of zinc administered per day from all sources.
Other considerations	The major adverse effect of higher zinc intake is on serum copper levels.	For every 8–15 mg zinc, 1 mg of copper can help prevent zinc-induced copper deficiency.[6]

INTRODUCTION

The skin is the third most zinc-abundant tissue in the body.[26] The regulatory functions of zinc ions, together with its function as a cofactor in thousands of zinc metalloproteins, impacts virtually all aspects of cell biology, including development, differentiation, and cell growth, making it important for skin renewal and repair and hair growth.

DIGESTION, ABSORPTION AND STORAGE

Digestion and Absorption

- Zinc absorption in the small intestine is one of the main mechanisms regulating its systemic homeostasis, along with the pancreas and liver. Endogenous zinc is continuously excreted into the intestinal lumen, from which parts are reabsorbed, while the remainder, is excreted with feces.[2]

- Fractional absorption of dietary zinc in humans is typically in the range of 16–50%, which is inversely related to oral zinc intake. Accordingly, human zinc absorption is more efficient from low zinc diets.[2] In instances of zinc deficiency, intestinal absorption can near 100%,[27] while fecal and urinal zinc losses decrease.[2]

- Zinc absorption is also affected by the form in which it is administered.[2] Dietary protein levels positively correlate with zinc uptake. The addition of protein to vegetable-based food significantly improves its zinc bioavailability in vivo.[2]

Storage

- The total zinc content in the human body amounts to 2–4 g (skeletal muscle 60%, bones 30%, liver 5%, and skin 5%),[28] with a plasma concentration of 12–16 µM. While it is a small plasma pool, it is rapidly exchangeable and mobile due to the several transporters of zinc.[27]

- Sufficient daily intake of zinc is necessary to maintain a steady state because, unlike iron, the body has no specialized zinc storage system.[27]

MECHANISM OF ACTION

Due to its role in cellular activities and enzymatic reactions, zinc plays an important role in skin's structure, function, as well as its immune system, both as a proinflammatory and anti-inflammatory mediator. It is no wonder that many disorders accompanied with skin and hair manifestations are caused by mutations or dysregulation of zinc transporters.[26] The potential benefits derived from supplementation with zinc seem to be at least partly attributable to zinc's anti-inflammatory and antioxidant properties.

Structural Role

Zinc plays a structural and functional role in all cell types found in the skin, and the processes that govern extracellular matrix production. For example, matrix metalloproteinases (MMPs) are one of enzyme families that contain zinc, and can degrade and remodel the proteins that form the extracellular matrix during turnover and wound healing.[26]

Catalytic and structural functions occur due to about 3,000 human zinc metalloproteins, a number that translates into approximately every tenth protein being a zinc protein.[29] A finger-like structure, known as a zinc finger motif, stabilizes the structure of several proteins. Examples include the superfamily of nuclear receptors that bind and respond to steroids and other molecules, such as estrogens, thyroid hormones, vitamin D, and vitamin A.

Zinc finger motifs are also involved in interactions of proteins with other proteins, ribonucleotides, and lipids. Its involvement in lipid synthesis and metabolism makes it important for barrier function as well.

Antioxidant Role

Zinc exerts its antioxidant properties by four mechanisms.[30]

- Zinc competes with iron (Fe) and copper (Cu) ions for binding to cell membranes and proteins, displacing these redox active metals, which catalyze the production of hydroxyl radicals from H_2O_2.

- Zinc binds to (SH) sulfhydryl groups of biomolecules protecting them from oxidation.

- Zinc increases the activation of antioxidant proteins, molecules, and enzymes such as glutathione (GSH), catalase, and superoxide dismutase (SOD)[31] and also reduces the activities of oxidant-promoting enzymes such as inducible nitric oxide synthase (iNOS) and NADPH oxidase and inhibits the generation of lipid peroxidation products.

- Zinc induces the expression of a metal-binding protein metallothionein (MT), which is very rich in cysteine and is an excellent scavanger of OH ions.[32,33]

Zinc finger motifs in the structure of nuclear receptors allow them to bind to DNA and act as transcription factors to regulate gene expression, and exert its anti-inflammatory role.

Regulatory Role

Zinc plays a role in cell signalling via the metal-response element (MRE)-binding transcription factor 1 (MTF1); MTF1 has a zinc finger domain that allows its binding to MRE sequences in the promoter of target genes and the subsequent expression of zinc-responsive genes. Zinc may also have a direct regulatory function, modulating the activity of cell-signalling enzymes and transcription factors.[26] For example, zinc has been shown to have antiandrogenic properties. It specifically inhibits 5α-reductase type 1 and 2 activity, which play a role in dihydrotestosterone (DHT) production, thus promoting hair growth.[34]

MOLECULAR TARGETS	MODE OF ACTION
Increase expression of the peroxisome proliferator-activated receptor PPARα.[35]	These inhibit the nuclear factor kappa B (NF-κB) pathway NF-κB and its targets, such as TNF-α, IL6 and IL-1β, increase inflammation.
Inhibitor of cyclic nucleotide phosphodiesterase (PDE).[36,37]	
Inhibitor A20, also known as the TNFα-induced protein 3; TNFAIP3.[38]	
Tristetraprolin (TTP) a known zinc finger protein,[39] also known as ZFP36 and ZFP36L1v.[40]	TTP is known to bind to elements of mRNAs, specifically encoding TNF-α and granulocyte/macrophage colony-stimulating factor.
Increases nuclear factor erythroid 2-related factor 2 (Nrf2).[41]	Regulates the gene expression of antioxidant proteins and enzymes such as GSH and SOD, as well as detoxifying enzymes such as glutathione-S-transferase-1 (GSTA1) and hemeoxygenase-1 (HO-1)
Increases KLF4 that is mainly expressed in suprabasal layers.[40]	Modulates the expression of genes involved in keratinocyte differentiation (ECM1, SPINK5, CDSN, FLG, and LCE3)

The research on the use of zinc for various dermatosis like psoriasis, atopic dermatitis, pityriasis alba, androgenetic alopecia areata, telogen effluvium, vitiligo, melasma, acne, seborrheic dermatitis and hidradenitis suppurativa may be scarce. However, research suggests a predominance of low serum zinc levels in all the dermatoses. Given its key role in skin's immune system and its antioxidant activities, zinc supplementation can be used as an adjuvant therapy in the management of chronic inflammatory and autoimmune skin diseases.[42]

▶ REFERENCES

1. Nitzan YB, Cohen AD. Zinc in skin pathology and care. J Dermatolog Treat. 2006;17:205-10.
2. Maares M, Haase H. A Guide to Human Zinc Absorption: General Overview and Recent Advances of In Vitro Intestinal Models. Nutrients. 2020;12.
3. Akhtar S. Zinc Status in South Asian Populations—An Update. J Health Popul Nutr. 2013;31(2):139-49.
4. Smith MR, DeFries R, Chhatre A, Ghosh-Jerath S, Myers SS. Inadequate Zinc Intake in India: Past, Present, and Future. Food Nutr Bull. 2019;40(1):26-40.
5. National Institute of Nutrition Indian Council of Medical Research. Recommended Dietary Allowances and Estimated Average Requirements for Indians - 2020. RDA Full Report 2020.
6. Zhang L, Guo Q, Duan Y, Lin X, Ni H, Zhou C, et al. Comparison of the Effects of Inorganic or Amino Acid-Chelated Zinc on Mouse Myoblast Growth in vitro and Growth Performance and Carcass Traits in Growing-Finishing Pigs. Front Nutr. 2022;9:857393.
7. Karashima T, Tsuruta D, Hamada T, Ono F, Ishii N, Abe T, et al. Oral zinc therapy for zinc deficiency-related telogen effluvium. Dermatol Ther. 2012;25(2):210-3.
8. Bor Naci M, Karabiyikoglu A. Zinc in Treatment of Psoriasis. Journal of Islamic Academy of Sciences.1991;4:78-82.
9. Lin PH, Sermersheim M, Li H, Lee PHU, Steinberg SM, Ma J. Zinc in Wound Healing Modulation. Nutrients. 2017;10(1):16.
10. Lim Y, Levy M, Bray TM. Dietary zinc alters early inflammatory responses during cutaneous wound healing in weanling CD-1 mice. J Nutr. 2004;134(4):811-6.
11. Yee BE, Richards P, Sui JY, Marsch AF. Serum zinc levels and efficacy of zinc treatment in acne vulgaris: A systematic review and meta-analysis. Dermatol Ther. 2020;33(6):e14252.
12. Rebell T, Atherton DJ, Holden C. The Effect of Oral Zinc Administration on Sebum Free Fatty Acids in Acne vulgaris. Acta Derm Venereol. 1986;66(4):305-10.
13. Dreno B, Foulc P, Reynaud A, Moyse D, Habert H, Richet H. Effect of zinc gluconate on propionibacterium acnes resistance to erythromycin in patients with inflammatory acne: in vitro and in vivo study. Eur J Dermatol. 2005;15(3):152-5.
14. Sharquie KE, Najim RA, Al-Salman HN. Oral zinc sulfate in the treatment of rosacea: a double-blind, placebo-controlled study. Int J Dermatol. 2006;45(7):857-61.
15. Karabay AE, Çerman AA. Serum zinc levels in seborrheic dermatitis: a case-control study. Turk J Med Sci. 2019;49(5):1503-8.
16. Sharma S, Barman KD, Sarkar R, Manjhi M, Garg VK. Efficacy of oral zinc therapy in epidermodysplasia verruciformis with squamous cell carcinoma. Indian Dermatol Online J. 2014;5(1):55-8.
17. Mun J-H, Kim S-H, Jung D-S, Ko H-C, Kim B-S, Kwon K-S, et al. Oral zinc sulfate treatment for viral warts: an open-label study. J Dermatol. 2011;38(6):541-5.
18. Sharquie KE, Najim RA, Farjou IB, Al-Timimi DJ. Oral zinc sulphate in the treatment of acute cutaneous leishmaniasis. Clin Exp Dermatol. 2001;26(1):21-6.
19. Brocard A, Knol AC, Khammari A, Dréno B. Hidradenitis suppurativa and zinc: a new therapeutic approach. A pilot study. Dermatology. 2007;214(4):325-7.
20. Mirnezami M, Rahimi H. Serum zinc level in vitiligo: A case-control study. Indian J Dermatol. 2018;63(3):227-30.
21. Sharquie KE, Najim RA, Al-Dori WS, Al-Hayani RK. Oral zinc sulfate in the treatment of Behcet's disease: a double blind cross-over study. J Dermatol. 2006;33(8):541-6.
22. Wegmüller R, Tay F, Zeder C, Brnić M, Hurrell RF. Zinc Absorption by Young Adults from Supplemental Zinc Citrate Is Comparable with That from Zinc Gluconate and Higher than from Zinc Oxide. J Nutr. 2014;144(2):132-6.
23. Liu FF, Azad MAK, Li Z-H, Li J, Mo K-B, Ni K-J. Zinc Supplementation Forms Influenced Zinc Absorption and Accumulation in Piglets. Animals (Basel). 2020;11(1):36.
24. Xiaoming XC, Zafra-Stone S, Bagchi M, Bagchi D. Bioavailability, antioxidant and immune-enhancing properties of zinc methionine. Biofactors. 2006;27(1-4):231-44.
25. Saper RB, Rash R. Zinc: An Essential Micronutrient. Am Fam Physician. 2009;79(9):768-72.
26. Ogawa Y, Kinoshita M, Shimada S, Kawamura T. Zinc and Skin Disorders. Nutrients. 2018;10(2):199.
27. Gammoh NZ, Rink L. Zinc in Infection and Inflammation. Nutrients. 2017;9(6):624.
28. Jackson, Malcolm J. "Physiology of Zinc: General Aspects. Zinc in Human Biology, edited by C.F. Mills, Springer, 1989, pp. 1-14.
29. Maret W. Zinc in Cellular Regulation: The Nature and Significance of "Zinc Signals". Int J Mol Sci. 2017;18(11):2285.
30. Prasad AS. Zinc is an Antioxidant and Anti-Inflammatory Agent: Its Role in Human Health. Front Nutr. 2014:1:14.
31. Iuchi Y, Roy D, Okada F, Kibe N, Tsunoda S, Suzuki S, et al. Spontaneous skin damage and delayed wound healing in SOD1-deficient mice. Mol Cell Biochem. 2010;341(1-2):181-94.
32. Atrián-Blasco E, Santoro A, Pountney DL, Meloni G, Hureau C, Fallerl P. Chemistry of mammalian metallothioneins and their interaction with amyloidogenic peptides and proteins. Chem Soc Rev. 2017;46(24):7683-93.
33. Hijova E. Metallothioneins and zinc: their functions and interactions. Bratisl Lek Listy. 2004;105(5-6):230-4.
34. Dhaher SA, Yacoub AA, Jacob AA. Estimation of Zinc and Iron Levels in the Serum and Hair of Women with Androgenetic Alopecia: Case–control Study. Indian J Dermatol. 2018;63(5):369-74.
35. von Bülow V, Dubben S, Engelhardt G, Hebel S, Plümäkers B, Heine H, et al. Zinc-dependent suppression of TNF-alpha production is mediated by protein kinase A-induced inhibition of Raf-1, I kappa B kinase beta, and NF-kappa B. J Immunol. 2007;179(6):4180-6.
36. Nishida K, Hasegawa A, Nakae S, Oboki K, Saito H, Yamasaki S, et al. Zinc transporter Znt5/Slc30a5 is required for the mast cell-mediated delayed-type allergic reaction but not the immediate-type reaction. J Exp Med. 2009;206(6):1351-64.

37. Brieger A, Rink L, Haase H. Differential regulation of TLR-dependent MyD88 and TRIF signaling pathways by free zinc ions. J Immunol. 2013;191(4):1808-17.
38. Jarosz M, Olbert M, Wyszogrodzka G, Młyniec K, Librowski T. Antioxidant and anti-inflammatory effects of zinc. Zinc-dependent NF-κB signaling. Inflammopharmacology. 2017;25(1):11-24.
39. Prasad AS, Bao B. Molecular Mechanisms of Zinc as a Pro-Antioxidant Mediator: Clinical Therapeutic Implications. Antioxidants (Basel). 2019;8(6):164.
40. Cassandri M, Smirnov A, Novelli F, Pitolli C, Agostini M, Malewicz M, et al. Zinc-finger proteins in health and disease. Cell Death Discov. 2017:3:17071.
41. Prasad AS, Bao B. Molecular Mechanisms of Zinc as a Pro-Antioxidant Mediator: Clinical Therapeutic Implications. Antioxidants (Basel). 2019;8(6):164.
42. Al Abadie M, Sharara Z, Abadie MA, Ball PA, Morrissey H. Possible relationship between poor skin disorders prognosis and serum zinc level: A narrative review. Dermatol Reports. 2022;14(4):9512.

12

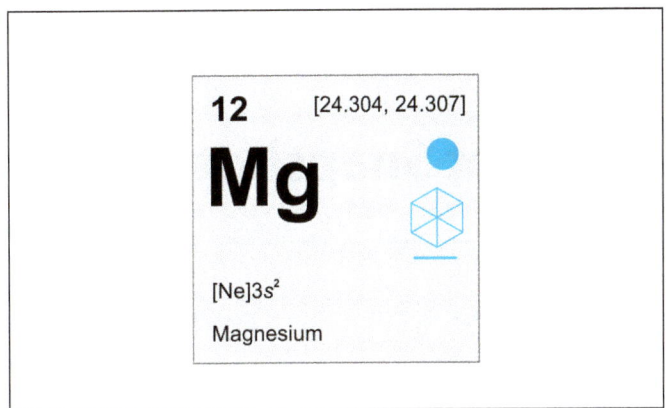

Magnesium

Magnesium

✎ Abhishek De

CONTENTS

MAGNESIUM: NUTRIENT SNAPSHOT

- ▶ REQUIREMENT IN THE INDIAN CONTEXT | 118
- ▶ ACTIVE FORMS | 119
- ▶ SAFETY AND DOSAGE | 119
- ▶ CLINICAL CONDITIONS | 119
- ▶ SUPPLEMENTATION | 122

INTRODUCTION | 124

DIGESTION, ABSORPTION AND STORAGE | 124

MECHANISM OF ACTION | 124

KEY TOPICS

- ACNE VULGARIS
- ATOPIC DERMATITIS
- ATOPIC ECZEMA/DERMATITIS SYNDROME (AEDS)
- FIBROBLASTS SENESCENCE

Nutrient Snapshot

▶ **REQUIREMENT IN THE INDIAN CONTEXT**

- At the cellular level, magnesium is one of the most abundant inorganic elements, befitting its paramount role. Magnesium is a cofactor for hundreds of enzymatic reactions that sustain life.[1]

- As the metal ion in chlorophyll, plant foods are a major dietary source of magnesium. It is also found in meat and legumes, which is why magnesium was believed to be sufficient in our diet. But as for any other mineral, absorption is limited to 13–50% due to various factors, such as intake of dietary fiber, and other minerals.[2] A depletion may also occur due to gastrointestinal issues and renal loss (due to alcohol and many commonly used drugs). Furthermore, a deficiency is multifactorial in nature, making its detection difficult.

- Magnesium deficit diets have been reported in children, even those from affluent households. In adults, increased fractional excretion has been reported in those with type-2 diabetes mellitus, hypertension and obesity, all of which are common in India. Diet surveys from most industrialized countries show a suboptimal intake of magnesium, and thus marginal deficiencies or insufficiencies may be more common in India than is believed.[3] That's why it is frequently called the forgotten mineral.[4]

- Magnesium is involved in skin cell growth and differentiation, skin remodeling, and hair growth. Magnesium improves barrier function by reducing transepidermal water loss (TEWL) and lowering inflammation, and therefore, exhibits favorable effects in inflammatory diseases. It is often used in topical agents, skin biomaterials, and patches.[5,6] Supplementation may be useful for promoting wound healing, hair growth and in the treatment regimen of inflammatory dermatoses. Even marginal magnesium deficiency is believed to cause inflammatory stress.[7]

- Taking large doses of vitamin D can induce severe depletion of Mg. Its supplementation should be considered during vitamin D therapy, which, due to the severe vitamin D deficiency, is a common practice in India. Magnesium is often given to individuals on isotretinoin, and those who experience migraine or psychological stress.[8]

▶ ACTIVE FORMS

ACTIVE FORMS	SUPPLEMENT SOURCES	SALIENT FEATURES
Magnesium	Organic and inorganic salts, chelated form, algal magnesium	Normally, the chelated form may have a slightly lower purity but has better bioavailability and tolerance over organic and inorganic salt forms.

▶ SAFETY AND DOSAGE

GENERAL REQUIREMENTS	
Indian recommendations	RDA 2020: Male—440 mg/day, Female—370 mg/day
	TUL: 350 mg/day (TUL value given here is only for nondietary pharmacological doses)
Global recommendations and limits	NIH RDA: Male—420 mg/day, Female—320 mg/day
	TUL for supplemental magnesium: 350 mg
	EFSA AI: Men—350 mg/day, Female—300 mg/day
	NOAEL: 250 mg/kg[9]
	LOAEL: 360 mg from supplemental sources[2]
Notes:	Calcium to magnesium ratios <1.7 and >2.8 can be detrimental, and optimal ratio may be approximately 2.0.[10]

▶ CLINICAL CONDITIONS

EVIDENCE LEVEL	CONDITION OR USE CASE	DOSAGE	BENEFIT OR MECHANISM OF ACTION
++++	Acne vulgaris	N/A (observational study)	Patients with acne and connective tissue dysplasia had reduced magnesium ions level in blood (compared to the group without connective tissue dysplasia).[11]

▶ **CLINICAL CONDITIONS** (*Continued*)

EVIDENCE LEVEL	CONDITION OR USE CASE	DOSAGE	BENEFIT OR MECHANISM OF ACTION
++	Acne vulgaris	N/A (observational study)	Serum magnesium and zinc concentrations were lower in the severe acne group compared with the mild acne group. With regard to serum copper levels, there was no difference between patient groups and control groups.[12]
+++	Acne vulgaris	Subjects received topical antibiotic treatment and ingested normocaloric diet with or without a supplement composed of myo-inositol 2,000 mg, liposomal magnesium (56.25 mg) and folic acid (duration unavailable)	The study showed that patients with a poor metabolic profile and insulin resistance saw an improvement in acne severity with supplementation. There was a reduction in global acne grading system (GAGS) levels in this group. They also saw an improvement in their metabolic profile as recorded by decreases in insulinemia (high levels of insulin in blood) and HOMA-IR (test for diabetes).[13]
++	Fibroblasts senescence	Human fibroblasts cells were cultured in magnesium deficient medium (in vitro)	The study suggested that the long-term inadequate magnesium availability in human fibroblast cultures lead to accelerated cellular senescence. This may be a mechanism through which chronic magnesium inadequacy could promote or exacerbate age-related disease.[14]

CLINICAL CONDITIONS (Continued)

EVIDENCE LEVEL	CONDITION OR USE CASE	DOSAGE	BENEFIT OR MECHANISM OF ACTION
+++	Atopic dermatitis	In this mouse study, one group was fed with a standard diet containing 0.25 g/100 g of magnesium and 6–7 mg/100 g zinc while other group were fed with 0.14 g/100 g of magnesium and 3–4 mg/100 g of zinc for 6 weeks	In the reduced Mg-Zn diet group, the following changes were seen (vs. standard diet group): • Skin drying and wrinkle-like changes and scratching behavior were observed 3–4 weeks after starting the diet. These changes increased with time. • There was thickening of the epidermis and dermis, with infiltration of many types of cells including mast cells and eosinophils. • After 6 weeks, the skin's water content decreased and TEWL increased. • Blood IgE levels began to increase at about 2–3 weeks and further increased after 6 weeks[15]
+++	Atopic eczema/dermatitis syndrome (AEDS)	Subjects ingested 500 mL of deep sea water daily for 6 months. Composition of water was as follows: Mg (100 mg), sodium (37 mg), calcium (35 mg), postassium (34 mg), zinc (2 mg), copper (2.2 mg), iodine (1.4 mg), phosphorus (4.5 mg), selenium (0.2 mg)	The skin symptoms of AEDS were improved in 27 out of 33 patients.[16] There was an improvement in skin symptoms and mineral imbalance and a decrease in serum IgE levels and IgE-inducing cytokines such as IL-4, IL-13 and IL-18 in patients with AEDS.[17]

▶ SUPPLEMENTATION

	BASIS	WHAT TO LOOK OUT FOR
Supplementation form	Inorganic salts: • Magnesium oxide (purity ≈60%) • Magnesium sulfate, magnesium chloride (purity ≈12%) • Magnesium gluconate, magnesium aspartate (purity ≈25%,) • Magnesium hydroxide Organic salts: • Magnesium citrate (purity ≈16%) • Magnesium ascorbate, magnesium orotate (purity ≈6%), magnesium lactate • Magnesium fumarate (purity ≈76%) • Magnesium malate (purity ≈11%), magnesium carbonate Magnesium phosphate dibasic (magnesium hydrogen phosphate) magnesium phosphate tribasic (trimagnesium phosphate) Amino acid chelated form: Magnesium glycinate/bisglycinate or, magnesium taurate, magnesium triglycine Chelate form has better tolerability as it reduces laxation and increases solubility, resulting in greater bioavailability.[18]	The form is stated in the ingredients section of the product packaging. Bioavailability/low side effects: Amino acid chelate> organic salts> inorganic salts[8,19]
Administration form	Capsules, tablets, syrups, powders, gummies, effervescent tablets, chewable tablets, strips, caplets	N/A
Purity considerations	Inorganic salts have a higher concentration of magnesium but have poor bioavailability, while organic ones have better bioavailability but purity may be comparatively low.[20,21]	Elemental dose per serving is stated on the nutritional information of the product packaging.

▶ SUPPLEMENTATION (Continued)

	BASIS	WHAT TO LOOK OUT FOR
Patient considerations	Magnesium should not be taken at the same time of the day as other mineral supplements (such as calcium, phosphorus, iron, copper, manganese and zinc) or fiber supplements as they may interfere with magnesium absorption.[19,22]	Supplementation of magnesium can be taken after a different meal than other mineral/fiber supplements.
	Magnesium may cause a laxative effect in some individuals.	A low dose of magnesium (approximately 100 mg) or using a chelate may help prevent laxation.
Safety considerations	Adverse effects of magnesium supplementation are associated with cardiovascular and neuromuscular health. These effects may vary depending on the exact formulation. Common adverse effects are: Flushing, hypotension, vasodilation, impaired reflexes, abdominal pain diarrhea, flatulence, nausea/vomiting, respiratory depression, electrolyte disorders, (hypocalcemia, hyperkalemia), and hypermagnesemia.[23] High doses of magnesium may lead to laxative effects.	Biochemical tests are not a good indicator of magnesium status. High doses must be avoided.
Other considerations	Individuals with irritable bowel syndrome should exercise caution before taking magnesium supplements. Individuals with renal issues and neuromuscular gravis, and pregnant women should avoid magnesium supplements.[23]	Individuals with chronic disorders should check with their doctors before starting any nutritional supplementation.

INTRODUCTION

As the second most abundant intracellular divalent cation, magnesium (Mg^{2+}) is indispensable for human health. It is required for energy transfer reactions involving high energy compounds like ATP and creatine phosphate. It plays a vital role in metabolic reactions as a cofactor (like DNA and RNA formation, protein synthesis and mitochondrial membrane stabilization. Thus, it is also involved in the functioning of muscles, nerves, the heart, bone and many more tissue.[4]

Epidemiological studies suggest that a low magnesium status is associated with chronic diseases such as cardiovascular disease (CVD), type 2 diabetes mellitus, metabolic syndrome, and skeletal disorders. This has resulted in the conclusion that magnesium deficiency is a greater nutritional problem than currently recognized.[7]

Magnesium also needs to be looked at through the lens of it's synergistic and contraindicative relationship with calcium. Magnesium is nature's calcium channel blocker and is required for the transport of potassium and sodium across the plasma membrane, directly influencing cellular activity and function. The ratio of calcium to magnesium may be more important than intake of either alone.[10]

DIGESTION, ABSORPTION AND STORAGE

Digestion and Absorption

- Although magnesium is absorbed along the entire intestinal tract, maximum absorption occurs in the distal small intestine.

- An active Mg-transport system accounts for greater fractional absorption at low dietary intake. At high dietary intakes, Mg absorption occurs at a lower rate and is due to passive absorption.

- Magnesium absorption is lower in the presence of zinc, calcium, potassium, and phosphate and when protein intake is < 30 g/day.[24]

Storage

The normal adult body content is approximately 20–25 g and the majority of it is stored in bone, muscle, and liver.[4]

MECHANISM OF ACTION

01 | Cell Growth and Metabolism

The hair follicle has one of the highest rates of cell division in the body, which is why hair growth is a highly energy-consuming process. Glycolysis and fatty acid oxidation in mitochondria generate ATP. Magnesium is required by enzymes for glycolysis, which is the preferred energy pathway for hair follicle cells.[2,25,26]

Mg^{2+} ion-ATP complexes are required for phosphate transfer reactions for mitochondria to carry out oxidative phosphorylation, another major metabolic pathway to provide energy for cells. DNA replication and repair are dependent on Mg^{2+} ions. Therefore, it plays a role in the proliferation of cells in skin regeneration and repair.[14,24]

02 | Barrier Function and Anti-inflammatory Action

Other than regulating cell growth, calcium and magnesium gradients regulate terminal differentiation of keratinocytes and epidermal lipid metabolism, resulting in the constitution of the stratum corneum barrier.[1,27] Magnesium ions also affect migration of cells, therefore playing a key role in wound healing.

Low magnesium status is associated with excessive production of free radicals and increased inflammation. Magnesium ions can reduce the expression of inflammatory mediators such as tumor necrosis factor alpha (TNF-α) and nuclear factor kappa B (NFκB).[28] Studies have indicated an inverse relationship of magnesium intake and elevated serum or plasma C-reactive protein (CRP),

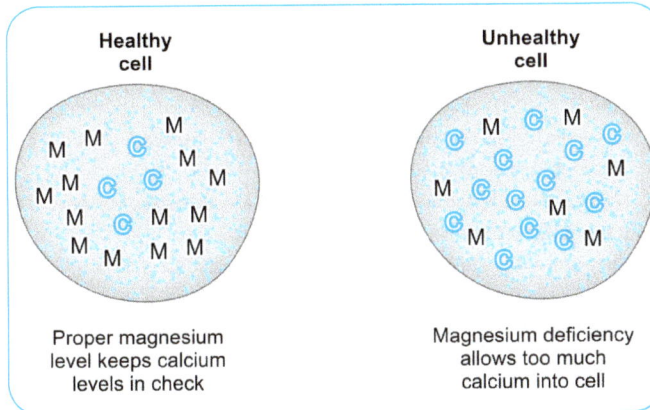

Figure 1: Magnesium is required to maintain the level of calcium in cells and tissue. Low Magnesium status leads to too much calcium in cells.

an established indicator of low-grade or chronic inflammation. A reduction in extracellular magnesium leads to the cellular entry of excess calcium and its signaling that results in the release of inflammatory neuropeptides, cytokines, prostaglandins, and leukotrienes.[7,29] This is perhaps the reason its deficiency is thought to cause hair loss[29] and its use has been postulated to improve skin allergies **Figure 1**.[30]

03 | Microcirculation

Microcirculatory dysfunction, which limits delivery of oxygen and nutrients, is a key element in the pathogenesis of many types of hair fall.[31] Magnesium supplementation improves endothelial function in two ways: (1) Indirectly by an endothelium-dependent release of nitric oxide and reducing inflammation; and (2) Directly via its ability to induce vasodilation by acting upon vascular smooth muscle as a calcium competitor.[32] Magnesium deficiency has shown a reduction in capillary, and venular blood flow. The greater the degree of deficiency, the greater the reductions in microvascular lumen sizes.[33]

▶ REFERENCES

1. Haftek M, Abdayem R, Guyonnet-Debersac P. Skin Minerals: Key Roles of Inorganic Elements in Skin Physiological Functions. Int J Mol Sci. 2022;23(11):6267.
2. National Institute of Nutrition Indian Council of Medical Research. Recommended Dietary Allowances and Estimated Average Requirements for Indians – 2020. RDA Full Report 2020.
3. Hartwig A. Role of magnesium in genomic stability. Mutat Res. 2001;475(1–2):113-21.
4. Shu S, Kobayashi M, Marunaka K, Yoshino Y, Goto M, Katsuta Y, et al. Magnesium Supplementation Attenuates Ultraviolet-B-Induced Damage Mediated through Elevation of Polyamine Production in Human HaCaT Keratinocytes. Cells. 2022;11(15):2268.
5. Gröber U, Werner T, Vormann J, Kisters K. Myth or Reality—Transdermal Magnesium? Nutrients. 2017;9(8):813.
6. Jang D, Shim J, Shin DM, Noh H, Oh SJ, Park J, et al. Magnesium microneedle patches for under-eye wrinkles. Dermatol Ther. 2022;35(9):e15732.
7. Nielsen FH. Magnesium, inflammation, and obesity in chronic disease. Nutrition Reviews. 2010;68(6):333-40.
8. Reddy P, Edwards LR. Magnesium Supplementation in Vitamin D Deficiency. Am J Ther. 2019;26(1):e124-32.
9. EFSA Panel on Dietetic Products, Nutrition and Allergies (NDA). Scientific Opinion on Dietary Reference Values for magnesium. EFSA Journal. 2015;13(7):4186.
10. Rosanoff A, Dai Q, Shapses SA. Essential Nutrient Interactions: Does Low or Suboptimal Magnesium Status Interact with Vitamin D and/or Calcium Status? Adv Nutr. 2016;7(1):25-43.
11. Koshel MV, Chebotarev VV. Acne treatment in patients with connective tissue dysplasia. Stavropol State Medical University, Russian Federation. UDC 616.53–002:616.33–008.3, doi:dx.doi.org/10.14300/mnnc.2014.09048.
12. Saleh BO, Anbar ZNH, Majid AY. Role of Some Trace Elements in Pathogenesis and Severity of Acne Vulgaris in Iraqi Male Patients. Journal of Clinical & Experimental Dermatology Research. 2013;4(1);1000169.
13. Gabriella F, Marianna D, Giuseppe R, Claudio M, Savastano S, Barrea L, et al. Effectiveness of supplementation with myo-inositol, folic acid and liposomal magnesium in male insulin-resistant patients with acne. Esperienze Dermatologiche. 2016;18(2):76-9
14. Killilea DW, Ames BN. Magnesium deficiency accelerates cellular senescence in cultured human fibroblasts. Proc Natl Acad Sci U S A. 2008;105(15):5768-73.
15. Makiura M, Akamatsu H, Akita H, Yagami A, Shimizu Y, Eiro H, et al. Atopic Dermatitis-Like Symptoms in HR-1 Hairless Mice Fed a Diet Low in Magnesium and Zinc. J Int Med Res. 2004;32(4):392-9.
16. Hataguchi Y, Tai H, Nakajima H, Kimata H. Drinking deep-sea water restores mineral imbalance in atopic eczema/dermatitis syndrome. Eur J Clin Nutr. 2005;59(9):1093-6.
17. Kimata H, Tai H, Nakagawa K, Yokoyama Y, Nakajima H, Ikegami Y. Improvement of skin symptoms and mineral imbalance by drinking deep sea water in patients with atopic eczema/dermatitis syndrome (AEDS). Acta Medica (Hradec Kralove). 2002;45(2):83-4.
18. Case DR, Zubieta J, Gonzalez R, Doyle RP. Synthesis and Chemical and Biological Evaluation of a Glycine Tripeptide Chelate of Magnesium. Molecules. 2021;26(9):2419.
19. Schuchardt JP, Hahn A. Intestinal Absorption and Factors Influencing Bioavailability of Magnesium-An Update. Curr Nutr Food Sci. 2017;13(4):260-78.
20. Blancquaert L, Vervaet C, Derave W. Predicting and Testing Bioavailability of Magnesium Supplements. Nutrients. 2019;11(7):1663.
21. Rylander R. Bioavailability of Magnesium Salts – A Review. Journal of Pharmacy and Nutrition Sciences. 2014;4(1):57-9.

22. Office of Dietary Supplements. Fact Sheet for Health Professionals - Magnesium. National Institute of Health.
23. Allen MJ, Sharma S. Magnesium. In: StatPearls. Treasure Island (FL): StatPearls Publishing; 2024.
24. Institute of Medicine (US) Standing Committee on the Scientific Evaluation of Dietary. Dietary Reference Intakes for Calcium, Phosphorus, Magnesium, Vitamin D, and Fluoride. Chapter 6: Magnesium. National Academies Press (US); 1997.
25. Kealey T, Williams R, Philpott MP. The human hair follicle engages in glutaminolysis and aerobic glycolysis: implications for skin, splanchnic and neoplastic metabolism. Skin Pharmacol. 1994;7(1–2):41-6.
26. Williams R, Philpott MP, Kealey T. Metabolism of freshly isolated human hair follicles capable of hair elongation: A glutaminolytic, aerobic glycolytic tissue. J Invest Dermatol. 1993;100(6):834-40.
27. Denda Mitsuhiro. New strategies to improve skin barrier homeostasis. Adv Drug Deliv Rev. 2002:54(Suppl 1):S123-30.
28. Chandrasekaran N, Weir C, Alfraji S, Grice J, Roberts M, Barnard R. Effects of magnesium deficiency - More than skin deep. Exp Biol Med (Maywood). 2014;239(10):1280-91.
29. John SN. The 'bald' phenotype (androgenetic alopecia) is caused by the high glycaemic, high cholesterol and low mineral 'western diet.' Trends in Food Science & Technology. 2021;116:1170-8.
30. Błach J, Nowacki W, Mazur A. Magnesium in skin allergy. Postepy Hig Med Dosw (Online). 2007;61:548-54.
31. Gerkowicz A, Krasowska D, Pietrzak A, Michalak-Stoma A, Bartosińska J, Juszkiewicz-Borowiec M, et al. Videocapillaroscopic Alterations in Alopecia Areata. Biomed Res Int. 2013:2013:160203.
32. Pranskunas A, Vellinga NA, Pilvinis V, Koopmans M, Boerma EC. Microcirculatory changes during open label magnesium sulphate infusion in patients with severe sepsis and septic shock. BMC Anesthesiol. 2011;11:12.
33. Altura BM, Altura BT, Asefa G, Hartmut I, Theo G. Magnesium Deficiency and Hypertension: Correlation Between Magnesium-Deficient Diets and Microcirculatory Changes in Situ. Science. 1984;223(4642):1315-7.

13

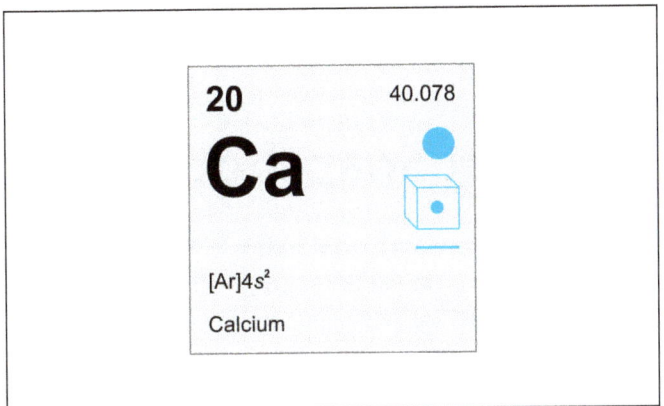

Calcium

Calcium

✍ Abhishek De

CONTENTS

CALCIUM: NUTRIENT SNAPSHOT

▶ REQUIREMENT IN THE INDIAN CONTEXT | **128**

▶ ACTIVE FORMS | **129**

▶ SAFETY AND DOSAGE | **129**

▶ CLINICAL CONDITIONS | **130**

▶ SUPPLEMENTATION | **131**

INTRODUCTION | **133**

DIGESTION, ABSORPTION AND STORAGE | **133**

MECHANISM OF ACTION | **133**

KEY TOPICS

- PREMATURE GRAYING OF HAIR
- PUSTULAR PSORIASIS
- SQUAMOUS CELL CARCINOMA [(SCC); NONMELANOMA SKIN CANCERS]
- VON ZUMBUSCH PSORIASIS–GENERALIZED PUSTULAR PSORIASIS

Nutrient Snapshot

▶ **REQUIREMENT IN THE INDIAN CONTEXT**

- Calcium is abundant in the human body, and is mostly stored in bone. This is why it is usually linked with bone metabolism. However, it is required by every cell in the body. Calcium promotes haemostatis, but also is a key regulator of epithelialization. Of critical importance to the skin is its role in regulating cell differentiation and migration, which is important for barrier function and wound healing.[1,2] Calcium also aids hair growth and hormone and enzyme secretion.

- A complex interplay of vitamin D and hormones tightly regulate the plasma and extracellular calcium pool.[3,4] It is lost through stool, urine, bile and sweat.[4] During low intake, calcium in bone helps maintain the blood level. That's why the body can adapt to different levels of calcium intake.

- Since milk is a major source of calcium, populations that consume plenty of milk get a sufficient amount. Animal protein also limits the loss of calcium in urine.[4] The intake of animal protein is not sufficient in many communities in India. Furthermore, through food or supplements, the average absorption rate is only 10–30%.[4]

- As the skin ages, the calcium epidermal gradient goes down, causing an increase in pH of the epidermis and a rearrangement of the cornified envelope. This eventually leads to an increased prevalence of infections, reduced resistance against mechanical stress and reduced wound healing.[2] Calcium loss from skin and hair also occurs due to detergents and shampoos.

- Besides low intake of vitamin D, low calcium intake may be responsible for the high prevalence of osteopenia and osteoporosis in India, especially in women.[4] Calcium can be supplemented if signs of low calcium intake are presented, and in balance with magnesium supplements.

▶ ACTIVE FORMS

ACTIVE FORMS	SUPPLEMENT SOURCES	SALIENT FEATURES
Calcium	Organic, inorganic salts, coral calcium, algal calcium	Calcium carbonate (calcite) from limestone is normally used in supplements, which is dense and has poor solubility in the digestive tract. Some sources of calcium (algae and coral) are largely composed of calcite, but also contain vaterite and aragonite, which have better solubility than calcite. They also have traces of other minerals, which likely do not affect our nutritional status. Calcium citrate malate is water soluble, and has better bioavailability than calcite.[5,6]

▶ SAFETY AND DOSAGE

GENERAL REQUIREMENTS	
Indian recommendations	ICMR-NIN RDA 2020: 1,000 mg/day[4] TUL: 2,500 mg/day
Global recommendations and limits	NIH RDA: Male—1,000 mg and Female—1,200 mg/day TUL: 2,000 mg/day EFSA dietary reference value: 1,000 mg/day[7] LOAEL: 2,000 mg/day[8]
Notes:	Ca: Mg optimum ratio is in the range of 1.7–2.6. Low magnesium intakes coupled with high calcium intakes (high Ca: Mg) have been associated with increased risk for chronic conditions such as cardiovascular disease and metabolic syndrome, as well as some cancers and total mortality. A high dietary Ca:Mg ratio (>2.6) may affect body magnesium status while, on the other hand, high intakes of magnesium could adversely impact individuals with an exceedingly low dietary Ca:Mg ratio (<1.70). Thus, a Ca:Mg ratio range of 1.7–2.6 (weight-to-weight) has been proposed as an optimum range.[9] Calcium absorption is inversely proportional to the dose. With daily calcium intake of <500 mg, the absorption is about 60–80%, which can easily supply the daily needs of calcium, whereas calcium intake of >900 mg is about 25–35%. The highest absorption was seen at 250 mg[10]

▶ **CLINICAL CONDITIONS**

EVIDENCE LEVEL	CONDITION OR USE CASE	DOSAGE	BENEFIT OR MECHANISM OF ACTION
+	Pustular psoriasis	Intravenous calcium followed by cholecalciferol dose (vitamin D) along with antibiotics treatment (dose and duration not available)	The case study of febrile pustular psoriasis, associated with severe hypocalcemia, showed an improvement with calcium supplementation alone.[11]
+	von Zumbusch psoriasis- generalized pustular psoriasis	Intravenous calcium and cholecalciferol, with regular use of oral levothyroxine (dose and duration not available)	The case study of severe von Zumbusch psoriasis with life-threatening complications triggered by severe hypocalcemia secondary to hypoparathyroidism was successfully treated with aggressive calcium reposition.[12]
++	Psoriasis	N/A (observational study)	Of all the psoriasis patients, 37.2% were hypocalcemic and 63.7% had normal serum calcium, whereas in the control group 89% were normocalcemic. This study suggests that hypocalcemia is a risk factor of psoriasis.[13]
+++++	Squamous cell carcinoma (SCC) (nonmelanoma skin cancers)	Participants ingested either only vitamin D3 (1,000 IU), only calcium (1,200 mg), both vitamin D and calcium, or placebo for 3–5 years	SCC incidence was unrelated to treatment with vitamin D3 compared with no vitamin D3, but there was suggestive evidence of beneficial treatment effects for calcium compared with no calcium.[14]
++	Premature graying of hair	N/A (observational study)	Serum calcium and vitamin D3 levels were found to be low in participants with premature graying of hair.[15]

▶ SUPPLEMENTATION

	BASIS	WHAT TO LOOK OUT FOR
Supplementation form	**Inorganic forms:** Calcium carbonate (purity ≈40%), calcium chloride, calcium hydroxide, calcium oxide, calcium phosphate, monobasic (purity ≈38%); calcium phosphate, dibasic calcium phosphate; tribasic calcium sulfate **Organic forms:** Calcium salts of citric acid (purity ≈21%), calcium gluconate (purity ≈9%), calcium lactate (purity ≈13%), calcium citrate malate (purity≈30%) Calcium from algae including red seaweed natural forms of calcium obtained from corals, shells, pearls, conch, oysters and milk[10,16-18] Calcium carbonate appears to cause more side effects than calcium citrate, especially in older adults who have lower levels of stomach acid.	The form of calcium is stated on the ingredients list of the product packaging
Administration form	Capsules, tablets, syrups, powders gummies, chewable tablets, effervescent tablets, caplets	N/A
Purity considerations	Calcium carbonate and citrate are commonly used and to a lesser extent, calcium lactate and gluconate is used. Calcium carbonate has high elemental calcium content (40%) while calcium citrate provides less elemental calcium (21%). The latter has better bioavailability.[17]	The elemental calcium is often mentioned on the product packaging. If not, it can be provided by the product manufacturer.

▶ SUPPLEMENTATION (Continued)

	BASIS	WHAT TO LOOK OUT FOR
Patient considerations	Depending on the form, calcium supplements can be taken with or without meals. Calcium carbonate can cause constipation. It has very low solubility in water, and should be taken with meals, since gastric acidity is required for sufficient absorption.[17] Calcium citrate is the most easily absorbed calcium supplement, and it may be taken with or without meals, since its absorption is not dependent on gastric acidity.[17]	It is important to consider instructions for use given on the package. For people experiencing constipation, switching calcium forms or taking smaller calcium doses at a time, or taking the supplement with meals can help manage the symptoms.[16]
Safety considerations	Some individuals who take calcium supplements might experience gastrointestinal side effects such as gas, bloating, constipation, or a combination of these symptoms.[16]	Calcium concentration in hair represents intracellular calcium levels.[19,20] However, this is not a common test. Normally, if a patient exhibits other symptoms of calcium insufficiency (like osteopenia), then supplementation can be given. Menopausal or postmenopausal women can be given calcium and magnesium supplementation.
Other considerations	Individuals with kidney stones or a history of it should exercise caution while consuming calcium supplements.[21] Individuals undergoing or at the risk of cardiovascular health issues should be cautious before taking calcium supplements.[19,20] Calcium may interfere with other mineral absorption so the consumption time should be spaced out from other supplements.	Individuals with clinical issues should seek medical consultation before starting any nutritional supplementation.

INTRODUCTION

Calcium is required and used throughout the body, due to its role in intracellular signalling, and hormonal secretion. It is therefore involved in bone health, vascular and muscle function, nerve transmission, and cardiac health. Its role in skin and hair health however is often overlooked.[4]

Calcium and magnesium share a competitive relationship and both are critical for life. The two cations compete in the modulation of muscular contraction, and in the regulation of a number of enzymatic reactions involved in energy metabolism and signal transduction.[9]

Calcium supplementation has been controversial due to the concern of mineralization of soft tissue and blood vessels. However, mineralization is a complex, multifaceted process, and the calcium level in the blood is tightly regulated. It is not a concern for healthy individuals, especially under the guidance of a healthcare professional.

DIGESTION, ABSORPTION AND STORAGE

Digestion and Absorption

- Calcium in humans is absorbed by 2–3 different pathways. (1) vitamin D-dependent active transport across the intestinal epithelium, mainly through the duodenum and jejunum; (2) passive paracellular transport of free calcium ions, which depends on the free calcium concentration in the small intestine; and (3) passive absorption of calcium complexes such as calcium oxalate.[22]

- Other minerals like iron may interfere with calcium absorption. They can be taken at different times of the day.

- Caffeine should be avoided immediately before/after calcium supplements. Daily intake of ≤400 mg of caffeine is unlikely to interfere with overall calcium homeostasis.[23]

Storage

- More than 99% (1.2–1.4 kg) is stored in the bones and teeth while less than 1% is found in blood, muscle and other tissue.

- The epidermis has a characteristic calcium gradient. Low calcium levels are found in the lower, basal, and spinous layers, whereas calcium levels increase progressively toward the outer stratum granulosum, and decline again in the stratum corneum.[24]

MECHANISM OF ACTION

01 | Cellular Activity and Barrier Function

Calcium is a key modulator of directional locomotion of keratinocytes and fibroblasts, and is a well-known regulator of keratinocyte differentiation to corneocytes and cellular adhesion. Changes in calcium levels regulate the transcription of many unique proteins required for keratinocyte differentiation, such as involucrin, small proline-rich proteins, loricrin, filaggrin, and keratins (**Figure 1**).[24,25] Evidence suggests that the proper combination of calcium and magnesium enhances barrier repair.

Calcium levels also affect melanogenesis and sweat production. Depletion of intracellular calcium (Ca^{2+}) stores triggers an influx of Ca^{2+} across the plasma membrane, which is central to the

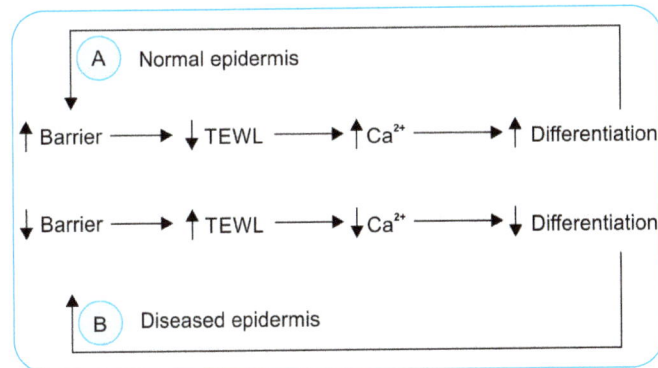

Figure 1: Relationship of epidermal Ca^{2+} with skin barrier properties.
(TEWL: transepidermal water loss, Ca^{2+}: calcium ion)
Source: Adapted from Elias (2022).[24]

normal physiology of these cells. Emerging evidence suggests that numerous skin pathologies including dermatitis, anhidrotic ectodermal dysplasia, hyperhidrosis, and hair loss may be related to improper calcium homeostasis.[26]

02 | Promoting Hair Growth

Despite their clear impact on keratinocyte differentiation, the role of vitamin D and calcium in hair follicle cycling is not entirely clear. Calcium is believed to affect hair growth directly via hormone and enzyme secretion, and indirectly by affecting cell signalling and mediating vasoconstriction and vasodilation. Low dietary intake may disrupt the hair follicle cycle.[27]

▶ REFERENCES

1. Polefka TG, Bianchini RJ, Shapiro S. Interaction of mineral salts with the skin: a literature survey. International Journal of Cosmetic Science. 2012;34(5):416-23.
2. Rinnerthaler M, Richter K. The Influence of Calcium on the Skin pH and Epidermal Barrier During Aging. 2018.
3. Narayanan V, Pallewar S, Mane A, Bhargava A. A Randomized, Volunteer, Pharmacokinetic Study Comparing Absorption and Bioavailability of Coral Calcium with Calcium Carbonate and Calcium Citrate Malate Supplements. EJPMR. 2018;5:341.
4. National Institute of Nutrition Indian Council of Medical Research. Recommended Dietary Allowances and Estimated Average Requirements for Indians – 2020. RDA Full Report 2020.
5. Scientific Opinion of the Panel on Food Additives, Flavourings, Processing aids and Materials in Contact with food (AFC). Calcium citrate malate as source for calcium for use in foods for Particular Nutritional Uses and in foods for the general population (including food supplements). The EFSA Journal. 2007;5(12):612.
6. Patrick L. Comparative absorption of calcium sources and calcium citrate malate for the prevention of osteoporosis. Altern Med Rev. 1999;4(2):74-85.
7. EFSA Panel on Dietetic Products, Nutrition and Allergies (NDA). Scientific Opinion on Dietary Reference Values for calcium. EFSA Journal 2015;13(5):4101
8. Institute of Medicine (US) Committee to Review Dietary Reference Intakes for Vitamin D and Calcium. Dietary Reference Intakes for Calcium and Vitamin D. ACatharine Ross et. al. (eds), National Academies Press (US), 2011. doi:10.17226/13050
9. Costello RB, Rosanoff A, Dai Q, Saldanha LG, Potischman NA. Perspective: Characterization of Dietary Supplements Containing Calcium and Magnesium and Their Respective Ratio—Is a Rising Ratio a Cause for Concern? Adv Nutr. 2020;12(2):291-7.
10. Garg MK, Mahalle N. Calcium Supplementation: Why, Which, and How? Indian J Endocrinol Metab. 2019;23(4):387-90.
11. Masson L, Saillard C, Ping Man SL, Baggio R, Kammerer-Jacquet SF, Adamski H, et al. A pustular psoriasis flare treated with calcium supplementation. JAAD Case Rep. 2021 23;12:40-5.
12. Guerreiro de Moura CAG, de Assis LH, Góes P, Rosa F, Nunes V, Gusmão ÍM, et al. A Case of Acute Generalized Pustular Psoriasis of von Zumbusch Triggered by Hypocalcemia. Case Rep Dermatol. 2015;7(3):345-51.
13. Qadim HH, Goforoushan F, Nejad SB, Goldust M. Studying the calcium serum level in patients suffering from psoriasis. Pak J Biol Sci. 2013;16(6):291-4.
14. Passarelli MN, Karagas MR, Mott LA, Rees JR, Barry EL, Baron JA. Risk of keratinocyte carcinomas with vitamin D and calcium supplementation: a secondary analysis of a randomized clinical trial. Am J Clin Nutr. 2020;112(6):1532-9.
15. Bhat RM, Sharma R, Pinto AC, Dandekeri S, Martis J. Epidemiological and Investigative Study of Premature Graying of Hair in Higher Secondary and Pre-University School Children. Int J Trichology. 2013;5(1):17-21.
16. Fact Sheet for Health Professionals. Calcium [Online]. Available from: https://ods.od.nih.gov/factsheets/calcium-HealthProfessional/
17. Wiria M, Tran HM, Nguyen PHB, Valencia O, Dutta S, Pouteau E. Relative bioavailability and pharmacokinetic comparison of calcium glucoheptonate with calcium carbonate. Pharmacol Res Perspect. 2020;8(2):e00589.
18. Bourassa MW, Abrams SA, Belizán JM, Boy E, Cormick G, Quijano CD, et al. Interventions to improve calcium intake through foods in populations with low intake. Ann N Y Acad Sci. 2022;1511(1):40-58.
19. Park SJ, Lee SH, Cho DY, Kim KM, Lee DJ, Kim BT. Hair Calcium Concentration is Associated with Calcium Intake and Bone Mineral Density. International Journal for Vitamin and Nutrition Research. 2013;83(3):154-61.
20. Park JM, Lee B, Kim YS, Hong KW, Park YC, Shin DH, et al. Calcium Supplementation, Risk of Cardiovascular Diseases, and Mortality: A Real-World Study of the Korean National Health Insurance Service Data. Nutrients. 2022;14(12):2538.
21. Sorensen MD. Calcium intake and urinary stone disease. Transl Androl Urol. 2014;3(3):235-40.
22. Meiron OE, Bar-David E, Aflalo ED, Shechter A, Stepensky D, Berman A, et al. Solubility and bioavailability of stabilized amorphous calcium carbonate. Journal of Bone and Mineral Research. 2011;26(2):364-72.
23. Wikoff D, Welsh BT, Henderson R, Brorby GP, Britt J, Myers E, et al. Systematic review of the potential adverse effects of caffeine consumption in healthy adults, pregnant women, adolescents, and children. Food Chem Toxicol. 2017;109(Pt 1):585-648.
24. Elias PM, Brown BE, Crumrine D, Feingold KR, Ahn SK. Origin of the Epidermal Calcium Gradient: Regulation by Barrier Status and Role of Active vs Passive Mechanisms. J Invest Dermatol. 2002;119(6):1269-74.
25. Nopriyati, Suherman AL, Yahya YF, Devi M. The Role of Calcium in the Skin Barrier. Bioscientia Medicina : Journal of Biomedicine and Translational Research. 2022;6(7):1976-88.
26. Manning D, Dart C, Evans RL. Store-operated calcium channels in skin. Front Physiol. 2022;13:1033528.
27. Mady LJ, Ajibade DV, Hsaio C, Teichert A, Fong C, Wang Y, et al. The Transient Role for Calcium and Vitamin D during the Developmental Hair Follicle Cycle. J Invest Dermatol. 2016;136(7):1337-45.

14

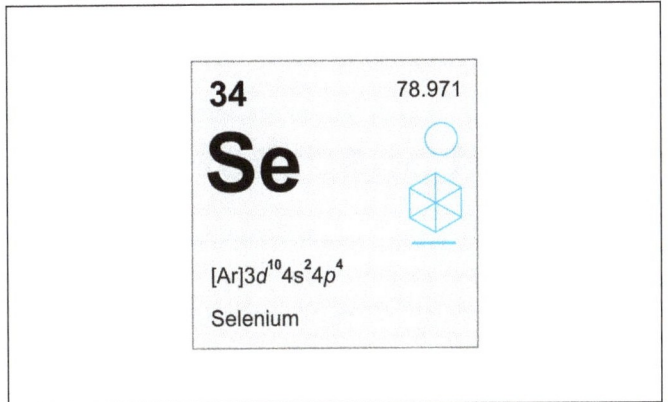

Selenium

Selenium

✒ Abhishek De

CONTENTS

SELENIUM: NUTRIENT SNAPSHOT

- ▶ REQUIREMENT IN THE INDIAN CONTEXT | 136
- ▶ ACTIVE FORMS | 137
- ▶ SAFETY AND DOSAGE | 137
- ▶ CLINICAL CONDITIONS | 138
- ▶ SUPPLEMENTATION | 144

INTRODUCTION | 145

DIGESTION, ABSORPTION AND STORAGE | 145

MECHANISM OF ACTION | 145

KEY TOPICS

- ACNE VULGARIS
- ALOPECIA AND PSEUDOALBINISM
- ALOPECIA WITH POLIOSIS
- ALOPECIA AREATA
- ATOPIC DERMATITIS
- CHLORIC ACNE VULGARIS
- DIABETES-RELATED SKIN DAMAGE
- PHOTOPROTECTION
- PSORIASIS
- SKIN ALLERGY
- SKIN DEVELOPMENT
- SKIN HYPERSENSITIVITY
- VITILIGO

Nutrient Snapshot

▶ **REQUIREMENT IN THE INDIAN CONTEXT**

- Selenium is an essential trace mineral, but like all minerals, it can be toxic at high levels. By acting as a cofactor for various enzymes known as selenoproteins, it is involved in redox, immune and thyroid function. These intrinsic functions have a major impact on skin and hair health.[1]

- Insufficient selenium intake may negatively affect the activity of several selenium-responsive enzymes, like glutathione peroxidases. Therefore, low selenium levels have been reported (in India) to occur after an infection caused by the SARS-CoV-2 virus (COVID-19).[2] This can be expected post an infection, due to its key role in our immunity, and supplementation can be useful for hair fall caused by infections.

- In healthy individuals, selenium is believed to be sufficient as it is found in many foods via the soil. It's level in plants and in the livestock that consume those plants vary considerably throughout the country.[3] That may account for the variability of reported levels in Indian populations, with some studies suggesting suboptimal selenium status, while others suggest the intake is sufficient.[4,5]

- The limit between safe and toxic amounts of selenium is small and has yet to be standardized. The recommendation for selenium intake has been set at the amount needed to achieve a plateau of plasma glutathione peroxidase.[6] As a rule of thumb, taking selenium in supplements higher than recommended daily intake should be done with caution.[7]

▶ ACTIVE FORMS

ACTIVE FORMS	SUPPLEMENT SOURCES	SALIENT FEATURES
Selenium	Organic and inorganic salts	Organic forms of selenium are more potent than inorganic forms.
	Selenium-enriched yeast	It is capable of increasing the activity of the selenoenzymes and its bioavailability has been found to be higher than that of inorganic selenium sources.[8] However, these are often not found in supplements.

▶ SAFETY AND DOSAGE

GENERAL REQUIREMENTS	
Indian recommendations	AI 2020: 40 µg/day[3]
	TUL: N/A
Global recommendations and limits	NIH RDA: 55 µg/day
	TUL: 400 µg/day[9]
	EFSA 2014: AI—70 µg/day[10]
	TUL: 255 µg/day
	LOAEL: 330 µg/day[11]
	Dose descriptors describing selenium toxicity were as low as 2–3 µg/kg body weight/day[12]
Notes:	Selenium is a "dual-surface" element, maintaining a very thin line between a level of necessity and harmfulness. A deficiency or excess of this element is dangerous and causes health-related problems, both physically and mentally.[13]
	Selenosis may occur when selenium's daily intake is higher than 400 µg. In this case, arthralgia, fatigue, headache, nausea, vomiting, diarrhea and telogen effluvium have been reported.[14]

▶ **CLINICAL CONDITIONS**

EVIDENCE LEVEL	CONDITION OR USE CASE	DOSAGE	BENEFIT OR MECHANISM OF ACTION
+++++	Alopecia areata (AA)	N/A (meta-analysis)	The results of this meta-analysis found that patients with AA had a lower serum level of zinc and selenium than the healthy controls thus, suggesting that low serum levels of zinc and selenium may be important risk factors for AA.[15]
+++	Alopecia with poliosis	Mice received diets providing excessive (2.0 µg/g), adequate (0.2 µg/g, or deficient <0.03 µg/g) amounts of selenium for 24 weeks	Alopecia with poliosis was observed in the groups receiving either excessive or deficient selenium. Skin biopsy from alopecia patches showed increased telogen hair follicles with epidermal atrophy. There was a decrease in antiapoptotic Bcl-2 and an increase in proapoptotic Bax in the excessive-selenium diet group compared with the adequate group. The study results suggest that alopecia with poliosis is caused due to the selenium imbalance and partially influenced by the decrease of the ratio of Bcl-2/Bax, which is associated with the induction of apoptosis of keratinocytes.[16]

▶ CLINICAL CONDITIONS (Continued)

EVIDENCE LEVEL	CONDITION OR USE CASE	DOSAGE	BENEFIT OR MECHANISM OF ACTION
+++++	Skin diseases (psoriasis, acne vulgaris, chloric acne, and atopic dermatitis)	N/A (meta-analysis)	A lower selenium level was found in patients with psoriasis, acne vulgaris, chloric acne, and atopic dermatitis. For disease severity, severe patients had a higher selenium level than in patients with mild psoriasis, but no difference was found in vitiligo and alopecia areata.[17]
+++	Skin damage related to diabetes	Rats were divided into 4 groups: 2 groups of healthy controls with/ without antioxidants the other 2 groups with induced diabetes with or without antioxidants (composed of vitamin C (250 mg/kg), vitamin E (250 mg/kg) and selenium (0.2 mg/kg)) for 30 days	In the diabetic group with and without antioxidants, the levels of serum urea and creatinine, skin lipid peroxidation and nonenzymatic glycosylation levels increased, but skin glutathione levels decreased. The diabetic group receiving treatment with antioxidants reversed these effects.[18]
+++	Psoriasis	Severe erythrodermic (EP) and arthropathic (PsA) forms of psoriasis patients received either coenzyme Q10 50 mg, vitamin E 50 mg, and selenium 48 μg or placebo for 30–35 day.	Plasma levels of oxidative stress markers were greater than normal in psoriatic patients. Supplementation resulted in an improvement of clinical conditions, which corresponded to the faster normalization of the oxidative stress markers compared to placebo.[19]

▶ **CLINICAL CONDITIONS** (*Continued*)

EVIDENCE LEVEL	CONDITION OR USE CASE	DOSAGE	BENEFIT OR MECHANISM OF ACTION
+++	Atopic dermatitis (AD)	Selenomethionine (SeMet) was orally administered daily for 23 days in the AD induced mice daily (dose not available).	Ear thickness was remarkably increased by repeated induction of dermatitis, and SeMet suppressed ear thickness. SeMet inhibited epidermal hyperplasia and dense infiltration of inflammatory cells. The number of induced mast cells was decreased by SeMet. The results demonstrated that SeMet supplementation suppressed AD-like skin lesions in mice and inhibited the expression of IgE and IL-4 in the ear with dermatitis.[20]
+++++	Glutathione peroxidase in platelets of atopic dermatitis patients.	Group 1 took 600 μg of selenium alone, group 2 600 μg of selenium plus 600 IU of vitamin E and group 3 was given a placebo for 12 weeks.	After 12 weeks, there was an increase in the concentration of selenium in whole blood and the activity of selenium-dependent glutathione peroxidase in platelets in groups 1 and 2 and the concentration of vitamin E in plasma in group 2. There was no significant difference between the three groups in the severity of eczema.[21]
+++++	Vitiligo	N/A (meta-analysis)	The overall selenium levels were similar between vitiligo patients and healthy controls, but the subgroup analysis showed decreased levels of selenium in Asian vitiligo patients.[22]

▶ CLINICAL CONDITIONS (*Continued*)

EVIDENCE LEVEL	CONDITION OR USE CASE	DOSAGE	BENEFIT OR MECHANISM OF ACTION
+++	Skin allergy	Mice were randomly assigned to one of four treatment groups and given a diet containing 0, 1, 2 or 3 µg/g selenomethionine.	Spontaneous dermatitis and the active cutaneous anaphylaxis, a Type-I allergic response of mice, was enhanced in mice given a diet containing 1 µg/g selenomethionine and suppressed in mice given a diet containing 3 µg/g selenomethionine. Thus suggesting that allergies seem to be aggravated in the presence of light selenium deficiency but inhibited when the diet is sufficient in or supplemented with selenomethionine.[23]
+++	Skin development	A mouse was generated with targeted removal of selenoproteins in keratin 14 (K14) expressing cells and their differentiated descendents.	The knockout progeny from this had a runt (unusually small) phenotype, it developed skin abnormalities and experienced premature death. Lack of selenoproteins in epidermal cells led to the development of hyperplastic epidermis and aberrant hair follicle morphogenesis, accompanied by progressive alopecia after birth. The analyses revealed that selenoproteins are essential antioxidants in the skin and have a role in keratinocyte growth and viability.[24]

▶ **CLINICAL CONDITIONS** *(Continued)*

EVIDENCE LEVEL	CONDITION OR USE CASE	DOSAGE	BENEFIT OR MECHANISM OF ACTION
+	Alopecia and pseudoalbinism	Infants received an elemental diet for 2–5 months or parenteral nutrition containing selenite for 15 months.	The resolution of hair symptoms corresponded to serum selenium levels after 1–2 months and there was rapid improvement in growth in all patients after the administration of selenite. The study concludes that early clinical symptoms of selenium deficiency in infants include growth retardation and alopecia with pseudoalbinism, and are reversible with selenite.[25]
+++	Skin cancer and pigmentation induced by UV irradiation	Mice were treated with either (1) lotion vehicle, (2) 0.02% L-selenomethionine (SeMet) lotion, or (3) vehicle and 1.5 ppm SeMet in the drinking water for 15 weeks.	Results showed that the skin selenium concentrations in areas of application of the lotion containing SeMet were greater than those of animals given comparable oral doses, while the selenium concentrations of untreated skin and liver were similar to those of animals receiving oral selenium. Mice treated with both selenium showed no signs of toxicity and had less skin damage by UV irradiation.[26]

► CLINICAL CONDITIONS (Continued)

EVIDENCE LEVEL	CONDITION OR USE CASE	DOSAGE	BENEFIT OR MECHANISM OF ACTION
++	Protection of skin cell apoptosis from UV-induced damage	Human keratinocytes and melanocytes were treated with sodium selenite or selenomethionine in vitro	Selenoprotein expression by human fibroblasts, keratinocytes and melanocytes increased. Proteins such as thioredoxin reductase and phospholipid glutathione peroxidase were identified. Sodium selenite or selenomethionine protected both cultured human keratinocytes and melanocytes from UVB-induced cell death.[27]
+++	Skin hypersensitivity	300 μg of selenium (Se) a day was given as high-Se Baker's yeast, or low-Se yeast for 48 weeks.	Tests of delayed-type hypersensitivity (DTH) skin responses to mumps, candida, trichophyton, tuberculin-purified protein, and tetanus were performed. Supplementation of the low-Se yeast induced anergy in DTH skin responses and increased counts of natural killer (NK) cells and T lymphocytes expressing both subunits of the high affinity interleukin-2 receptor (IL2R). DTH skin responses and IL2R+ cells did not change in the high-Se group, suggesting Se supplementation blocked induction of DTH anergy.[28]

▶ **SUPPLEMENTATION**

	BASIS	**WHAT TO LOOK OUT FOR**
Supplementation form	Inorganic form: Sodium selenate, sodium selenite, sodium hydrogen selenite, selenious acid Organic form: Selenomethionine, selenocysteine, selenium enrich yeast, selenium nanoparticles Selenium in the form of selenomethionine is better absorbed than selenite[9,13,29]	The form of selenium is stated in the ingredients list of the product packaging.
Administration form	Capsules, tablets, strips, syrups, powders, gummies, effervescent tablets	N/A
Purity considerations	No known purity-related concerns.	The elemental selenium is often mentioned on the packaging and if not, it can be provided by the product company.
Patient considerations	Selenium supplements are to be taken with or after meals.	
Safety considerations	Selenium in excess intake can show many symptoms. Early signs of excess intake are a garlic odor in the breath and a metallic taste in the mouth. The most common clinical signs of chronically high selenium intakes, or selenosis, are hair and nail loss or brittleness. Other signs and symptoms include nausea, diarrhea, skin rashes, mottled teeth, fatigue, irritability, and nervous system abnormalities.[9]	It is recommended to not exceed the dose of recommended dietary allowance as excess may be harmful and enough of it is available in our diet.
Other considerations	N/A	Individuals with medical conditions should seek doctor's advice before starting nutritional supplementation.

INTRODUCTION

Selenium is functionally important for several aspects of human health including the central nervous, reproductive, cardiovascular, muscular and endocrine systems, and for immunity.[1]

Selenium exerts its biological activity by selenol-amino acids, either as selenocysteine or selenomethionine.[30] During protein synthesis (translation), selenocysteine is incorporated into elongating proteins at specific locations in the amino acid sequence to form functional selenoproteins. Selenomethionine cannot be synthesized by humans; only by plants. It can be nonspecifically incorporated into proteins in place of methionine. Only selenocysteine-containing proteins are regarded as selenoproteins.[31]

At least 25 selenoproteins have been identified and their metabolic functions are being investigated. Among these, the most well characterized ones are glutathione peroxidases (GPx), iodothyronine deiodinases, selenoprotein W, and methionine-R-sulfoxide reductase B1.[32]

DIGESTION, ABSORPTION AND STORAGE

Digestion and Absorption

- Selenium absorption is very efficient (70–90%), especially for its major dietary form, selemethionine, which is absorbed by the same mechanism as methionine. Selenocysteine is acquired from animal sources.[3]

- Selenium absorption is not regulated.[6]

- Both, inorganic and organic forms of selenium can be metabolized to selenocysteine by the body and incorporated into selenoenzymes. However, they do not equally contribute to selenium status.[6]

- Selenate and selenite are not major dietary constituents, but are commonly used in selenium supplements (about 50% absorption).[6]

Storage

Two pools of reserve selenium are present in humans and animals. One of them, the selenium present as selenomethionine, which may not be made available to the body for selenoprotein synthesis. The second reserve pool is the selenium present in liver glutathione peroxidase, which is downregulated during an insufficiency.[6]

MECHANISM OF ACTION

01 | Antioxidant Activity

Along with copper, zinc and iron, selenium is a critical component of antioxidant enzymes. In this context, selenoproteins are required for three types of antioxidant enzymes: the glutathione (GSH) system, the thioredoxin system and the methionine sulfoxide reduction system.[31]

In mammals, five selenocysteine-containing GPx and three selenocysteine-containing thioredoxin reductase (TrxR) enzymes have been identified.

GSH is involved in the direct interception of pro-oxidants. GPx and TrxRs also serve as electron donors for the regeneration of other antioxidants, like vitamin C, vitamin E and coenzyme Q10 from their oxidized forms.[30]

Further to this, methionine sulfoxide reductase B1 is a selenoprotein critical for the regeneration of proteins damaged by oxidative stress.[31]

02 | Cell Growth and Signaling

Selenium is required for the metabolism of thyroid hormones. The reaction where one iodine atom from thyroxine (T4) is removed to make the biologically active triiodothyronine (T3) is catalyzed by selenium-dependent iodothyronine deiodinase enzymes. Thyroid activity is very important in skin homeostasis and the regulation of hair growth:

- It stimulates keratinocyte proliferation. Hypothyroid patients have a thin epidermis and they frequently develop alopecia. Most actions of the thyroid hormones are mediated by binding to nuclear thyroid hormone receptors (TRs).[33]

- Thyroid hormones also affect the mobilization of hair bulge stems cells, which divide several times during anagen, thereby maintaining hair cycling.[33]

- Thyroid hormones also influence hair pigmentation.[34]

Further to this, selenoproteins have numerous functions in metabolism, cell signaling, and protein interactions, making it essential for renewal of tissue.

03 | Regulating Immune Function

Selenium plays essential roles in regulating the migration, proliferation, differentiation, and activation of immune cells, thus influencing innate immunity, T-cell immunity and B-cell dependent antibody production. Research also suggests selenoproteins may be involved in the production of eicosanoids involved in inflammatory responses. Dysregulation of these processes may lead to inflammation or immune-related diseases. Topical selenium has shown benefits in psoriasis patients by reducing inflammation.

▶ REFERENCES

1. Avery JC, Hoffmann PR. Selenium, Selenoproteins, and Immunity. Nutrients. 2018;10(9):1203.
2. Majeed M, Nagabhushanam K, Gowda S, Mundkur L. An exploratory study of selenium status in healthy individuals and in patients with COVID-19 in a south Indian population: The case for adequate selenium status. Nutrition. 2021;82:111053.
3. National Institute of Nutrition Indian Council of Medical Research. Recommended Dietary Allowances and Estimated Average Requirements for Indians – 2020. RDA Full Report 2020.
4. Yadav S, Singh I, Singh D, Han SD. Selenium status in soils of northern districts of India. J Environ Manage. 2005;75(2):129-32.
5. Mehmood S, Velumani A, Iyer S, Sinkar P. Micronutrient Selenium: A Pan-India Report on Borderline High. Asian Journal of Biological and Life Sciences. 2019;8(1):41-3.
6. Institute of Medicine (US) Panel on Dietary Antioxidants and Related Compounds. Dietary Reference Intakes for Vitamin C, Vitamin E, Selenium, and Carotenoids. Chapter 7: Selenium. National Academies Press (US); 2000.
7. Hossain A, Skalicky M, Brestic M, Maitra S, Sarkar S, Ahmad Z, et al. Selenium Biofortification: Roles, Mechanisms, Responses and Prospects. Molecules. 2021;26(4):881.
8. Rayman MP. The use of high-selenium yeast to raise selenium status: how does it measure up? Br J Nutr. 2004;92(4):557-73.
9. Fact Sheet for Health Professionals. Selenium [Online]. Available from: https://ods.od.nih.gov/factsheets/Selenium-HealthProfessional/
10. EFSA Panel on Dietetic Products, Nutrition and Allergies (NDA). Scientific Opinion on Dietary Reference Values for selenium. EFSA Journal. 2014;12(10):3846.
11. EFSA Panel on Nutrition, Novel Foods and Food Allergens (NDA); Turck D, Bohn T, Castenmiller J, de Henauw S, Hirsch-Ernst KI, et al. Scientific opinion on the tolerable upper intake level for selenium. EFSA Journal. 2023;21(1):e07704.
12. Hadrup N, Ravn-Haren G. Toxicity of repeated oral intake of organic selenium, inorganic selenium, and selenium nanoparticles: A review. Journal of Trace Elements in Medicine and Biology. 2023;79:127235.
13. Bodnar M, Szczyglowska M, Konieczka P, Namiesnik J. Methods of Selenium Supplementation: Bioavailability and Determination of Selenium Compounds. Crit Rev Food Sci Nutr. 2016;56(1):36-55.
14. Tortelly Costa VD, Melo DF, Matsunaga AM. The Relevance of Selenium to Alopecias. Int J Trichology. 2018;10(2):92-3.
15. Jin W, Zheng H, Shan B, Wu Y. Changes of serum trace elements level in patients with alopecia areata: A meta-analysis. J Dermatol. 2017;44(5):588-91.
16. Hwang SW, Lee HJ, Suh KS, Kim ST, Park SW, Hur DY, et al. Changes in murine hair with dietary selenium excess or deficiency. Experimental Dermatology. 2011;20(4):367-9.
17. Lv J, Ai P, Lei S, Zhou F, Chen S, Zhang Y. Selenium levels and skin diseases: systematic review and meta-analysis. J Trace Elem Med Biol. 2020;62:126548.
18. Sokmen BB, Basaraner H, Yanardag R. Combined effects of treatment with vitamin C, vitamin E and selenium on the skin of diabetic rats. Hum Exp Toxicol. 2013;32(4):379-84.
19. Kharaeva Z, Gostova E, Luca CD, Raskovic D, Korkina L. Clinical and biochemical effects of coenzyme Q10, vitamin E, and selenium supplementation to psoriasis patients. Nutrition. 2009;25(3):295-302.
20. Arakawa T, Sugiyama T, Matsuura H, Okuno T, Ogino H, Sakazaki F, et al. Effects of Supplementary Seleno-L-methionine on Atopic Dermatitis-Like Skin Lesions in Mice. Biol Pharm Bull. 2018;41(9):1456-62.
21. Fairris GM, Perkins PJ, Lloyd B, Hinks L, Clayton BE. The effect on atopic dermatitis of supplementation with selenium and vitamin E. Acta Dermato-Venereologica. 1989;69(4):359-62.
22. Dai T, Xiaoying S, Li X, Hongjin L, Yaqiong Z, Bo L. Selenium Level in Patients with Vitiligo: A Meta-Analysis. Biomed Res Int. 2020 Jun 11;2020:7580939.

23. Sakazaki F, Arakawa T, Shimizu R, Ogino H, Okuno T, Ueno H. Allergies are aggravated by mild selenium deficiency and abrogated by supplementation with selenomethionine. Food and Agricultural Immunology. 2014;25(4):477-85.
24. Sengupta A, Lichti UF, Carlson BA, Ryscavage AO, Gladyshev VN, Yuspa SH, et al. Selenoproteins Are Essential for Proper Keratinocyte Function and Skin Development. PLoS One. 2010;5(8):e12249.
25. Masumoto K, Nagata K, Higashi M, Nakatsuji T, Uesugi T, Takahashi Y, et al. Clinical features of selenium deficiency in infants receiving long-term nutritional support. Nutrition. 2007;23(11–12):782-7.
26. Burke KE, Combs GF, Gross EG, Bhuyan KC, Abu-Libdeh H. The effects of topical and oral L-selenomethionine on pigmentation and skin cancer induced by ultraviolet irradiation. Nutr Cancer. 1992;17(2):123-37.
27. Rafferty TS, McKenzie RC, Hunter JA, Howie AF, Arthur JR, Nicol F, et al. Differential expression of selenoproteins by human skin cells and protection by selenium from UVB-radiation-induced cell death. Biochem J. 1998;332(Pt 1):231-6.
28. Hawkes WC, Hwang A, Alkan Z. The effect of selenium supplementation on DTH skin responses in healthy North American men. J Trace Elem Med Biol. 2009;23(4):272-80.
29. Burk RF, Norsworthy BK, Hill KE, Motley AK, Byrne DW. Effects of chemical form of selenium on plasma biomarkers in a high-dose human supplementation trial. Cancer Epidemiol Biomarkers Prev. 2006;15(4):804-10.
30. Arteel GE, Sies H. The biochemistry of selenium and the glutathione system. Environ Toxicol Pharmacol. 2001;10(4):153-8.
31. Kim HY. The Methionine Sulfoxide Reduction System: Selenium Utilization and Methionine Sulfoxide Reductase Enzymes and Their Functions. Antioxid Redox Signal. 2013;19(9):958-69.
32. Mariotti M, Ridge PG, Zhang Y, Lobanov AV, Pringle TH, Guigo R, et al. Composition and evolution of the vertebrate and mammalian selenoproteomes. PLoS One. 2012;7(3):e33066.
33. Contreras-Jurado C, Lorz C, García-Serrano L, Paramio JM, Aranda A. Thyroid hormone signaling controls hair follicle stem cell function. Mol Biol Cell. 2015;26(7):1263-72.
34. van Beek N, Bodó E, Kromminga A, Gáspár E, Meyer K, Zmijewski MA, et al. Thyroid Hormones Directly Alter Human Hair Follicle Functions: Anagen Prolongation and Stimulation of Both Hair Matrix Keratinocyte Proliferation and Hair Pigmentation. J Clin Endocrinol Metab. 2008;93(11):4381-8.

15

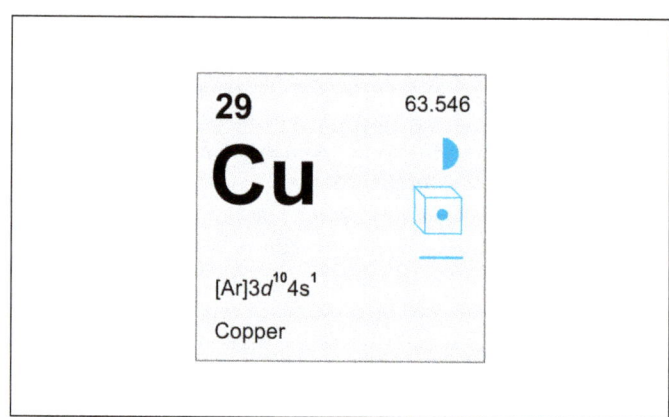

Copper

Copper

✍ Rasya Dixit

CONTENTS

COPPER: NUTRIENT SNAPSHOT

- ▸ REQUIREMENT IN THE INDIAN CONTEXT | 149
- ▸ ACTIVE FORMS | 150
- ▸ SAFETY AND DOSAGE | 150
- ▸ CLINICAL CONDITIONS | 150
- ▸ SUPPLEMENTATION | 151

INTRODUCTION | 152

DIGESTION, ABSORPTION AND STORAGE | 152

MECHANISM OF ACTION | 152

KEY TOPICS

- ACQUIRED PERFORATING DERMATOSIS
- ALOPECIA UNIVERSALIS
- ANTI-AGING

Nutrient Snapshot

▶ **REQUIREMENT IN THE INDIAN CONTEXT**

- Copper is an essential trace element for humans and animals. The biochemical role for copper is primarily catalytic; cuproenzymes, or those that require copper as a cofactor, play a role in energy production, iron metabolism, connective tissue maturation, and neurotransmission.

- In dermatology, copper is known for its importance in collagen, elastin and melanin synthesis and in reduction-oxidation (redox) reactions.

- Copper is found in a variety of foods, and is normally sufficient in the Indian diet. There are very few studies in India looking at copper status in healthy individuals. Copper deficiency has been reported in one study on a low-income group in India.[1,2]

- While it is difficult to get an excess of copper through food, toxicity can occur through excess supplementation. However, it is added to zinc-containing supplements to offset high supplemental zinc intake, which can lead to a decreased ability to absorb and use copper from the diet.[3-6]

- For every 8–15 mg zinc, 1 mg of copper can help prevent zinc-induced copper deficiency.[7] It is important to maintain the ratio of zinc and copper supplementation when picking any zinc-containing supplement like a multivitamin and mineral supplement or a multinutrient hair supplement, where this can be often overlooked.

▶ ACTIVE FORMS

ACTIVE FORMS	SUPPLEMENT SOURCES	SALIENT FEATURES
Copper	Inorganic copper salts, chelated lysine complex.	Chelated copper has higher bioavailability as compared to inorganic copper salts.

▶ SAFETY AND DOSAGE

GENERAL REQUIREMENTS	
Indian recommendations	NIN-ICMR RDA 2020: 1.7 mg[18]
	TUL: Not available
Global recommendations and limits	IOM, Food and Nutrition Board–RDA: 900 μg.[8]
	Upper limit: 10 mg/day
	NOAEL: 10 mg/day
Side effects	No known side effects for RDA doses
Notes:	For every 8–15 mg of supplemental zinc, 1 mg of copper can help prevent zinc-induced copper deficiency.[7]
	Studies show that individuals with celiac disease may have a copper deficiency due to malabsorption of copper due to the disease.[8]

▶ CLINICAL CONDITIONS

EVIDENCE LEVEL	CONDITION OR USE CASE	DOSAGE	BENEFIT OR MECHANISM OF ACTION
++	Anti-aging	Skin graft exposed to saline containing 0.02 or 1 μmol/L of copper ions for 6 days	There was an increase in elastin and pro-collagen 1 concentrations as compared to the control explants.[9]
+	Acquired perforating dermatosis (APD)	4 mg of copper supplementation for approximately 3 months	Patients having low serum copper concentration were supplemented with oral copper and their APD resolved completely.[10]
++	Alopecia universalis	N/A	Patients with alopecia universalis had low levels of serum copper.[11]

▶ SUPPLEMENTATION

	BASIS	WHAT TO LOOK OUT FOR
Supplementation form—inorganic salts	Cupric carbonate Cupric citrate Cupric gluconate Cupric sulphate Copper oxide As per animal studies copper carbonate, sulphate, and gluconate have a better bioavailability as compared to copper oxide.[12] Copper sulfate and gluconate are preferred for food fortification over any other form, but gluconate is more stable than copper sulfate.[13]	The form of copper is mentioned in the ingredients section of the product packaging.
Amino acid chelated form	Copper lysine complex Animal studies show that copper lysine complex has the highest bioavailability as compared to salts.[14]	
Administration form	Multivitamin-mineral supplements in capsule, tablet, and gummies forms	For every 8–15 mg zinc, 1 mg of copper can help prevent zinc-induced copper deficiency.[7]
Purity considerations	N/A	The elemental copper is often mentioned on the packaging and if not, can be provided by the product company.
Patient considerations	Copper is a fat soluble mineral so should be taken after meals.	N/A
Safety considerations	Chronic supplementation of copper above upper limits (10 mg/d) can cause liver damage, abdominal pain, cramps, nausea, diarrhea, and vomiting.[8] Individuals with a known case of Wilson's disease should stay away from copper supplements as they are at the risk of toxicity.[15,16]	The dose is mentioned on the nutritional table of the label (back).
Other considerations	N/A	

▶ INTRODUCTION

Copper is an essential trace element critical for normal human metabolism. In dermatology, copper has found recent fame in topical applications in the form of copper peptides. Nutritionally, copper plays important roles in skin health and hair growth.

Copper is a cofactor in several important enzymes like cytochrome oxidase (mitochondrial electron transport chain), superoxide dismutase [(SOD); protective against reactive oxygen species] and lysyl oxidase (cross-linking of collagen and elastin).[17]

Indian diets show a wide variation in copper intake (1.6–5.2 mg/day), but surveys suggest most people are at the higher end of the spectrum. In addition, copper homeostasis is very efficient as more copper is absorbed, turnover is faster, and biliary copper excretion is adjusted to maintain balance.[18] Yet, caution must be exercised with supplementation.[19]

▶ DIGESTION, ABSORPTION AND STORAGE

Digestion and Absorption

- The human gastrointestinal system can absorb 30–40% of ingested copper from typical diets.[20] The rate of copper absorption varies inversely with copper intake and can be as low as 12%. Absorption of copper salts has been found to vary between 25–60%.[21]

- Copper absorption occurs primarily in the small intestine by copper transport protein 1 (CTR1) in enterocytes and a small fraction from the stomach.[1,22]

- Following absorption, copper is secreted into the bloodstream and bound to soluble chaperones, such as albumin, transcuprein, histidines, and macroglobulins.[23]

- Upon reaching the liver, the hepatocytes mediate the uptake of copper via CTR1. Inside the cytoplasm, copper is then either delivered by copper chaperones to specific proteins or chelated by metallothionein (MT) for storage.[19]

- Copper-ATPases (Cu-ATPases) pump copper ions from the liver back into the blood, where soluble chaperones transport it to target tissue.[19]

- Zinc supplementation interferes with absorption of copper.

Storage

- Only small amounts of copper are typically stored in the body, most of it being in the liver, muscle and the skeleton, and the excess is eliminated in feces.[23]

- Intracellular copper concentration is kept at a relatively low range, and moderate increases can cause cytotoxicity and even lead to cell death.[23]

▶ MECHANISM OF ACTION

01 | Collagen and Elastin Formation

The importance of copper in extracellular matrix (ECM) structure is defined by its role as a cofactor to lysyl oxidase, which oxidizes lysine and hydroxylysine residues in collagen and elastin for the formation of crosslinks.[24]

Copper stimulates dermal fibroblast proliferation and upregulates collagen (types I, II, and V) and elastin fiber components production. This occurs through the induction of transforming growth factor-beta (TGF-β), the primary stimulator of these extracellular structures. TGF-β also plays a significant role in scar formation.[25]

Copper also stimulates heat shock protein-47 (HSP-47), a stress protein that acts as a collagen-specific chaperone needed for the formation of the collagen triple helical structure.[24]

With skin aging, there is loss/atrophy of structural ECM and reduced expression of TGF-β, which is why copper is used as an anti-aging ingredient.

02 | Melanin Synthesis

Copper serves as a cofactor of tyrosinase, an essential enzyme required for biosynthesis of melanin by melanocytes.[26]

03 | Protection from Reactive Oxygen Species

Copper participates in redox reactions as a cofactor to the antioxidant enzyme, SOD. Human skin contains copper/zinc, Cu/Zn superoxide dismutase, known as SOD1, resides in the cytoplasm of keratinocytes, where up to 90% of cellular reactive oxygen species (ROS) are produced. It catalyzes the conversion of the superoxide anion, O_2^-, to hydrogen peroxide, H_2O_2.[27]

Furthermore, in response to oxidative stress, high levels of H_2O_2 promote Cu/Zn SOD nuclear translocation, and as a transcription factor, the enzyme regulates the expression of oxidative resistance and repair genes.[27,28]

▶ REFERENCES

1. Radhika P, Bhushanam K, Anbarasu K, Rangaraju A, Reddy Putta S, Daga S, et al. Low copper containing diet for Wilson disease patients. Journal of Medical and Scientific Research. 2016;4:147-9.
2. Ma J, Betts NM. Zinc and copper intakes and their major food sources for older adults in the 1994-96 Continuing Survey of Food Intakes by Individuals (CSFII). J Nutr. 2000;130(11): 2838-43.
3. Duncan A, Yacoubian C, Watson N, Morrison I. The risk of copper deficiency in patients prescribed zinc supplements. J Clin Pathol. 2015;68(9):723-5.
4. Hoffman HN, Phyliky RL, Fleming CR. Zinc-induced copper deficiency. Gastroenterology. 1988;94:508-12.
5. Wahab A, Mushtaq K, Borak SG, Bellam N. Zinc-induced copper deficiency, sideroblastic anemia, and neutropenia: A perplexing facet of zinc excess. Clin Case Rep. 2020;8(9):1666-71.
6. Fischer PWF, Giroux A, L'Abbe MR. Effects of zinc on mucosal copper binding and on the kinetics of copper absorption. J Nutr. 1983;113(2):462-9.
7. Zhang W, Fan M, Wang C, Mahawar K, Parmar C, Chen W, et al. Importance of Maintaining Zinc and Copper Supplement Dosage Ratio After Metabolic and Bariatric Surgery. Obes Surg. 2021;31(7):3339-40.
8. Copper - Health Professional Fact Sheet. [Online] Available from https://ods.od.nih.gov/factsheets/ Copper-HealthProfessional/#en3.
9. gen-Shtern N, Chumin K, Cohen G, Borkow G. Increased pro-collagen 1, elastin, and TGF-β1 expression by copper ions in an ex-vivo human skin model. J Cosmet Dermatol. 2020;19(6):1522-27.
10. Varghese JA, Quan VL, Colavincenzo ML, Zheng L. Acquired perforating dermatosis in patients with copper deficiency. JAAD Case Rep. 2021;15:110.
11. Mussalo-Rauhamaa H, Lakomaa EL, Kianto U, Lehto J. Element concentrations in serum, erythrocytes, hair and urine of alopecia patients. Acta Derm Venereol. 1986;66(2):103-9.
12. Wapnir RA. Copper absorption and bioavailability. Am J Clin Nutr. 1998;67(5 Suppl):1054S-60S.
13. Rosado JL. Zinc and copper: Proposed fortification levels and recommended zinc compounds. J Nutr. 2003;133(9):2985S-9S.
14. Apgar GA, Kornegay ET, Lindemann MD, Notter DR. Evaluation of copper sulfate and a copper lysine complex as growth promoters for weanling swine. J Anim Sci. 1995;73(9):2640-6.
15. Bhattacharya K, Thankappan B. Wilson's Disease Update: An Indian Perspective. Ann Indian Acad Neurol. 2022;25(1):43-53.
16. Burkhead JL, Collins JF. Nutrition Information Brief—Copper. Adv Nutr. 2022;13(2):681-3.
17. Borkow G. Using Copper to Improve the Well-Being of the Skin. Curr Chem Biol. 2014;8(2):89-102.
18. National Institute of Nutrition Indian Council of Medical Research. Recommended Dietary Allowances and Estimated Average Requirements for Indians - 2020. RDA Full Report 2020.
19. Institute of Medicine (US) Panel on Micronutrients. Dietary Reference Intakes for Vitamin A, Vitamin K, Arsenic, Boron, Chromium, Copper, Iodine, Iron, Manganese, Molybdenum, Nickel, Silicon, Vanadium, and Zinc. National Academies Press (US), 2001.
20. Wapnir RA. Copper absorption and bioavailability. Am J Clin Nutr. 1998;67 (5 Suppl):1054S-60S.
21. Joint FAO/WHO Expert Committee of Food Additives (JECFA). "Copper." Evaluation of Certain Food Additives and Contaminants, World Health Organisation, 1982. WHO Food Additives Series No. 17.
22. Linder MC, Hazegh-Azam M. Copper biochemistry and molecular biology. Am J Clin Nutr. 1996;63(5):797S-811S.
23. Chen L, Min J, Wang F. Copper homeostasis and cuproptosis in health and disease. Signal Transduct Target Ther. 2022;7(1):378.
24. Philips N, Philips S, Parakandi H, Gopal S, Siomyk H, Ministro A, et al. Beneficial regulation of fibrillar collagens, heat shock protein-47, elastin fiber components, transforming growth factor-β1, vascular endothelial growth factor and oxidative stress effects by copper in dermal fibroblasts. Connect Tissue Res. 2012;53(5):373-8.
25. Kiani AK, Dhuli K, Donato K, Aquilanti B, Velluti V, Matera G, et al. Main nutritional deficiencies. J Prev Med Hyg. 2022;63(2 Suppl 3):E93-101.
26. Solano F. On the Metal Cofactor in the Tyrosinase Family. Int J Mol Sci. 2018;19(2):633.
27. Altobelli GG, Van Noorden S, Balato A, Cimini V. Copper/Zinc Superoxide Dismutase in Human Skin: Current Knowledge. Front Med (Lausanne). 2020;7:183.
28. Tsang CK wan, Liu Y, Thomas J, Zhang Y, Zheng XFS. Superoxide dismutase 1 acts as a nuclear transcription factor to regulate oxidative stress resistance. Nat Commun. 2014;5:3446.

16

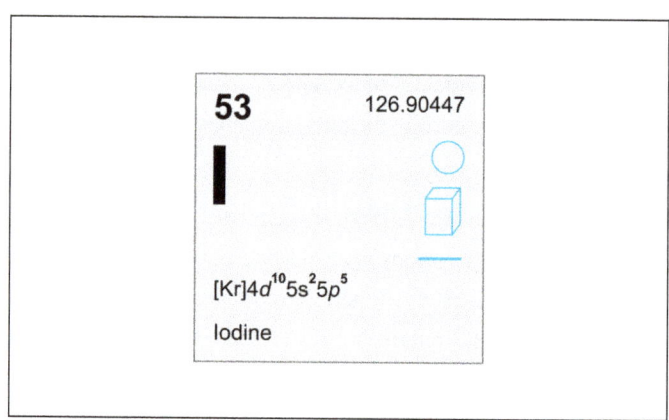

Iodine

Iodine

✍ Abhishek De

CONTENTS

IODINE: NUTRIENT SNAPSHOT

- ▶ REQUIREMENT IN THE INDIAN CONTEXT | 155
- ▶ ACTIVE FORMS | 156
- ▶ SAFETY AND DOSAGE | 156
- ▶ CLINICAL CONDITIONS | 157
- ▶ SUPPLEMENTATION | 159

INTRODUCTION | 160

DIGESTION, ABSORPTION AND STORAGE | 160

MECHANISM OF ACTION | 160

KEY TOPICS

- CUTANEOUS INFLAMMATORY DISORDERS
- CUTANEOUS SPOROTRICHOSIS
- PHOTOPROTECTION
- SKIN APPEARANCE
- SPOROTRICHOSIS

Nutrient Snapshot

▶ **REQUIREMENT IN THE INDIAN CONTEXT**

- Iodine is the limiting substrate for thyroid hormones, which are required throughout life for normal growth and development, and metabolism. About 120 countries worldwide have introduced programs of iodine-fortification in salt in order to correct iodine deficiency in populations and reduce the incidence of goiter and other iodine deficiency disorders.

- It has been known for decades that thyroid disorders lead to altered skin and hair features.[1] Thyroid hormone is an important regulator of skin homeostasis and its immunity.[2] Furthermore, thyroid hormones directly affect hair follicles, particularly anagen, and hypothyroidism and hyperthyroidism have been linked to different types of alopecia.[3,4]

- Today, a lack of iodine is one of the most common nutritional deficiencies in the world.[5] The population in India is particularly prone to a deficiency due to low levels of iodine in the soil. Of these, many are consuming salt with inadequate iodine,[6] or perceived "healthier" alternatives to iodized salt (like Himalayan pink salt or sea salt). Furthermore, iodine can be lost with storage and upon cooking.[7]

- The problem is further compounded with vegetarians and vegans, as its main sources, other than iodized salt, are dairy, seafood and seaweed.[8-11] Vegans may also consume high amounts of soy and cruciferous vegetables (cabbage, broccoli, and cauliflower). While these are largely health promoting, they have small amounts of compounds (goitrogens) that inhibit iodine uptake, making vegans and vegetarians more vulnerable to iodine deficiency.[11] Environmental contaminants like perchlorate and those found in cigarette smoke (thiocyanate) can also block iodine uptake.[11]

- Too much iodine can also be harmful. Several studies suggest that the benefits of iodine greatly outweigh any concerns iodine may cause.[12] Assuming that some iodine is coming from the diet, subrecommended doses can help achieve sufficiency, especially where dermatological symptoms like hair fall are experienced.

▶ ACTIVE FORMS

ACTIVE FORMS	SUPPLEMENT SOURCES	SALIENT FEATURES
Iodine	Inorganic and organic salts, natural-sea kelp	According to one study, the bioavailability of potassium iodide was found to be excellent (96.4%).[13] Potassium iodide is commonly used for nutraceuticals with a concentration of iodine of about 76%.[14]

▶ SAFETY AND DOSAGE

GENERAL REQUIREMENTS	
Indian recommendations	RDA 2020: 140 µg/day[28] TUL: 1,100 µg/day
Global recommendations and limits	NIH RDA: 150 µg/day TUL: 1100 µg/day[15]
	EFSA 2014: 150 µg/day
	LOAEL: 1,700 µg/day NOAEL by Council of Responsible Nutrition: 500 µg/day for supplements and 1,000 µg for total intake.
Notes:	Assuming some intake from the diet, iodine intake from supplements should be at sub-recommended levels to avoid an excess.

▶ CLINICAL CONDITIONS

EVIDENCE LEVEL	CONDITION OR USE CASE	DOSAGE	BENEFIT OR MECHANISM OF ACTION
+++	Skin appearance	Subjects were divided into groups: Active and placebo receiving 3 tablets in the morning and at night for 12 weeks. Morning tablet of the active group was composed of 225 µg of iodine along with many vitamins, minerals, omega-3 fats and plant extracts.	The subjects in the active group noted an improvement in skin firmness, healing rate, hydration, dullness, roughness, pigmentation, and overall appearance at week 8, and further at week 12, over placebo. The quality of life evaluation, showed an improvement from placebo in all attributes at week 12. There was also a reduction in wrinkle breadth in the active group versus placebo at week 12.[16]
++	UVB irradiated photoprotection	Strong iodine solution and potassium iodide solutions were topically applied on human keratinocytes from human skin ex vivo, either prior to irradiation or immediately after irradiation	The prior treatment with strong iodine solution resulted in a decrease in cell apoptosis and approximately 60% of epidermal cells survived compared to the control (irradiated untreated). The postirradiation treatment resulted in a decrease in cell apoptosis and there was epidermal cell survival compared to the control (irradiated untreated). These results also demonstrate a possible role of the Nrf2 (regulator of antioxidant response) pathway by activation in UVB-induced cytotoxicity in the skin.[17] A prior in vitro study suggested that iodine solution treatment of keratinocytes prior to UVB exposure resulted in enhanced cell survival and ~90% of the cells were viable.

▶ **CLINICAL CONDITIONS** (*Continued*)

EVIDENCE LEVEL	CONDITION OR USE CASE	DOSAGE	BENEFIT OR MECHANISM OF ACTION
+	Sporotrichosis	Case study: Subject was treated with oral potassium iodide (600 mg/day) and/or itraconazole and topical heat therapy for 4 weeks. It was stopped due to discomfort but again started after the recurrence of lesions.	The subject had three recurrences after treatment and her facial plaque was eventually excised and then grafted. After the surgical procedure, oral medication was continued for two months. A few years later, new lesions appeared on her left hand and forearm, confirming reinfection with sporotrichosis. She was again treated with potassium iodide. The cutaneous lesions completely resolved after 26 weeks without surgical treatment.[18]
+	Sporotrichosis	Case study: After ineffective therapy of itraconazole for 12 weeks, the patient was started on the saturated solution of potassium iodide (in drops) for 5 weeks. The patient continued it for one more month after complete clearance of the lesion. Dose not available	The patient responded dramatically with over 90% regression of the lesions within a period of 5 weeks. The patient tolerated the drug well and had slight gastrointestinal discomfort and a headache. There was no relapse after a follow-up period of more than 5 months.[19]
++ (Retrospective study)	Cutaneous inflammatory disorders	Potassium iodide (KI) was ingested by patients for 5–7 weeks and the dose varied from 300–1800 mg/day (900 mg/day was commonly prescribed)	KI was prescribed for various skin conditions: Erythema nodosum, disseminated granuloma annulare, necrobiosis lipoidica, nodular vasculitis, cutaneous sarcoidosis, and granulomatous perioral dermatitis/rosacea. The global assessment of efficacy showed an improvement in disease in about a third of all patients.[20]

▶ SUPPLEMENTATION

	BASIS	WHAT TO LOOK OUT FOR
Supplementation form	Sodium iodide Sodium iodate Potassium iodide (concentration: 76%) Potassium iodate Iodine from sea kelp (seaweed)	The form of iodine added in the supplement is mentioned in the ingredients list on the product packaging.
Administration form	Multivitamin-mineral supplement in capsules, soft gels, tablets, gummies, syrups	N/A
Purity considerations	N/A	N/A
Patient considerations	Iodine can be added in multivitamin-mineral supplements, thus recommended to be taken with or after meals.	The main biochemical indicator that is widely used for the assessment of iodine deficiency disorders is urinary iodine concentration (mUIC). However, this is not routinely done. Thyroid function tests are used to identify hypo/hyperthyroidism. Biochemical tests are unnecessary for sub-RDA doses, which can be prescribed as part of a hair multivitamin-mineral supplement.
Safety considerations	Cases of acute iodine poisoning are rare and are usually caused by doses of many grams.[15]	The dose per serving is stated on the nutritional label. It is recommended to not exceed the RDA.
Other considerations	Individuals with thyroid disorders should first consult their endocrinologists before they start a supplement containing iodine in it. Iodine supplementation may not only interfere with thyroid medication but also with hypertension medication [diuretics and angiotensin-converting enzyme (ACE) inhibitors].[15]	Individuals with medical conditions and those on medications should consult their doctor before starting any nutritional supplement. Especially, those with thyroid disorders should be careful while taking multivitamins as it may contain iodine in it.

▶ **INTRODUCTION**

Iodine is a nonmetallic trace element, and is required by humans for the synthesis of thyroid hormones, triiodothyronine (T3) and thyroxine (T4). T3 is the physiologically active thyroid hormone that can bind to thyroid receptors in the nuclei of cells and regulate gene expression. T4 is the abundant circulating form, which can be converted to T3 by selenium-containing enzymes, iodothyronine deiodinases.

Thyroid hormones regulate a number of physiologic processes, including growth, development, metabolism, and reproductive function. The immunomodulatory activity of iodine has been utilized topically to treat inflammatory dermatoses and fungal infections.[14]

In our diet, iodine is present in several chemical forms including sodium and potassium salts, inorganic iodine (I2), iodate (normally an additive to salt), and iodide (the reduced form of iodine).[15]

▶ **DIGESTION, ABSORPTION AND STORAGE**

Digestion and Absorption

- Most ingested iodine is reduced in the gut and almost completely absorbed.[21]

- Once in circulation, iodide is removed principally by the thyroid gland and the kidney.[21,22]

Storage

- A healthy adult body contains 15–20 mg of iodine, 70–80% of which is stored in the thyroid gland.[22]

▶ **MECHANISM OF ACTION**

Thyroid activity is very important in skin homeostasis and the regulation of hair growth:

01 | Cell Growth and Signaling

Thyroid hormones exert their action through the thyroid hormone receptor (TR) found on many cell types in skin tissue. T3 regulates keratinocyte and fibroblast proliferation and differentiation, as well as promotes proteoglycan and hyaluronic acid production by dermal fibroblasts, therefore playing a key role in wound healing. T3 is also involved in the physiology of sebaceous, eccrine and apocrine glands.

The thyroid-skin neuroendocrine connection encompasses many layers of complexity, as it is controlled by the hypothalamic-pituitary-thyroid (HPT) axis, with various endocrine feedback loops that maintain homeostasis. A lot of this currently remains unclear, and its understanding will aid in the treatment of skin disorders, particularly in autoimmune conditions.[24,25]

02 | Promoting Barrier Function

T3 promotes barrier formation by increasing the activity of enzymes in the cholesterol sulfate cycle. T3 is also involved in the formation of the cornified envelope, the development of the lamellar granules, which are vital in the maintenance of the epidermal barrier and its antimicrobial properties. Thus, hypothyroidism hinders epidermal barrier function.[2]

03 | Regulating Hair Cycling and Pigmentation

Both hypo- and hyperthyroid states are associated with substantial hair loss. Research has demonstrated that thyroid hormones can prolong the duration of anagen. They affect the mobilization of hair bulge stems cells, helping maintain hair cycling.[24]

Further to this, thyroid hormones participate in hair growth by stimulating keratinocyte proliferation and hair pigmentation.[24,25] They even stimulate the expression of selected keratins, a process that slows down as we age.[24]

04 | Regulating Immune Function

The skin is an active immune organ, where the thyroid hormones play a key role in protecting skin from external and internal insults.

T3 can exert responses in various immune cells, like monocytes, macrophages, natural killer cells, and lymphocytes, affecting several inflammation-related processes (like chemotaxis, phagocytosis and cytokine production).[26]

The thyroid gland is a common target of autoimmune dysregulation, and is sensitive to nutritional variables, like iodine intake. This can be exploited for managing autoimmune conditions.[3,12] For example, alopecia areata is thought to result from a collapse of the relative immune privilege enjoyed by hair follicles.[27] Many other autoimmune skin disease are associated with thyroid dysfunction including dermatitis, vitiligo, pernicious anemia, bullous disorders, connective tissue diseases (lupus erythematosus, scleroderma), and many more.[4,27]

▶ REFERENCES

1. Creswell JE, Michael BZ. Feingold KR, Anawalt B, Blackman MR, Boyce A, et al. The Iodine Deficiency Disorders. Endotext. South Dartmouth (MA): MDText.com, Inc.; 2000.
2. Safer Joshua D. Thyroid hormone action on skin. Dermatoendocrinol. 2011;3(3):211-5.
3. Piyu PN, Syed NF. Association between alopecia areata and thyroid dysfunction. Postgrad Med. 2021;133(8):895-8.
4. Enikö B, Arno K, Tamás B, István B, Gáspár E, Zmijewski MA, et al. Human Female Hair Follicles Are a Direct, Nonclassical Target for Thyroid-Stimulating Hormone. J Invest Dermatol. 2009;129(5):1126-39.
5. Berislav M, Juraj P, Vjeran V, Margarita SG, Mimica N, Drmić S, et al. Hair Iodine for Human Iodine Status Assessment. Thyroid. 2014;24(6):1018-26.
6. Pandav CS, Yadav K, Srivastava R, Pandav R, Karmarkar MG. Iodine deficiency disorders (IDD) control in India. Indian J Med Res. 2013;138(3):418-33.
7. Rana R, Raghuvanshi R. Effect of different cooking methods on iodine losses. J Food Sci Technol. 2013;50:1212-6.
8. Krajcovicová-Kudláčková M, Buková K, Klimes I, Seboková E. Iodine deficiency in vegetarians and vegans. Ann Nutr Metab. 2003;47(5):183-5.
9. Lightowler HJ, Davies GJ. Iodine intake and iodine deficiency in vegans as assessed by the duplicate-portion technique and urinary iodine excretion. Br J Nutr. 1998;80(6):529-35.
10. Fallon N, Dillon SA. Low Intakes of Iodine and Selenium Amongst Vegan and Vegetarian Women Highlight a Potential Nutritional Vulnerability. Front Nutr. 2020;7:72.
11. Leung AM, LaMar A, He X, Braverman LE, Pearce EN. Iodine Status and Thyroid Function of Boston-Area Vegetarians and Vegans. J Clin Endocrinol Metab. 2011;96(8):E1303-7.
12. Kalarani IB, Veerabathiran R. Impact of iodine intake on the pathogenesis of autoimmune thyroid disease in children and adults. Ann Pediatr Endocrinol Metab. 2022;27(4):256-64.
13. Aquaron R, Delange F, Marchal P, Lognoné V, Ninane L. Bioavailability of seaweed iodine in human beings. Cell Mol Biol (Noisy-le-grand). 2002;48(5):563-9.
14. Costa RO, de Macedo PM, Carvalhal A, Bernardes-Engemann AR. Use of potassium iodide in Dermatology: updates on an old drug. An Bras Dermatol. 2013;88(3):396-402.
15. Fact Sheet for Health Professionals. Iodine [Online]. Available from: https://ods.od.nih.gov/factsheets/Iodine-HealthProfessional/
16. Draelos ZD. An Oral Supplement and the Nutrition–Skin Connection. J Clin Aesthet Dermatol. 2019;12(7):13-6.
17. Ben-Yehuda Greenwald M, Frušić-Zlotkin M, Soroka Y, Ben-Sasson S, Bianco-Peled H, Kohen R. A novel role of topical iodine in skin: Activation of the Nrf2 pathway. Free Radic Biol Med. 2017;104:238-48.
18. Shinogi T, Misago N, Narisawa Y. Cutaneous sporotrichosis with refractory and reinfectious lesions in a healthy female. J Dermatol. 2004;31(6):492-6.
19. Sandhu K, Gupta S. Potassium iodide remains the most effective therapy for cutaneous sporotrichosis. J Dermatolog Treat. 2003;14(4):200-2.
20. Anzengruber F, Mergenthaler C, Murer C, Dummer R. Potassium Iodide for Cutaneous Inflammatory Disorders: A Monocentric, Retrospective Study. Dermatology. 2019;235(2):137-43.
21. Institute of Medicine (US) Panel on Micronutrients. Dietary Reference Intakes for Vitamin A, Vitamin K, Arsenic, Boron, Chromium, Copper, Iodine, Iron, Manganese, Molybdenum, Nickel, Silicon, Vanadium, and Zinc. Chapter 8: Iodine. National Academies Press (US); 2001
22. Ahad F, Ganie SA. Iodine, Iodine metabolism and Iodine deficiency disorders revisited. Indian J Endocrinol Metab. 2010;14(1):13-7.
23. Slominski A, Wortsman J, Kohn L, Ain KB, Venkataraman GM, Pisarchik A, et al. Expression of Hypothalamic–Pituitary–Thyroid Axis Related Genes in the Human Skin. J Invest Dermatol. 2002;119(6):1449-55.
24. Paus R. Exploring the "Thyroid–Skin Connection": Concepts, Questions, and Clinical Relevance. J Invest Dermatol. 2010;130(1):7-10.
25. van Beek N, Bodó E, Kromminga A, Gáspár E, Meyer K, Zmijewski MA, et al. Thyroid Hormones Directly Alter Human Hair Follicle Functions: Anagen Prolongation and Stimulation of Both Hair Matrix Keratinocyte Proliferation and Hair Pigmentation. The J Clin Endocrinol Metab.. 2008;93(11):4381-8.
26. Jara EL, Muñoz-Durango N, Llanos C, Fardella C, González PA, Bueno SM, et al. Modulating the function of the immune system by thyroid hormones and thyrotropin. Immunol Lett. 2017;184:76-83.
27. Ito T, Ito N, Saatoff M, Hashizume H, Fukamizu H, Nickoloff BJ, et al. Maintenance of Hair Follicle Immune Privilege Is Linked to Prevention of NK Cell Attack. J Invest Dermatol. 2008;128(5):1196-206.
28. National Institute of Nutrition Indian Council of Medical Research. Recommended Dietary Allowances and Estimated Average Requirements for Indians - 2020. RDA Full Report 2020.

SECTION 03

Protein and Peptides

17. Protein — *Rajat Kandhari*
18. Collagen Peptides — *Rajat Kandhari*
19. Hyaluronic Acid — *Aseem Sharma*
20. Lactoferrin and Colostrum — *Aseem Sharma*

17

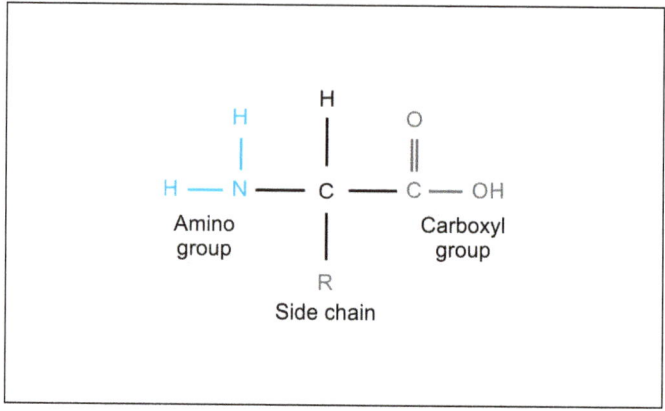

Amino Acid Structure (R is a side-chain that varies with amino acids)

Protein

✍ Rajat Kandhari

CONTENTS

PROTEIN: NUTRIENT SNAPSHOT
- ▸ REQUIREMENT IN THE INDIAN CONTEXT | 165
- ▸ ACTIVE FORMS | 166
- ▸ SAFETY AND DOSAGE | 167
- ▸ CLINICAL CONDITIONS | 167
- ▸ SUPPLEMENTATION | 170

INTRODUCTION | 172

DIGESTION, ABSORPTION AND STORAGE | 172

MECHANISM OF ACTION | 172

KEY TOPICS
- ATOPIC DERMATITIS
- HAIR GROWTH
- HAIR LOSS
- NAIL QUALITY
- PHOTOAGING
- SKIN AGING
- SKIN TEXTURE
- TELOGEN EFFLUVIUM
- WOUND HEALING

Nutrient Snapshot

▶ **REQUIREMENT IN THE INDIAN CONTEXT**

- Protein is an essential nutrient for the normal growth and development of the body. It plays many roles, from muscle growth, tissue maintenance and the production of certain hormones.

- Our skin, hair and nails are almost entirely made of protein. So a protein deficient diet can affect our health. In dermatology, protein not only plays a structural role; specific amino acids also have functional roles in their maintenance.

- According to a recent survey, 'Protein Consumption in Diet of Adult Indians: A General Consumer Survey'[1] 9 out of 10 urban Indians do not get sufficient protein in their diet, i.e., a minimum of 0.8 g protein per kg body weight per day.[1] This is because the Indian diet is cereal rich, so much, so that studies show it derives 60% of protein from cereal sources that are low in quality and digestibility.[2] The protein insufficiency was higher in vegetarians, perhaps due to the lower proportions of protein in vegetarian foods. This is likely worse in vegan diets.[1]

- Protein insufficiency leads to skin and hair issues, and amino acid supply is prioritized for critical functions for survival.

- Improving protein intake, can improve the absorption of minerals and promote gut health, resulting in better skin and hair health.

- Hair supplements often contain only a few amino acids, and in very minute quantities. Providing sufficient levels of a spectrum of amino acids through our diet or protein supplements can help prevent protein inadequacy.

▶ ACTIVE FORMS

ACTIVE FORMS	SUPPLEMENT SOURCES	SALIENT FEATURES*
Plant proteins	Soybean, pea, brown rice, oats, peanuts	Vegan option PDCAA score: Soy—0.92–1.00, Pea—0.66–0.93.[3] DIAA score: Brown rice—42,[4,5] soy – 98, peas—64, oats—75.[6] Pea protein and brown rice protein are often mixed together as their amino acids complement each other.
Other animal protein	Egg, poultry, fish	Animal sources offer biological value and excellent quality proteins. PDCAA score of animal proteins is very near or at 1.[7] DIAA score of all animal proteins >100.[6]
Dairy protein (mix)	Fermented dairy products	High biological value protein, which is a mix of whey and casein. and is easy on the gut as compared to lactose-containing dairy products.
Whey (dairy protein)	Milk (cow)	PDCAA score 1, DIAA score of whey protein >100.[6] There are three types in the market: 1. Concentrate – inexpensive; contains lactose; slow absorbing 2. Isolate – low levels of lactose as compared to concentrate; fast absorbing 3. Hydrolyzed – predigested; bitter; often added to protein blends or elemental formulas
Casein (dairy protein)	Milk (cow)	PDCAA score 1, DIAA score of casein protein >100 Casein is a normally a micellar protein, which makes it slow digesting. That is why it is normally recommended at night for muscle recovery (during fasting). The hydrolyzed form is fast digesting as it is predigested. Casein is the main cause of milk allergies.[8]
Skim milk powder	Milk (cow)	Skim milk powder contains milk protein (whey and casein) along with the fats and carbohydrates (lactose).

*PDCAA score: Protein digestibility corrected amino acid score (maximum score 1).
 DIAA score: Digestible indispensable amino acid score (score >100 is excellent quality).

▶ SAFETY AND DOSAGE

GENERAL REQUIREMENTS	
Indian recommendations	ICMR-NIN EAR 2020: 0.66 g/kg body weight (BW) per/day for both adult male and female considering high biological value protein. ICMR-NIN RDA 2020: 0.83 g/kg BW per/day for both adult male and female. ICMR-NIN TUL 2020: <40% of protein-to-energy ratio.
Global recommendations and limits	IOM: 0.8 g/kg BW/day. TUL: 3.5 g/kg BW/day.[9] EFSA average requirement (AR): 0.66 g/kg BW/day.[10] Population reference intake (PRI): 0.83 g/kg BW/day
Side effects	Chronic high protein intake >2 g/kg BW/day for adults may result in digestive, renal, and vascular abnormalities and should be avoided.[9] Chronic excessive protein intake (>35% of total energy) can lead to hyperaminoacidemia, hyperammonemia, hyperinsulinemia, nausea, and diarrhea.[11] Chronic intake of high amounts of individual amino acids or their derivatives may cause imbalance and thus may alter various biochemical pathways and cellular functions.[12]
Notes:	Both essential and nonessential amino acids play important roles in our body, so we need to take both in our diet.[13] As a general rule of thumb, protein requirement is calculated by 1 g/kg BW, and distributed between meals.

▶ CLINICAL CONDITIONS

EVIDENCE LEVEL	CONDITION OR USE CASE	DOSAGE	BENEFIT OR MECHANISM OF ACTION
+++	Skin texture	Amino-acid supplement containing 600 mg L-leucine, 250 mg L-arginine, and 300 mg L-glutamine for 6 weeks	There was an increase in skin moisture content, a and decrease in the TEWL levels, and an improvement in texture from baseline in the treatment group, which were not seen in placebo. There was also improvement seen in the skin texture after taking the amino acid supplement.[14]
+++++	Age-related skin changes	Supplement containing three types of amino acids [leucine, glutamine and arginine (LGA)] and 11 types of vitamins given twice daily for 8 weeks	The LGA group showed an improvement in the grade and number of the wrinkles in the corners of the eyes, and the stratum corneum cell area declined (which indicates improvement in epidermal turnover), compared to the placebo group.[15]

▶ **CLINICAL CONDITIONS** (*Continued*)

EVIDENCE LEVEL	CONDITION OR USE CASE	DOSAGE	BENEFIT OR MECHANISM OF ACTION
+++	Skin photoaging	UV irradiated mice were fed with a combination of different amino acids in a solution or single amino acid solution (1 gm/mL/kg BW)	Essential amino acids mixtures (BCAA + Arg + Gln, BCAA + Gln, and BCAA + Pro) significantly increased the fractional synthesis rate (FSR) of skin tropocollagen. This result suggests that the combinations of BCAA and glutamine or proline are important for restoring dermal collagen protein synthesis impaired by UV irradiation.[16]
+++	Atopic dermatitis (AD)	Patients were divided into 2 groups receiving 4 g of L-histidine or placebo for 8 weeks	Daily oral L-histidine reduced AD disease severity by 34% (physician assessment using the SCORing AD tool) and 39% (patient self-assessment using the Patient-Oriented Eczema Measure tool) after 4 weeks of treatment. No improvement was noted with the placebo. The clinical effect of oral L-histidine in AD was similar to that of mid-potency topical corticosteroids.[17]
+++++	Wound healing	N/A (meta-analysis)	Five studies on arginine and 39 studies on glutamine supplementation suggest that there is a beneficial effect of these amino acids on wound healing.[18]
+++	Telogen effluvium	Supplement containing L-cystine 20 mg, keratin 20 mg, medicinal yeast 100 mg, calcium pantothenate 60 mg, thiamine nitrate 60 mg, PABA 20 mg. One capsule 3 times a day for 6 months	The treatment showed improvement and normalization of the mean anagen hair rate within 6 months of the treatment. The appearance of hair growth in the global photographic assessment was better in the treatment group than placebo.[19]
++++	Hair loss and nail quality	Two capsules containing 250 mg Cynatine (keratin peptide), zinc, copper and some B vitamins	The treatment showed a 12.5% reduction in hair loss over placebo at day 30 and a 34.5% and 34.4% reduction at days 60 and 90, respectively. It also showed improvement in their anagen/telogen ratio. The active group showed a 5.9% improvement in hair strength at day 90 compared to baseline over placebo. There was an improvement in nail strength and texture.[20]

▶ CLINICAL CONDITIONS (Continued)

EVIDENCE LEVEL	CONDITION OR USE CASE	DOSAGE	BENEFIT OR MECHANISM OF ACTION
+++	Hair growth	Rabbits were divided into 4 groups; were fed varying levels of methionine- supplemented diets (0, 0.30%, 0.60%, 0.90%)	The addition of methionine increased hair follicle density on the dorsal skin and enhanced expression level of Wnt10β/β-catenin (master regulator of hair follicle morphogenesis). *in vitro* methionine stimulation also prolonged hair shaft growth.[21]
+++	Hair and nail growth	Rodents were fed various combinations of arginine salicylate inositol complex (ASI) and magnesium biotinate (MgB) for 42 days	As a result, ASI and MgB were effective in hair growth by stimulating insulin-like growth factor-1, fibroblast growth factor, keratinocyte growth factor, hepatocyte growth factor, vascular endothelial growth factor, sirtuin-1, Wnt, and β-catenin signaling pathways. It was also found that ASI did not affect nail growth, whereas the combination of MgB was effective when higher doses of biotin were used.[22]
++	Hair growth	L-cystine, thiamine, calcium D-pantothenate, and folic acid on human hair follicular keratinocytes (HHFK) in vitro	The oral hair-growth formulation enhanced proliferation and metabolic activity of HHFKs compared to HHFKs cultivated without the formulation. Functional grouping of differentially expressed genes confirmed the regulation of cell cycle-/proliferation-associated genes (cdk1, HJURP) and revealed regulation of cell death and oxidative stress-associated gene groups. L-cystine dependent changes in the expression of the anti-oxidative gene hmox1 were found. The combination of all four compounds gave optimal protection from UV radiation.[23]

▸ SUPPLEMENTATION

	BASIS	WHAT TO LOOK OUT FOR
Supplementation form	Whey (concentrate, whey isolate, or whey hydrolysate) Casein (micellar or casein hydrolysate) Skim milk powder Plant protein (concentrate or plant protein isolate; soy, pea, rice and combinations) Egg albumin BCAA, a blend of plant and animal proteins	Label ingredients will have information about the composition of the supplement, whether it is a blend of plant and animal protein forms or just amino acids. Some forms of whey and carbohydrates as gainers can be selected for patients trying to put on weight. For patients with a normal or high BMI, a purer protein source may be recommended.
Administration form	Powders, breakfast/workout bars, chips, biscuits, ice cream	Amino acids found in capsules may likely be in very small amounts to have any effect.
Purity considerations	PDCAA score of whey/casein supplements is 1 while that of plant proteins may vary based on source (except for soy the PDCAA is 1). DIAA score of whey/casein supplements is ≥ 100 while that of plant proteins may vary as the source. DIAA score of pea protein is 100. Sugar-content may be high in certain protein supplements. This can also be in the form of maltodextrin. Some amino acid fortification (especially in vegan proteins) might be used. Unfortunately, amino acid spiking may also happen to inflate protein quantity.	It is best to check the ingredients section of the product label as it gives information about the content of the type of whey proteins. The brand front label might say whey isolate but may also contain whey concentrate in it. One can ask for an amino acid profiling test report from the company to confirm that there is no amino acid spiking.

SUPPLEMENTATION (Continued)

	BASIS	WHAT TO LOOK OUT FOR
Patient considerations	Protein supplements containing lactose (a sugar found in milk) that may cause GI disturbances such as bloating, flatulence, etc. Plant proteins may have an aftertaste (like soy protein), a grainy texture (like pea protein) and a high satiety. Companies may put many additives to counteract these issues.	A protein supplement containing whey isolate (with very little lactose) can be used. The lactose content may not be mentioned on the label but the manufacturer can provide that information. A plant protein can be used as an alternative.
Safety considerations	There are correlation studies on whey supplements and acne. While there are many confounding factors, whey protein is thought to increase the IGF-1 levels in the body so individuals prone to acne should exercise caution.[24] A plant protein supplements can be suggested. Individuals with chronic kidney disease (but not on dialysis) have, not on dialysis have to limit their protein intake. Thus, protein supplement can be risky.	

▶ INTRODUCTION

Protein is not just for those who want to build muscle; it is an important macronutrient for everyone. Nine of the twenty amino acids needed to make all the proteins found in the human body are deemed 'essential' as they cannot be made by our body and must be acquired by our diet.[25]

While all amino acids may not be essential, nonessential amino acids also play important roles in our body. They can become 'conditionally essential' because of elevated needs during pathological conditions. In these instances, our metabolism may not be able to maintain their concentrations at sufficient levels to match metabolic requirements.[25]

In addition to the primary function as protein building blocks, amino acids serve multiple other purposes, even in our skin, hair and nails. The protein quantity and quality in our diet has a direct effect on the growth, maintenance and quality of our skin and hair, and insufficient supply can make tissue more susceptible to aging.

▶ DIGESTION, ABSORPTION AND STORAGE

Digestion and Absorption

- Protein is denatured and broken down into amino acids and peptides by proteases in the stomach, followed by further breakdown in the small intestine.[25]

- Transporters are used to absorb amino acids and peptides into enterocytes, which are eventually released into the bloodstream.[25]

Storage

Amino acids are used to form new proteins, energy, and other biological molecules. The free amino acid pool in cells is derived from dietary amino acids, de novo synthesis and proteolysis of body proteins.

▶ MECHANISM OF ACTION

01 | Direct Structural and Functional Roles of Protein

The amino acids we get from protein intake play countless structural and functional roles in skin and hair health, especially glutamine and the sulfur-containing amino acids, methionine, cysteine and taurine.

i] Sulfur-containing Amino Acids

Keratin has a high content of cysteine, about 7–20% of the total amino acid residues. This conditionally essential amino acid contains sulfur, due to which cysteine can form intramolecular and intermolecular disulfide bonds.[26] These bonds confer strength and rigidity to keratin. Active form of B6 vitamin (pyridoxal phosphate) increases L-cysteine incorporation into keratin.[27]

Cysteine upregulates keratins expression in keratinocytes and its supplementation has shown to counteract the adverse effect of iron deficiency on keratin expression.[28] Hair growth rate and diameter depend on the availability of cysteine. It is also the rate-limiting factor in the synthesis of glutathione, an important antioxidant.

Methionine is another sulfur-containing amino acid that is essential, i.e., it must be acquired from the diet. Methionine is vital for both keratin and procollagen synthesis.[29] Our body produces cysteine and taurine from methionine. An in vitro study suggested that taurine is taken up by the connective tissue sheath, the proximal outer root sheath and the hair bulb, and prevents TGF-β1-induced deleterious effects on the hair follicle.[30] Taurine can improve hair density.[31]

Furthermore, methionine (and arginine) counteract hydrogen peroxide-mediated oxidative stress[29], which means they can protect our hair from the deleterious effects of hair color.

ii] Lysine and Proline

Lysine is one of 9 essential amino acids that cannot be made in the body, that's low in cereals. Proline can be made in the body, but low-protein/vegetarian diets may not always promote optimal L-proline production.

Lysine and proline play important roles in the growth of hair follicles. Lysine is important for iron uptake, an important nutrient for countless reactions in our body.[29] Supplementing iron with lysine, improves mean serum ferritin concentrations.[31] As part of the hair root, lysine governs hair shape and volume. Insufficient supply causes brittle and thin hair.[27]

Proline serves as an important building block for collagen production. Vitamin C and iron participate in collagen fiber synthesis via hydroxylation of proline and lysine,[32] to produce hydroxyproline and hydroxylysine, amino acids that are unique to collagen and collagen-like proteins.[33]

iii] Glycine

Glycine accounts for a third of the sequence of collagen. It is has the smallest R-group and is thus able to enable the folding of the collagen triple helix.

iv] Glutamine and Arginine

Glutamine and glutamate with proline, histidine, arginine and ornithine, comprise 25% of the dietary amino acid intake and constitute the "glutamate family" of amino acids, which are disposed of through conversion to glutamate.[34]

Glutamine serves as an essential metabolic precursor in nucleotide, glucose and amino sugar biosynthesis, glutathione homeostasis, protein synthesis, and a source of oxidative energy.[34] Glutamine supports the growth of cells that have high energy demands and synthesize large amounts of proteins and nucleic acids. That's why it is an energy source for hair follicles and is required for repopulating hair follicle stem cells after their mobilization at the onset of anagen.[8,35,36] Glutamine is an important metabolite for the transcription and production of IL-1β, which can stimulate wound-induced hair follicle neogenesis, where functional hair follicles reemerge during healing of large cutaneous wounds.[36] Proline synthesis from glutamine and arginine is also important for collagen synthesis.[37,25] Glutamine, arginine (and its precursor citrulline) and protein supplements, in general, are therefore often employed for wound healing.[25,38]

Glutamate and its receptors have been identified in the skin and hair follicles and their role is currently being explored.[39]

v] Branched-chain Amino Acids (BCAAs)

BCAAs (leucine, isoleucine and valine) have been the subject of extensive research for their role in muscle protein synthesis. An animal study showed that essential amino acid mixtures (BCAAs with arginine, glycine and proline) significantly increased the synthesis rate of dermal tropocollagen after UVB irradiation. This suggests that these amino acids are important for restoring collagen synthesis impaired by UV radiation.[16]

vi] Other Amino Acids

Histidine, an essential amino acid, forms a skin barrier protein (filaggrin). It has beneficial effects on atopic dermatitis patients.[17] It is converted to urocanic acid, which acts as a sunscreen.[40]

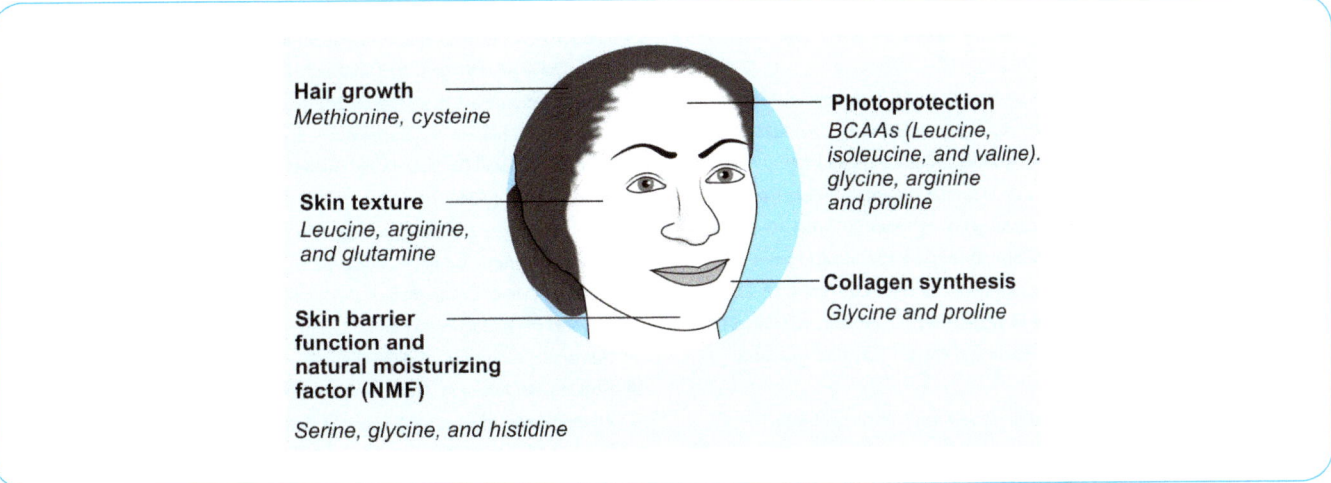

Figure 1: The various roles of amino acids in skin and hair health.

Serine, glycine, pyrrolidone-5-carboxylic acid, arginine, ornithine, citrulline, alanine, histidine and urocanic acid are the main components of natural moisturizing factor (NMF) that keeps skin moist.[41]

Tyrosine is converted to DOPAquinone as a first step in the process of melanogenesis, for both the brown-black eumelanin and the yellow-red pheomelanin.[42,43]

02 | Indirect Benefits of Protein Intake

In general, protein consumption has shown to positively correlate with overall microbial diversity in the gut.[44] The gut microbiota composition regulates the immune system, and communicates with skin in a bidirectional manner, conceptualized as the gut-skin axis. The kind of protein intake may have indirect effects on skin through this modulation.[44] For example, intake of whey and pea protein has been reported to increase beneficial gut-commensals, Bifidobacterium and Lactobacillus, whilst also reducing pathogenic strains.[44–46] This can increase intestinal levels of bacterial metabolites called short chain fatty acids (SCFAs),[45] which are anti-inflammatory and important for maintenance of the skin's barrier.[47] A reduced capacity to produce SCFA has been implicated in inflammatory diseases like atopic dermatitis.[47] More information about this can be found in Probiotics and Prebiotics.

▶ REFERENCES

1. Marathe M, Padmanabh P. A study on Quality of Life in Indian adults-Outcomes and role of nutrition. International Journal of Advance Research, Ideas and Innovations in Technology. 2021;7(4):V7I4-1370.
2. Swaminathan S, Vaz M, Kurpad AV. Protein intakes in India. Br J Nutr. 2012:108(Suppl 2):S50-8.
3. Qin P, Wang T, Luo Y. A review on plant-based proteins from soybean: Health benefits and soy product development. J Agric Food Res. 2022;7:100265.
4. Joye I. Protein Digestibility of Cereal Products. Foods. 2019;8(6):199.
5. Han F, Han F, Wang Y, Fan L, Song G, Chen X. et al. Digestible indispensable amino acid scores of nine cooked cereal grains. Br J Nutr. 2019;121:30-41.
6. Bailey HM, Stein HH. Can the digestible indispensable amino acid score methodology decrease protein malnutrition. Anim Front. 2019;9(4):18-23.
7. Hertzler SR, Lieblein-Boff JC, Weiler M, Allgeier C. Plant Proteins: Assessing Their Nutritional Quality and Effects on Health and Physical Function. Nutrients. 2020;12(12):3704.
8. Kim J. Pre-sleep casein protein ingestion: new paradigm in post-exercise recovery nutrition. Phys Act Nutr. 2020;24(2):6-10.
9. Wu G. Dietary protein intake and human health. Food Funct. 2016;7(3):1251-65.
10. EFSA Panel on Dietetic Products, Nutrition and Allergies (NDA). Scientific Opinion on Dietary Reference Values for Protein. EFSA Journal. 2012;10(2): 2557.
11. Bilsborough S, Mann N. A review of issues of dietary protein intake in humans. Int J Sport Nutr Exerc Metab. 2006 Apr;16(2):129-52.
12. Holeček M. Side Effects of Amino Acid Supplements. Physiol Res. 2022;71(1):29-45.
13. Hou Y, Yin Y, Wu G. Dietary essentiality of "nutritionally non-essential amino acids" for animals and humans. Exp Biol Med (Maywood). 2015;240(8):997-1007.
14. Takaoka M, Okumura S, Seki T, Ohtani M. Effect of amino-acid intake on physical conditions and skin state: a randomized, double-blind, placebo-controlled, crossover trial. J Clin Biochem Nutr. 2019;65(1):52-8.
15. Yamashita R, Ooe M, Saya Y, Sugisawa N, Murakami N, Matsunaka H. Effect of Vitamin-Containing Amino Acid Supplements on Menopausal Symptoms and Age-Related Skin Changes: A Randomised, Double-Blind, Placebo-Controlled Study. Dermatol Ther (Heidelb). 2021;11(5):1681-92.
16. Murakami H, Shimbo K, Inoue Y, Takino Y, Kobayashi H. Importance of amino acid composition to improve skin collagen protein synthesis rates in UV-irradiated mice. Amino Acids. 2012;42(6):2481-9.
17. Tan SP, Brown SB, Griffiths CEM, Weller RB, Gibbs NK. Feeding filaggrin: effects of l-histidine supplementation in atopic dermatitis. Clin Cosmet Investig Dermatol. 2017:10:403-11.
18. Arribas-López E, Zand N, Ojo O, Snowden MJ, Kochhar T. The Effect of Amino Acids on Wound Healing: A Systematic Review and Meta-Analysis on Arginine and Glutamine. Nutrients. 2021;13(8):2498.
19. Lengg N, Heidecker B, Seifert B, Trüeb RM. Dietary supplement increases anagen hair rate in women with telogen effluvium: results of a double-blind, placebo-controlled trial. Therapy. 2007;4:59-65.
20. Beer C, Wood S, Veghte RH. A Clinical Trial to Investigate the Effect of Cynatine HNS on Hair and Nail Parameters. ScientificWorldJournal. 2014:2014:641723.
21. Zhu Y, Wu Z, Liu H, Liu G, Li F. Methionine promotes the development of hair follicles via the Wnt/β-catenin signalling pathway in Rex rabbits. J Anim Physiol Anim Nutr (Berl). 2020;104(1):379-84.
22. Demir B, Cicek D, Orhan C, Er B, Erten F, Tuzcu M, et al. Effects of a Combination of Arginine Silicate Inositol Complex and a Novel Form of Biotin on Hair and Nail Growth in a Rodent Model. Biol Trace Elem Res. 2023;201(2):751-65.
23. Riegel K, Hengl T, Krischok S, Schlinzig K, Abts HF. L-Cystine-Containing Hair-Growth Formulation Supports Protection, Viability, and Proliferation of Keratinocytes. Clin Cosmet Investig Dermatol. 2020:13:499-510.
24. Podgórska A, Puścion-Jakubik A, Markiewicz-Żukowska R, Gromkowska-Kępka KJ, Socha K. Acne Vulgaris and Intake of Selected Dietary Nutrients—A Summary of Information. Healthcare (Basel). 2021;9(6):668.
25. Lopez MJ, Mohiuddin SS. Biochemistry, Essential Amino Acids. StatPearls (2023).
26. Numata K, Kaplan DL. Biologically derived scaffolds. Advanced Wound Repair Therapies. 2011:524–51.
27. Goluch-Koniuszy ZS. Nutrition of women with hair loss problem during the period of menopause. Prz Menopauzalny. 2016;15(1):56-61.
28. Miniaci MC, Irace C, Capuozzo A, Piccolo M, Pascale AD, Russo A et al. Cysteine Prevents the Reduction in Keratin Synthesis Induced by Iron Deficiency in Human Keratinocytes. J Cell Biochem. 2016;117(2):402-12.
29. Hosking AM, Juhasz M, Atanaskova Mesinkovska N. Complementary and Alternative Treatments for Alopecia: A Comprehensive Review. Skin Appendage Disord. 2019;5(2):72-89.
30. Collin C, Gautier B, Gaillard O, Hallegot P, Chabane S, Bastien P, et al. Protective effects of taurine on human hair follicle grown in vitro. Int J Cosmet Sci. 2006;28(4):289-98.

31. Sardana K, Sachdeva S. Role of nutritional supplements in selected dermatological disorders: A review. J Cosmet Dermatol. 2022;21(1):85-98.
32. Rushton DH. Nutritional factors and hair loss. Clin Exp Dermatol. 2002;27(5):396-404.
33. Wang J, Gao C, Chen X, Liu L. Expanding the lysine industry: biotechnological production of L-lysine and its derivatives. Adv Appl Microbiol. 2021:115:1-33.
34. Tapiero H, Mathé G, Couvreur P, Tew KD. II. Glutamine and glutamate. Biomed Pharmacother. 2002;56(9):446-57.
35. Kim CS, Ding X, Allmeroth K, Biggs LC, Kolenc OI, L'Hoest N, et al. Glutamine Metabolism Controls Stem Cell Fate Reversibility and Long-Term Maintenance in the Hair Follicle. Cell Metab. 2020;32(4):629-42.e8.
36. Wang G, Sweren E, Andrews W, Li Y, Chen J, Xue Y, et al. Commensal microbiome promotes hair follicle regeneration by inducing keratinocyte HIF-1α signaling and glutamine metabolism. Sci Adv. 2023;9(1):eabo7555.
37. Karna E, Miltyk W, Wolczyński S, Palka JA. The potential mechanism for glutamine-induced collagen biosynthesis in cultured human skin fibroblasts. Comp Biochem Physiol B Biochem Mol Biol. 2001;130(1):23-32.
38. Ellinger S. Micronutrients, Arginine, and Glutamine: Does Supplementation Provide an Efficient Tool for Prevention and Treatment of Different Kinds of Wounds? Adv Wound Care (New Rochelle). 2014;3(11):691-707.
39. Jara CP, Berti BDA, Mendes NF, Engel DF, Zanesco AM, de Souza GFP, et al. Glutamic acid promotes hair growth in mice. Sci Rep. 2021;11(1):15453.
40. Gibbs NK, Norval M. Urocanic acid in the skin: A mixed blessing. J Invest Dermatol. 2011;131(1):14-7.
41. Caspers PJ, Lucassen GW, Carter EA, Bruining HA, Puppels GJ. In Vivo Confocal Raman Microspectroscopy of the Skin: Noninvasive Determination of Molecular Concentration Profiles. J Invest Dermatol. 2001;116(3):434-42.
42. Rzepka Z, Buszman E, Beberok A, Wrześniok D. From tyrosine to melanin: Signaling pathways and factors regulating melanogenesis. Postepy Hig Med Dosw (Online). 2016;70(0):695-708.
43. Watson A, Wayman J, Kelley R, Feugier A, Biourge V. Increased dietary intake of tyrosine upregulates melanin deposition in the hair of adult blackcoated dogs. Anim Nutr. 2018;4(4):422-28.
44. Singh RK, Chang H-W, Yan D, Lee KM, Ucmak D, Wong K, et al. Influence of diet on the gut microbiome and implications for human health. J Transl Med. 2017;15(1):73.
45. Dominika Ś, Arjan N, Karyn RP, Henryk K. The study on the impact of glycated pea proteins on human intestinal bacteria. Int J Food Microbiol. 2011;145(1):267-72.
46. Romond MB, Ais A, Guillemot F, Bounouader R, Cortot A, Romond C. Cell-free whey from milk fermented with Bifidobacterium breve C50 used to modify the colonic microflora of healthy subjects. J Dairy Sci. 1998;81(5):1229-35.
47. Trompette A, Pernot J, Perdijk O, A Alqahtani RA, Domingo JS, Camacho-Muñoz D, et al. Gut-derived short-chain fatty acids modulate skin barrier integrity by promoting keratinocyte metabolism and differentiation. Mucosal Immunol. 2022;15(5):908-26.

Nutrition in Dermatology

18

Gly-Pro-Hyp tripeptide   Pro-Hyp dipeptide

Collagen di- and tripeptides

Collagen Peptides

✍ Rajat Kandhari

CONTENTS

COLLAGEN PEPTIDES: NUTRIENT SNAPSHOT

- ▶ REQUIREMENT IN THE INDIAN CONTEXT | 177
- ▶ ACTIVE FORMS | 178
- ▶ SAFETY AND DOSAGE | 178
- ▶ CLINICAL CONDITIONS | 179
- ▶ SUPPLEMENTATION | 187

INTRODUCTION | 188

DIGESTION, ABSORPTION AND STORAGE | 188

MECHANISM OF ACTION | 188

KEY TOPICS

- ANTI-AGING
- ATOPIC DERMATITIS
- CELLULITIS
- HAIR GROWTH
- HAIR THINNING
- MICROCIRCULATION
- PHOTOAGING
- SKIN ELASTICITY
- SKIN MOISTURE
- TELOGEN EFFLUVIUM

Nutrient Snapshot

▶ **REQUIREMENT IN THE INDIAN CONTEXT**

- Collagen is the main component of skin's extracellular matrix. As skin ages, with time and due to internal and external factors (especially UV rays), there is a reduction in cell metabolism and a concomitant decrease in skin's matrix components like collagen, elastin and hyaluronic acid. This is accompanied by a gradual decline in skin's defences and an increase in oxidative stress.

- Bioactive peptides offer a great diversity of biological activities, and play an important role in the field of anti-aging, especially for preventing ultraviolet-induced photoaging. Until recently, they have mostly been explored for topical applications. Hydrolysates of collagen, known as collagen peptides or collagen hydrolysate, are becoming popular for oral consumption, as they can deliver bioactive peptides to active fibroblasts in the dermis.

- As the emergence of an aging population and the healthy consciousness gradually deepening, more attention is given to skin health treatments that aim to increase skin's matrix.[1] Indian skin is more prone to hyperpigmentation[2] and exhibits greater age-related changes in the face, such as nasolabial folds and tear troughs, amongst some other signs of aging, compared to other Asians and Caucasians.[3]

- Collagen peptides offer a dietary source of building blocks for matrix components, and also stimulate their production. Further to an anti-aging solution, it may be used alongside collagen-stimulating treatments, as well as, for wound healing and the management of skin conditions. This is because improving the structural integrity of skin can enhance its functions and defences.

▶ ACTIVE FORMS

ACTIVE FORMS	SUPPLEMENT SOURCES	SALIENT FEATURES
hydrolyzed collagen peptides	Marine, poultry, bovine, porcine source[4]	Bovine collagen is very cheap but due to cultural preferences individuals prefer marine collagen. But those with an allergy to fish can opt for bovine and poultry sources.
	Vegetarians sources	These peptides are not likely absorbed intact (due to low levels of hydroxyproline) and therefore, may not be bioactive. They are less effective than non-vegetarian collagen peptides.

▶ SAFETY AND DOSAGE

GENERAL REQUIREMENTS	
Indian recommendations	N/A
Global recommendations and limits	One of the studies suggests incorporating collagen peptides in the standard diet, while maintaining indispensable amino acid balance. The amounts of collagen peptides observed in the literature suggest intakes in the range of 2.5–15 g daily.[5]
Notes:	Collagen supplementation is generally safe with no reported adverse events.[6]
	A high grade of collagen peptides (average molecular weight of ≤ 8 kDa) should be used for efficacy.
	Food allergies for animal-sourced collagen peptides should be considered when selecting a collagen peptide supplement.

▶ CLINICAL CONDITIONS

EVIDENCE LEVEL	CONDITION OR USE CASE	DOSAGE	BENEFIT OR MECHANISM OF ACTION
+++++	Anti-aging	Indian women were first given a placebo daily for 30 days to establish a baseline, followed by a product containing hydrolyzed collagen peptide (5.5 g), lycopene (5 mg), grape seed extract, green tea extract, taurine, vitamin C and E for 60 days.	Based on instrumental evaluation, product reduced wrinkle width, open pores, skin roughness, and the color of hyperpigmented blemishes, while there was improvement in skin hydration, firmness and barrier function from baseline to day 30 and 60. Product also increased elasticity at day 30. Clinical evaluation showed that periorbital hyperpigmentation and wrinkles also reduced.[7]
+++++	Skin moisture	Subjects took a formulated powder drink in the morning before breakfast which contained either 10 g placebo or 10 g Peptan for 84 days.	The oral intake collagen peptides increased collagen density as early as 4 weeks after the start of the treatment when compared to the baseline, and this effect persisted after 12 weeks of treatment. After 12 weeks of Peptan intake, the treatment effect was higher than in the placebo group.[8]
++++	Anti-aging	Subjects received capsule containing marine collagen peptides (MCPs, 570 mg), grape-skin extract (10 mg), CoQ10 (10 mg), luteolin (10 mg), and selenium (0.05 mg) twice a day for 60 days	The supplementation improved skin elasticity, sebum production, and skin structure. Metabolic data showed increase of plasma hydroxyproline and ATP storage in erythrocytes.[9]

▶ CLINICAL CONDITIONS (Continued)

EVIDENCE LEVEL	CONDITION OR USE CASE	DOSAGE	BENEFIT OR MECHANISM OF ACTION
+++	Skin elasticity	Subjects received either astaxanthin 2 mg and collagen hydrolysate 3 mg or placebo for 12 weeks	The treatment group showed improvements in skin elasticity and TEWL in photoaged facial skin after 12 weeks compared to placebo. The treatment group also increased expression of procollagen type I mRNA and decreased MMP-1 and -12 mRNA compared to placebo group. There was no difference in UV-induced DNA damage between groups.[10]
+++++	Skin aging	Subjects received ampoules containing a blend of 2.5 g of collagen peptides, acerola fruit extract, vitamin C, zinc, biotin, and vitamin E or placebo for 12 weeks	There was an improvement in skin hydration, elasticity, roughness, and density between the treatment group and the placebo group.[11]
+++++	Skin aging	Subjects received a placebo or a supplement containing 1,000 mg of low molecular weight collagen peptide (LMWCP) along with vitamin C, and fruit concentrate mix once daily for 12 weeks.	Skin hydration and elasticity values were higher in the LMWCP group after 6 weeks and 12 weeks in the treatment group as compared to the placebo. After 12 weeks in the LMWCP group, the visual assessment score and three parameters of skin wrinkling were improved compared to the placebo group.[12]

▶ CLINICAL CONDITIONS (Continued)

EVIDENCE LEVEL	CONDITION OR USE CASE	DOSAGE	BENEFIT OR MECHANISM OF ACTION
+++++	Anti-aging	Subjects either received 2.5 or 5.0 g of collagen hydrolysate or placebo once daily for 8 weeks	The skin elasticity in both collagen groups showed an improvement in comparison to placebo. After 4 weeks of follow-up treatment, a higher skin elasticity level was determined in elderly women.[13]
++++	Anti-aging	Subjects consumed 10 g of hydrolyzed collagen or placebo powder daily, or placebo for 12 weeks.	The participants in the treatment group had a reduction in wrinkles after 12 weeks from baseline. A subgroup analysis based on age showed women 45–54 years had an improvement in cheek skin elasticity from baseline to weeks 6 and 12. At week 12, participants in the treatment group reported greater percentage improvements in overall skin score and wrinkle, elasticity, hydration, radiance, and firmness scores versus placebo.[14]
+++++	Anti-aging	Subjects received either a products containing 2.5 g specific short-chain collagen oligopeptides, 666 mg acerola fruit extract, 80 mg vitamin C, 3 mg zinc citrate, 2.3 mg vitamin E, and 50 µg biotin or placebo for 12 weeks	There was an improvement in the collagen structure of facial skin after intake of the test product compared to placebo. There was positive subjective evaluations of skin parameters such as elasticity, crinkliness/wrinkliness, and evenness in different body areas such as face, hands, décolleté, neck, backside, legs, and belly.[15]

▶ **CLINICAL CONDITIONS** (*Continued*)

EVIDENCE LEVEL	CONDITION OR USE CASE	DOSAGE	BENEFIT OR MECHANISM OF ACTION
+++++	Anti-aging	The subjects received a liquid supplement containing a hydrolyzed fish collagen type I (4,000 mg), molecular weight of 0.3–8 kDa, hyaluronic acid, glucosamine hydrochloride, L-carnitine, black pepper, and maca extracts, chondroitin sulphate, vitamins, and minerals for 90 days.	Subjects consuming the test product had an overall increase in skin elasticity when compared to placebo. Histological analysis of skin biopsies revealed positive changes in the skin architecture, with a reduction in solar elastosis and improvement in collagen fiber organization in the test product group. As reported in the self-perception questionnaires, participants agreed their skin was more hydrated and more elastic. The consumption of the test product also reduced joint pain and improved joint mobility.[16]
+++++	Skin aging	Subjects received syrup containing nutri cosmeceutical or a placebo for 90 days. Nutri cosmeceutical was composed of—hydrolyzed collagen type I (5,000 mg), hyaluronic acid, borage oil and N-acetylglucosamine along with vitamins and minerals and a blend of antioxidants	There was an overall increase in skin elasticity and an improvement in skin texture in the treatment group. The histological examinations in the test product group revealed an improvement in the structure and stratification of the epidermal layers and in the collagen and elastin fibers network in addition to a reduction in the photoaging parameters. Self assessment also recorded a positive feedback from the patients.[17]

▶ CLINICAL CONDITIONS (Continued)

EVIDENCE LEVEL	CONDITION OR USE CASE	DOSAGE	BENEFIT OR MECHANISM OF ACTION
+++	Anti-aging	Subjected received either 10 g of fish-derived collagen peptide with 400 mg of ornithine (CPO) or placebo for 8 weeks	There was improvement in skin elasticity and TEWL in the CPO group compared to placebo. The CPO group showed increased plasma IGF-1 levels after 8 weeks of supplementation compared with the baseline. The author suggests that improvement in skin condition is maybe due to increase in IGF-1 levels.[18]
+++	Anti-aging	In the first month (28 days), subjects were asked to intake either collagen or the maltodextrin once a day: 1 g per 10 kg BW, and for the second month, the dose to be taken was 5 g in total (total study period: 56 days)	Skin hydration and elasticity of the participants taking the hydrolyzed collagen increased on day 28 until the end of the treatment. Wrinkle depth decreased from baseline on day 28 and 56 days of treatment. Clinical evaluations showed improvements in skin softness, skin firmness, skin smoothness, and visibility of wrinkles.[19]
+++	Anti-aging	Subjects received a syrup either containing hydrolyzed fish collagen: 4,000 mg, water-soluble CoQ10: 50 mg, vitamin C: 80 mg, vitamin A: 920 µg, biotin: 150 µg or placebo group for 12 weeks	There was improvement in dermis density, and skin smoothness while there was reduction in periorbital wrinkle area and the total wrinkle score.[20]

▶ CLINICAL CONDITIONS (Continued)

EVIDENCE LEVEL	CONDITION OR USE CASE	DOSAGE	BENEFIT OR MECHANISM OF ACTION
+++++	Anti-aging	Subjects with either received high content dipeptide collagen product (HCP) or low content dipeptide collagen product or placebo for 8 weeks	There was improvement in skin moisture, elasticity, wrinkles, and roughness, compared with a placebo group at 4 and 8 weeks. HCP showed more improvement than LCP in facial skin moisture, elasticity (R2), wrinkles and roughness, compared with the placebo group.[21]
+++	Microcirculation and photoaging	Women received daily supplementation of 1 g BioCell Collagen® along with low-molecular-weight hyaluronic acid and chondroitin sulfate for 12 weeks	There was reduction of skin dryness/scaling and global lines/wrinkles as measured by visual/tactile score. There was also an increase in the content of hemoglobin and collagen in the skin dermis after 6 weeks of supplementation. At the end of the study, the increase in hemoglobin remained significant, while the increase in collagen content was maintained.[22]
++++	Skin elasticity	Subjects were divided into 3 groups. One group was asked to topically apply di- and tri-peptides of hydrolyzed rice protein on face twice daily, second group received oral supplement composed of 9 g hydrolyzed collagen along with vitamin A (600 μg), C (45 mg), E (10 mg), and zinc (7.0 mg) or placebo daily for 90 days.	The group with the topical application showed an increase in the stratum corneum water content and skin elasticity after 28 days, which reflected in the dermis echogenicity after 90 days. The oral supplementation after 90 days improved skin elasticity and showed more pronounced effect on dermis echogenicity and on reducing skin pores.[23]

► CLINICAL CONDITIONS (Continued)

EVIDENCE LEVEL	CONDITION OR USE CASE	DOSAGE	BENEFIT OR MECHANISM OF ACTION
+++	UV radiation-induced skin dehydration	The dorsal skin of mice exposed to UVB radiation with or without oral administration of collagen peptide (CP) at two doses (500 and 1,000 mg/kg) for 9 weeks.	The oral administration of CP increased skin hydration and decreased wrinkle formation compared to the UVB-irradiated group. Treatment of CP increased the mRNA and protein expression of hyaluronic acid synthases (HAS-1 and -2) with an increased hyaluronic acid production in skin tissue. The expression of hyaluronidase (HYAL-1 and 2) mRNA was downregulated in the CP-treated group. In addition, the protein expression of skin-hydrating factors, filaggrin and involucrin, was upregulated via oral administration of CP.[24]
+++++	Telogen effluvium	One group of women received a syrup for the first month and a tablet while other group received placebo for the following 5 months. The syrup was composed of hydrolyzed collagen (8 g), vitamin B5, vitamin B6, and zinc sulfate and tablet was composed of hydrolyzed collagen (300 mg), B-vitamins, L-cystine (100 mg), L-methionine (50 mg), ferric pyrophosphate, zinc sulfate, sodium selenite, and hyaluronic acid (10 mg)	The highest increase in the percentage of hairs in anagen phase was observed with the sequential combination treatment. The treatment of both nutritional supplements in combination with telogen effluvium showed the highest improvement with a reduction of the telogen phase.[25]
+++++	Thinning hair	Subjects received a supplement containing AminoMar, composed of a proprietary blend of shark powder and mollusk powder, and horsetail which contains a naturally occurring form of silica, acerola cherry which provides vitamin C, biotin, and zinc for 6 months	The hair shedding was reduced in the first 3–6 months of daily consumption of the supplement compared to placebo. The phototrichogram image analysis revealed an increase in the mean vellus-like hair diameter after 6 months of supplement consumption when compared to placebo.[26]

▶ **CLINICAL CONDITIONS** *(Continued)*

EVIDENCE LEVEL	CONDITION OR USE CASE	DOSAGE	BENEFIT OR MECHANISM OF ACTION
+++	Hair thinning	Subjects received a tablet containing vitamin C, zinc, AminoMar™ Marine Complex (shark powder and mollusk powder) 452.9 mg, horsetail (stem) extract 24.5 mg, and flax seed extract 50 mg or placebo for 6 months	After 180 days, there was increase in total hair count, total hair density, and terminal hair density. The investigator assessments revealed improvements in terminal and vellus hair count and terminal hair density. Fewer hair were removed in hair pull test as results were lower for treatment versus placebo after 90 and 180 days. Subjects reported overall improvement in their quality of life.
+++++	Hair growth in temporary thinning hair	Marine protein supplement (MPS) containing AminoMar, a marine complex (composed of a proprietary blend of shark powder and mollusk powder), *Equisetum arvense* species (horsetail which contains a naturally occurring form of silica), malpighia glabra, biotin, and zinc given twice daily for 90 days.	There was a increase in the mean number of terminal hairs and vellus hairs in treatment group compared to placebo. Hair shedding counts decreased in the MPS subjects, and higher total scores than placebo were obtained on the Self-assessment Questionnaire and Quality of Life Questionnaire.
+++	Atopic dermatitis	Subjects either received 3.9 g of a collagen tripeptide (CTP) or normal collagen peptides (CP) daily for 12 weeks.	The eruption area, severity scoring of atopic dermatitis (SCORAD), and TEWL at week 12 were reduced compared to baseline in the CTP but not CP group. There was a reduction in the serum thymus- and activation-regulated chemokine (TARC, inflammatory cytokines and chemokines) level only in the CTP group at week 12.[27]
+++++	Cellulitis	Normal and overweight women received daily dosage of 2.5 g collagen bioactive peptide or a placebo for 6 months	The treatment led to a decrease in the degree of cellulite and a reduced skin waviness on thighs in normal weight women. The dermal density was improved compared to placebo. The efficacy of treatment was also confirmed in overweight women, but the impact was less pronounced than normal weight women.[28]

▶ SUPPLEMENTATION

	BASIS	**WHAT TO LOOK OUT FOR**
Supplement form	Collagen is an animal protein. Therefore, there is no vegetarian source commercially available. Vegetarian collagen products are amino acids or collagen builders/boosters. The animal source or collagen type (I, II or III) don't likely affect efficacy. Collagen type I, II and III are very similar in their amino acid composition. Moreover, their structure is broken during hydrolysis, leaving only the peptides of the amino acids. Similarly, the animal source is relevant only in case of an allergy.	The source of collagen peptides is mentioned in the ingredients section of the product packaging. If not, it is normally from a bovine source.
Administration format	Powder, capsule, liquid As per studies, a 5 g dose of hydrolyzed collagen per day is found to be effective for improving skin, hair and nail parameters.	Powders normally provide the 5 g required dose for promoting skin, hair and nail health.
Purity considerations	Molecular weight: Presence of di- and tri-peptides of collagen's main amino acids (glycine, proline and hydroxyproline) is dependent on the average molecular weight of the hydrolyzed collagen peptides. Molecular weight ≤ 8 kDa has high amounts of di- and tri-peptides. Higher the amounts of di- and tri-peptides, higher is the bioactivity.	The product does not normally state the average molecular weight of collagen peptides on the packaging. This information can be obtained from the manufacturer, with a report of the same.
Patients consideration	Some collagen peptide supplements may not have a palatable taste.	Flavored collagen peptides can be used to mask the taste. Some high grade collagen peptides (made without solvents) can have a mild taste profile, so unflavoured variants can be added to beverages.
Safety consideration	Fish is recognized as one of the big eight allergens.	Bovine or poultry collagen can be used for those with fish allergies.

INTRODUCTION

Collagen is an ubiquitous animal protein, making up 30% of our body's protein and specifically 70–75% of skin's matrix. Various types of collagen exist, and contain at least one triple-helical domain. Collagens play structural roles and contribute to mechanical properties, organization, and shape of tissues. They interact with cells via several receptors and regulate their proliferation, migration, and differentiation. The abundance of the amino acids, glycine, proline and hydroxyproline, is a hallmark feature shared by members of this protein superfamily.[29]

In order to make collagen peptide supplements, collagen from animals is hydrolyzed into peptides to produce both oligopeptides (2–20 amino acids) and polypeptides (>20 amino acids).[1] A lower average molecular weight (MW) implies that the supplement has a larger amount of di- and tri-peptides, which are desirable due to their intact absorption in the peptide form.[30,31]

Collagen peptide supplements are mainly used for anti-aging purposes. UV radiation can increase reactive oxygen species (ROS) and activate matrix metalloproteinases (MMPs) that degrade extracellular matrix, resulting in damage to skin's cells and the collagenous matrix. Normally, ROS are effectively eliminated by innate antioxidant defence systems, such as antioxidant enzymes and nonenzymatic factors. However, the balance between the generation and elimination of ROS is increasingly destabilized as we age (leading to signs of aging) or under pathological conditions. Collagen hydrolysates or collagen peptide supplements are used to restore this balance by promoting the production of skin's matrix.

DIGESTION, ABSORPTION AND STORAGE

Digestion and Absorption

- Collagen peptides are often believed to be broken down into single amino acids, just like other protein. However, this is not entirely the case and dependant on the average MW of the peptides. Di- and tri-peptides are absorbed intact as digestive enzymes cannot specifically cleave hydroxyproline residues (Hyp) residues.[30,31] This has been shown by the presence of Hyp-containing di- and tri-peptides in human blood shortly after oral consumption.[32,33]

- They are transported across the intestinal epithelium via PEPT-1 peptides transporter, as well as by other passive transport mechanisms.[8,34,35]

- Hyp-containing peptides in plasma have shown to reach a peak level 0.5–2 hours after ingestion.[32,33]

- Animal studies with radiolabeled collagen peptides have shown peptides are delivered to tissue like bone, joints, liver, kidney and skin.[36,37]

Storage

Collagen peptides have shown to stay in the skin for up to 14 days.[36] They are possibly integrated into newly synthesized matrix or metabolized by the body.

MECHANISM OF ACTION

01 | Promoting Matrix Protein Synthesis

The amino acids that make up matrix proteins are acquired from our diet. Collagen peptides can provide the building blocks of collagen to fibroblasts. However, research suggests they can also trigger signal cascades (summarized in **Figure 1**), which can act as ligands to cell receptors and stimulate the synthesis of matrix components like collagen, elastin[38] and glycosaminoglycans like hyaluronic acid.[39] That's why these peptides are referred to as 'bioactive'.

Collagen peptides are believed to be perceived by fibroblasts as peptides produced from collagen degradation. This sends a deceptive signal in fibroblasts to synthesize new collagen fibers.[40] Furthermore, collagen peptides possess chemotactic properties, which can promote cell migration and proliferation, important processes in wound healing.[41,42]

Collagen peptides can also protect skin from photoaging. TGF-β/Smad and MAPK signaling regulate collagen synthesis in the dermis and also participate in the photoaging process. For example, UV exposure can interfere with the TGF-β/Smad signaling pathway and inhibit the synthesis of type I collagen.[43] UV can also induce the activation of NF-κB, PTEN/PKB, Hh and Wnt pathways, thereby causing photoaging, which may also be involved in the metabolism of collagen. Collagen peptides ameliorate photoaging skin by mediating these signaling pathways in mechanisms that are still being elucidated.[43]

02 | Inhibiting Enzymes

Matrix metalloproteinases are involved in the degradation process of the skin's matrix. For example, MMP-1 can degrade type I and type III collagen in the skin.[43] As shown in **Figure 1**, MMPs are upregulated by UV via MAPK-mediated activation of activator protein 1 (AP-1). Collagen peptides may reduce MMPs via this pathway.[44] This is consistent with collagen-peptide containing supplements reducing MMP expression in human, animal and in vitro models.[10,38,45]

Tyrosinase is the key enzyme of melanin formation, which can gradually transform tyrosine into melanin. Amino acids in collagen peptides can combine with the active part of tyrosinase leading to decreased tyrosinase activity. There are other possible mechanisms, which may involve MAPK and cyclic adenosine monophosphate (cAMP).[43] A reduction in hyperpigmentation has also been shown by supplements containing collagen peptides.[7]

03 | Reducing TEWL

By repairing skin's matrix, collagen peptides may be increasing skin's water holding capacity. The increase in hyaluronic acid synthesis may also contribute to reducing TEWL. Finally, amino acids in collagen peptides, and protein alike, can provide components of increase natural moisturizing factor (NMF).[43]

04 | Increasing Antioxidant Activity

Collagen peptides have the ability to scavenge excess free radicals. Some studies suggest that MW is the main factor for determining antioxidant capacity of collagen peptides, with smaller peptides (until 1400 Da) being more effective as they can expose more electronic donors.[46,47] They have also shown to increase the activity of antioxidant enzymes like superoxide dismutase (SOD), catalase (CAT), glutathione peroxidase (GSH-Px), and glutathione reductase (GSH-Rx).[48-50]

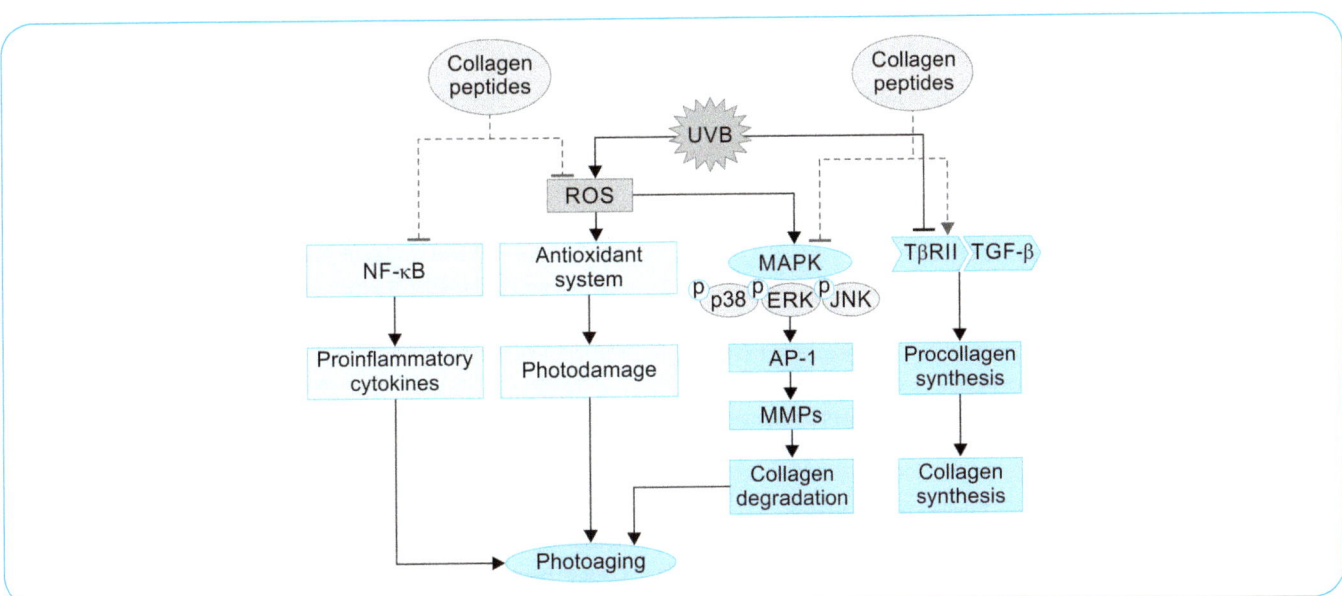

Figure 1: The protective mechanism of collagen peptides on UVB-induced photoaging skin. In addition to the above pathways, PTEN/PKB, Hh and Wnt pathways may also be involved in photoaging.
Source: Adapted from Li (2013).[47]

REFERENCES

1. Zhao X, Zhang X, Liu D. Collagen peptides and the related synthetic peptides: A review on improving skin health. Journal of Functional Foods. 2021;86:104680.
2. Hourblin V, Nouveau S, Roy N, de Lacharrière O. Skin complexion and pigmentary disorders in facial skin of 1204 women in 4 Indian cities. Indian J Dermatol Venereol Leprol. 2014;80(5):395-401.
3. Shome D, Vadera S, Khare S, Ram MS, Ayyar A, Kapoor R, et al. Aging and the Indian Face: An Analytical Study of Aging in the Asian Indian Face. Plast Reconstr Surg Glob Open. 2020;8(3):e2580.
4. León-López A, Morales-Peñaloza A, Martínez-Juárez VM, Vargas-Torres A, Zeugolis DI, Aguirre-Álvarez G. Hydrolyzed Collagen—Sources and Applications. Molecules. 2019;24(22):4031.
5. Paul C, Leser S, Oesser S. Significant Amounts of Functional Collagen Peptides Can Be Incorporated in the Diet While Maintaining Indispensable Amino Acid Balance. Nutrients. 2019;11(5):1079.
6. Choi FD, Sung CT, Juhasz MLW, Mesinkovsk NA. Oral Collagen Supplementation: A Systematic Review of Dermatological Applications. J Drugs Dermatol. 2019;18(1):9-16.
7. Motwani MS, Khan K, Pai A, Joshi R. Efficacy of a collagen hydrolysate and antioxidants-containing nutraceutical on metrics of skin health in Indian women. Journal of Cosmetic Dermatology. 2020;19(12):3371-82.
8. Asserin J, Lati E, Shioya T, Prawitt J. The effect of oral collagen peptide supplementation on skin moisture and the dermal collagen network: evidence from an ex vivo model and randomized, placebo-controlled clinical trials. Journal of Cosmetic Dermatology. 2015;14(4):291-301.
9. De Luca, Chiara, et al. "Skin Antiageing and Systemic Redox Effects of Supplementation with Marine Collagen Peptides and Plant-Derived Antioxidants: A Single-Blind Case-Control Clinical Study." Oxidative Medicine and Cellular Longevity, vol. 2016, 2016, p. 4389410. doi:10.1155/2016/4389410.
10. Yoon H-S, Cho HH, Cho S, Lee S-R, Shin M-H, Chung JH. Supplementing with Dietary Astaxanthin Combined with Collagen Hydrolysate Improves Facial Elasticity and Decreases Matrix Metalloproteinase-1 and -12 Expression: A Comparative Study with Placebo. Journal of medicinal food. 2014;17(7):810-6.
11. Bolke L, Schlippe G, Gerß J, Voss W. A Collagen Supplement Improves Skin Hydration, Elasticity, Roughness, and Density: Results of a Randomized, Placebo-Controlled, Blind Study. Nutrients. 2019;11(10):2494.
12. Kim DU, Chung HC, Choi J, Sakai Y, Lee BY. Oral Intake of Low-Molecular-Weight Collagen Peptide Improves Hydration, Elasticity, and Wrinkling in Human Skin: A Randomized, Double-Blind, Placebo-Controlled Study. Nutrients. 2018;10(7):826.
13. Proksch E, Segger D, Degwert J, Schunck M, Zague V, Oesser S. Oral supplementation of specific collagen peptides has beneficial effects on human skin physiology: a double-blind, placebo-controlled study. Skin Pharmacol Physiol. 2014;27(1):47-55.
14. Evans M, Lewis ED, Zakaria N, Pelipyagina T, Guthrie N. A randomized, triple-blind, placebo-controlled, parallel study to evaluate the efficacy of a freshwater marine collagen on skin wrinkles and elasticity. J Cosmet Dermatol. 2021;20(3):825-34.
15. Laing S, Bielfeldt S, Ehrenberg C, Wilhelm KP. A Dermonutrient Containing Special Collagen Peptides Improves Skin Structure and Function: A Randomized, Placebo-Controlled, Triple-Blind Trial Using Confocal Laser Scanning Microscopy on the Cosmetic Effects and Tolerance of a Drinkable Collagen Supplement. J Med Food. 2020;23(2):147-52.
16. Czajka A, Kania EM, Genovese L, Corbo A, Merone G, Luci C, et al. Daily oral supplementation with collagen peptides combined with vitamins and other bioactive compounds improves skin elasticity and has a beneficial effect on joint and general wellbeing. Nutr Res. 2018;57:97-108.
17. Genovese L, Corbo A, Sibilla S. An Insight into the Changes in Skin Texture and Properties following Dietary Intervention with a Nutricosmeceutical Containing a Blend of Collagen Bioactive Peptides and Antioxidants. Skin Pharmacology and Physiology. 2017;30(3):146-58.
18. Ito N, Seki S, Ueda F. Effects of Composite Supplement Containing Collagen Peptide and Ornithine on Skin Conditions and Plasma IGF-1 Levels—A Randomized, Double-Blind, Placebo-Controlled Trial. Mar Drugs. 2018;16(12):482.
19. Bianchi FM, Angelinetta C, Rizzi G, Praticò A, Villa R. Evaluation of the Efficacy of a Hydrolyzed Collagen Supplement for Improving Skin Moisturization, Smoothness, and Wrinkles. J Clin Aesthet Dermatol. 2022;15(3):48-52.
20. Žmitek K, Žmitek J, Rogl Butina M, Pogačnik T. Effects of a Combination of Water-Soluble Coenzyme Q10 and Collagen on Skin Parameters and Condition: Results of a Randomised, Placebo-Controlled, Double-Blind Study. Nutrients. 2020;12(3):618.
21. Inoue N, Sugihara F, Wang X. Ingestion of bioactive collagen hydrolysates enhance facial skin moisture and elasticity and reduce facial ageing signs in a randomised double-blind placebo-controlled clinical study. J Sci Food Agric. 2016;96(12):4077-81.
22. Schwartz SR, Park J. Ingestion of BioCell Collagen®, a novel hydrolyzed chicken sternal cartilage extract; enhanced blood microcirculation and reduced facial aging signs. Clin Interv Aging. 2012;7:267-73.
23. Maia Campos PMBG, Melo MO, Siqueira César FC. Topical application and oral supplementation of peptides in the improvement of skin viscoelasticity and density. J Cosmet Dermatol. 2019;18(6):1693-9.
24. Kang MC, Yumnam S, Kim SY. Oral Intake of Collagen Peptide Attenuates Ultraviolet B Irradiation-Induced Skin Dehydration In Vivo by Regulating Hyaluronic Acid Synthesis. International Journal of Molecular Sciences. 2018;19(11).
25. Arias EM, Floriach N, Moreno-Arias G, Camps A, Arias S, Trüeb RM. Targeted Nutritional Supplementation for Telogen Effluvium: Multicenter Study on Efficacy of a Hydrolyzed Collagen, Vitamin-, and Mineral-Based Induction and Maintenance Treatment. Int J Trichology. 2022 Mar-Apr;14(2):49-54.
26. Rizer RL, Stephens TJ, Herndon JH, Sperber BR, Murphy J, Ablon GR. A Marine Protein-based 8Dietary Supplement for Subclinical Hair Thinning/Loss: Results of a Multisite, Double-blind, Placebo-controlled Clinical Trial. Int J Trichology. 2015;7(4):156-66.
27. Hakuta A, Yamaguchi Y, Okawa T, Yamamoto S, Sakai Y, Aihara M. Anti-inflammatory effect of collagen tripeptide in atopic dermatitis. J Dermatol Sci. 2017;88(3):357-64.
28. Schunck M, Zague V, Oesser S, Proksch E. Dietary Supplementation with Specific Collagen Peptides Has a Body Mass Index-Dependent Beneficial Effect on Cellulite Morphology. J Med Food. 2015;18(12):1340-8.
29. Ricard-Blum S. The Collagen Family. Cold Spring Harb Perspect Biol. 2011;3(1):a004978.

30. Muhammad MA, Trajkovic S, Brayden DJ, Measuring the oral bioavailability of protein hydrolysates derived from food sources: A critical review of current bioassays. Biomedicine & Pharmacotherapy. 2021;144:112275.
31. Hong H, Fan H, Chalamaiah M, Wu J. Preparation of low-molecular-weight, collagen hydrolysates (peptides): Current progress, challenges, and future perspectives. Food Chem. 2019;301:125222.
32. Iwai K, Hasegawa T, Taguchi Y, Morimatsu F, Sato K, Nakamura Y, et al. Identification of food-derived collagen peptides in human blood after oral ingestion of gelatin hydrolysates. J Agric Food Chem. 2005;53(16):6531-6.
33. Ohara H, Matsumoto H, Ito K, Iwai K, Sato K. Comparison of quantity and structures of hydroxyproline-containing peptides in human blood after oral ingestion of gelatin hydrolysates from different sources. J Agric Food Chem. 2007;55(4):1532-5.
34. Aito-Inoue M, Lackeyram D, Fan MZ, Sato K, Mine Y. Transport of a tripeptide, Gly-Pro-Hyp, across the porcine intestinal brush-border membrane. J Pept Sci. 2007;13(7):468-74.
35. Sun X, Acquah C, Aluko R, Udenigwe C. Considering food matrix and gastrointestinal effects in enhancing bioactive peptide absorption and bioavailability. Journal of Functional Foods. 2020;64:103680.
36. Watanabe-Kamiyama M, Shimizu M, Kamiyama S, Taguchi Y, Sone H, Morimatsu F, et al. Absorption and effectiveness of orally administered low molecular weight collagen hydrolysate in rats. J Agric Food Chem. 2010;58(2):835-41.
37. Oesser S, Adam M, Babel W, Seifert J. Oral Administration of 14C Labeled Gelatin Hydrolysate Leads to an Accumulation of Radioactivity in Cartilage of Mice (C57/BL). The Journal of Nutrition. 1999;129(10):1891-5.
38. Edgar S, Hopley B, Genovese L, Sibilla S, Laight D, Shute J. Effects of collagen-derived bioactive peptides and natural antioxidant compounds on proliferation and matrix protein synthesis by cultured normal human dermal fibroblasts. Sci Rep. 2018;8(1):10474.
39. Ohara H, Ichikawa S, Matsumoto H, Akiyama M, Fujimoto N, Kobayashi T, et al. Collagen-derived dipeptide, proline-hydroxyproline, stimulates cell proliferation and hyaluronic acid synthesis in cultured human dermal fibroblasts. J Dermatol. 2010;37(4):330-8.
40. Sato K, Jimi S, Kusubata M. Generation of bioactive prolyl-hydroxyproline (Pro-Hyp) by oral administration of collagen hydrolysate and degradation of endogenous collagen. International Journal of Food Science & Technology. 2019;54(6):1976-80.
41. Banerjee P, Suguna L, Shanthi C. Wound healing activity of a collagen-derived cryptic peptide. Amino Acids. 2015;47(2):317-28.
42. Woonnoi W, Chotphruethipong L, Tanasawet S, Benjakul S, Sutthiwong N, Sukketsiri W. Hydrolyzed Collagen from Salmon Skin Increases the Migration and Filopodia Formation of Skin Keratinocytes by Activation of FAK/Src Pathway. Polish Journal of Food and Nutrition Sciences. 2021;71:323-32.
43. Chongyang Li, Yu F, Hongjie D, Wang Z, Gao R, Zhang Y. Recent progress in preventive effect of collagen peptides on photoaging skin and action mechanism. Food Science and Human Wellness. 2022;11(2):218-29.
44. Lu J, Hu Hou, Yan Fan, Yang T. Identification of MMP-1 inhibitory peptides from cod skin gelatin hydrolysates and the inhibition mechanism by MAPK signaling pathway. Journal of Functional Foods. 2017;33:251-60.
45. Zague V, de Freitas V, da Costa Rosa M, de Castro GÁ, Jaeger RG, Machado-Santelli GM. Collagen hydrolysate intake increases skin collagen expression and suppresses matrix metalloproteinase 2 activity. J Med Food. 2011;14(6):618-24.
46. Chi CF, Cao ZH, Wang B, Hu FY, Li ZR, Zhang B. Antioxidant and Functional Properties of Collagen Hydrolysates from Spanish Mackerel Skin as Influenced by Average Molecular Weight. Molecules. 2014;19(8):11211-30.
47. Li Z-R, Wang B, Chi C, Gong Y. Influence of average molecular weight on antioxidant and functional properties of cartilage collagen hydrolysates from Sphyrna lewini, Dasyatis akjei and Raja porosa. Food Research International. 2013;51(1):283-93.
48. Wang Z, Wang Q, Wang L, Xu W, He Y, Li Y, et al. Improvement of skin condition by oral administration of collagen hydrolysates in chronologically aged mice. J Sci Food Agric. 2017;97(9):2721-6.
49. Tao J, Zhao YQ, Chi CF, Wang B. Bioactive Peptides from Cartilage Protein Hydrolysate of Spotless Smoothhound and Their Antioxidant Activity In Vitro. Mar Drugs. 2018;16(4):100.
50. Zhang L, Zheng Y, Cheng X, Meng M, Luo Y, Li B. The anti-photoaging effect of antioxidant collagen peptides from silver carp (Hypophthalmichthys molitrix) skin is preferable to tea polyphenols and casein peptides. Food Funct. 2017;8(4):1698-707.

Hyaluronic acid

Hyaluronic Acid

✍ Aseem Sharma

CONTENTS

HYALURONIC ACID: NUTRIENT SNAPSHOT

- ▶ REQUIREMENT IN THE INDIAN CONTEXT | **193**
- ▶ ACTIVE FORMS | **194**
- ▶ SAFETY AND DOSAGE | **194**
- ▶ CLINICAL CONDITIONS | **194**
- ▶ SUPPLEMENTATION | **195**

INTRODUCTION | **197**

DIGESTION, ABSORPTION AND STORAGE | **197**

MECHANISM OF ACTION | **197**

KEY TOPICS

- ANTI-AGING
- DRY SKIN
- FACIAL SKIN ESTHETICS
- HAIR AND SKIN QUALITY
- SKIN MOISTURE
- WRINKLES

Nutrient Snapshot

▶ **REQUIREMENT IN THE INDIAN CONTEXT**

- The potential biological effects of extracellular matrix components (peptides or polysaccharides) have attracted attention for applications in skin health and appearance. One such component is hyaluronic acid (HA), a linear nonsulfated glycosaminoglycan. This long, linear polysaccharide is ubiquitous in connective tissue.[1]

- Hygroscopic in nature, HA controls tissue hydration and water transport. It also interacts with cell receptors and participates in cell signaling. These properties are entirely dependent on its chain length or molecular weight (MW).[2]

- The amount of HA in the skin decreases considerably with age. Furthermore, factors like UV light, and dryness, reduce the content of HA in the skin and the water content of the stratum corneum is decreased, leading to the formation of wrinkles and skin aging.[3] A study reported the HA content in the skin of individuals aged 75 years was less than a quarter of that measured in persons aged 19 years.[3,4]

- In dermatology, HA is often used in topical and injectable formulations to reduce the signs of aging. Due to its safety profile, HA is also becoming popular as a supplement, where some formulations have shown improvements in wrinkles, skin hydration and elasticity.[3,5] Whether all biological properties of endogenous HA will transcend to orally administered HA, and in which forms, is still under investigation. This will come to light as we understand more about HA and its functionally diverse chains. In the meantime, it is reasonable to assume that its benefits are ingredient-specific or MW-specific.

▶ ACTIVE FORMS

ACTIVE FORMS	SUPPLEMENT SOURCES	SALIENT FEATURES
Hyaluronic acid (HA)	Bacterial fermentation, chicken combs, synthetic	Exogenous HA obtained mainly by microbial fermentation (bio-HA) is structurally identical to the endogenous HA.[6]

▶ SAFETY AND DOSAGE

GENERAL REQUIREMENTS	
Indian recommendations	N/A
Global recommendations and limits	NOAEL: 48 mg/kg body weight/day.[5] Higher NOAEL's have been reported but the MW is unknown.[5,7]
Side effects	HA is well-tolerated, no known adverse effects found in the literature.
	Lowest recommended dose for skin health is 120 mg/day.
Notes:	Studies suggest that both high and low MW ingested HA are transferred to skin.[5] High-molecular-weight (HMW; >2000 kDa) and low-molecular-weight (LMW; <200 kDa), forms of HA have been reported to exhibit distinct biological effects, which may be mediated by their unique bindings with CD44 receptors. In vivo studies have shown that HMW-HA exhibits anti-inflammatory effects by inhibiting cell proliferation and mobility while, LMW-HA has been observed to stimulate cell proliferation and mobility, thus resulting in proinflammatory effects.[8-11]

▶ CLINICAL CONDITIONS

EVIDENCE LEVEL	CONDITION OR USE CASE	DOSAGE	BENEFIT OR MECHANISM OF ACTION
+++++	Dry skin and wrinkles	HA 120 mg/day or placebo for 12 weeks	There was significant improvement in wrinkles, stratum corneum water content, transepidermal water loss (TEWL) and skin elasticity in the treatment group versus the placebo group.[3]
+++++	Skin moisturizing	N/A (meta-analysis)	Meta-analysis shows that oral HA is proven to be effective in skin moisturizing.[12]
+++++	Wrinkles	120 mg of HA with MW 2 kDa or 300 kDa for 12 weeks	After 8 weeks, the 300 kDa group showed significantly diminished wrinkles compared to placebo. Skin luster and suppleness significantly improved after 12 weeks in both the MW groups.[13]

▶ CLINICAL CONDITIONS (Continued)

EVIDENCE LEVEL	CONDITION OR USE CASE	DOSAGE	BENEFIT OR MECHANISM OF ACTION
+++++	Dry skin	120 mg of HA with MW 300 kDa or 800 kDa or placebo for 6 weeks	The skin moisture content of the treatment groups increased more than those of the placebo group during the entire ingestion period. The group receiving 300 kDa of HA exhibited significant improvements in skin moisture content 2 weeks after ingestion ended compared to the placebo. A questionnaire survey method was done to evaluate subjective facial aging symptoms (wrinkles, skin luster and suppleness) which showed significant improvement in skin condition.[14]
++++	Hair and skin quality	450 mg hydrolyzed eggshell membrane (containing HA) or placebo for 12 weeks	Supplementation improved hair thickness and growth with a reduction in hair breakage from week 4 onwards. It had a positive impact on fine lines and wrinkles at week 4, and skin tone at week 8.[15]
++++	Facial skin esthetics	200 mg HA, 500 mg of L-carnosine, and 400 mg of methylsulfonylmethane or placebo for 60 days	Treatment group saw improvement in glabella skin hydration and elasticity, glabella sebaceous secretion decreased, skin hydration and elasticity increased. Wrinkle depth improved slightly.[16]
+++++	Anti-aging and improvement in skin profile	Food supplement containing biofermented HA (200 mg/day) of different MWs or placebo for 28 days	There was an improvement in skin hydration and protection from dehydration, with a decrease in both wrinkle depth and volume and an increase in elasticity and firmness.[17]

▶ SUPPLEMENTATION

	BASIS	WHAT TO LOOK OUT FOR
Supplemental form	Sodium hyaluronate[18] Potassium hyaluronate HA	The form of HA may not always be stated on the packaging but can be obtained from the product manufacturer.

▶ SUPPLEMENTATION (Continued)

	BASIS	WHAT TO LOOK OUT FOR
Administration form	Capsule, tablet, powders	N/A
Patients consideration	HA supplements should be taken with or after a meal.	N/A
Safety considerations	Patients given up to 200 mg of HA for 1 year for osteoarthritis did not show any side effects.[19] Patients having a history of cancer should be cautious about HA supplementation and should consult their oncologist.[20]	N/A
Other considerations	HA is heat and light sensitive so it is to be stored in dry, cool place, away from sunlight.	Storage conditions mentioned on the packaging should be followed.

INTRODUCTION

Hyaluronic acid serves as a structural component in different tissue and organs. For example, it serves as a lubricant in the synovial fluid of joints, gives jelly-like consistency to the eye and maintains the elastoviscosity of connective tissue, controlling tissue hydration and water transport.[1] Most cells in the body have the capability to synthesize HA during some point of their cell cycles, implicating its function in several fundamental biological processes.[2]

Hyaluronic acid performs its biological functions according to two primary mechanisms: tissue turnover and as a signaling macromolecule. Both mechanisms are dependent on the chain length. The topical use and oral administration of HA may be limited by the size that can be delivered to the site of tissue synthesis.[3]

The gradual inability to produce macromolecules like HA is a hallmark of aging. Studies have reported that oral ingestion of HA shows an improvement in wrinkles, hydration and elasticity.[3] However, this may be ingredient-specific due to the differences in MW affecting biological outcomes.

DIGESTION, ABSORPTION AND STORAGE

Digestion and Absorption

- Animal studies suggest that orally administered HA[20] is 90% absorbed and has an affinity for connective tissue.[21-23]

- High MW HA (300 kDa) has been shown to be distributed to skin by the blood and lymphatic transport systems. Depolymerized HA is absorbed by the gastrointestinal tract while intact HA is absorbed by the lymphatic system.[5,21] Another report suggested that an average MW of 2000 kDa was also absorbed.[22]

- While digestive enzymes do not degrade HA, it can be degraded by intestinal bacteria. This is thought to be a possible step in its absorption and elimination. Further studies need to elucidate the precise absorption mechanism of ingested HA.[5,24]

Storage

- The greatest amount of HA is present in the skin, synovial fluid and the vitreous body. Orally administered HA and its metabolites are possibly integrated into the extracellular matrix of skin and other tissue.[2]

- The metabolic halflife of HA varies from approximately 1.5 days in skin to 2–3 weeks in cartilage.[22]

- HA metabolism and excretion after migration into connective tissue have not been adequately examined.[23]

MECHANISM OF ACTION

Physiological roles of HA are well-characterized in body tissue and fluids. In general, HA is involved in physiological functions (lubrication, hydration balance, matrix structure, and steric interactions).[2]

01 | Skin Hydration

Due to its molecular structure at a neutral pH, HA attracts water molecules and can contain up to 10,000 times its weight in water. In aqueous solution, due to hydrophobic interactions and intermolecular hydrogen bonding, polymeric chains aggregate, with the formation of loose and elastic matrices, which facilitate cell migration.[25]

02 | Cellular Activity

HA is also involved in various cellular interactions (cell differentiation, proliferation, development, and recognition) by interaction between HA and its cell surface receptors, CD44, RHAMM (receptor for hyaluronan-mediated motility), and ICAM-1 (intercellular adhesion molecules-1).[2] HA fragments also bind to some toll-Like receptors (TLRs), which are involved in the activation of innate and adaptive immune responses and also play a role in inflammation.[25]

Orally administered HA is believed to promote cell proliferation. This increase of the cell number is thought to suppresses TEWL by filling the gaps of the skin cells and increasing the amount of HA synthesis by fibroblasts.[5] Therefore, HA may be a useful for wound healing and dry skin, and as a therapeutic agent for conditions like psoriasis and atopic dermatitis, where TEWL is exaggerated.[3,26]

03 | Prebiotic Effect

One theory of how HA exerts its biological effects is as a prebiotic, since it is readily fermented by the bacteria found in the gut microbiome. HA could significantly increase the relative abundance of beneficial bacteria, including those that produce short-chain fatty acids, which can regulate host immunity. Another interesting finding in this mouse model was the increase in the antioxidant, superoxide dismutase. This is possibly the reason for HA's antioxidant and anti-inflammatory effects previously reported. More research is required to understand these effects in humans and the biophysical properties of HA that are responsible for them.[1]

▶ REFERENCES

1. Huang G, Su L, Zhang N, Han R, Leong WK, Li X, et al. The prebiotic and anti-fatigue effects of hyaluronan. Front Nutr. 2022;9:977556.
2. Gupta RC, Lall R, Srivastava A, Sinha A. Hyaluronic Acid: Molecular Mechanisms and Therapeutic Trajectory. Front Vet Sci. 2019;6:192.
3. Hsu TF, Su ZR, Hsieh YH, Wang MF, Oe M, Matsuoka R, et al. Oral Hyaluronan Relieves Wrinkles and Improves Dry Skin: A 12-Week Double-Blinded, Placebo-Controlled Study. Nutrients. 2021;13(7):2220.
4. Longas MO, Russell CS, He XY. Evidence for structural changes in dermatan sulfate and hyaluronic acid with aging. Carbohydr Res. 1987;159(1):127-36.
5. Kawada C, Yoshida T, Yoshida H, Matsuoka R, Sakamoto W, Odanaka W, et al. Ingested hyaluronan moisturizes dry skin. Nutrition Journal. 2014;13:70.
6. Hyaluronic acid behavior in oral administration and perspectives for nanotechnology-based formulations: A review. Carbohydrate Polymers. 2019;222:115001.
7. Oe M, Yoshida T, Kanemitsu T, Matsuoka R, Masuda Y. Repeated 28-day oral toxicological study of hyaluronic acid in rats. 2011;81:11-21.
8. Jensen GS, Attridge VL, Lenninger MR, Benson KF. Oral Intake of a Liquid High-Molecular-Weight Hyaluronan Associated with Relief of Chronic Pain and Reduced Use of Pain Medication: Results of a Randomized, Placebo-Controlled Double-Blind Pilot Study. J Med Food. 2015;18(1):95-101.
9. Cyphert JM, Trempus CS, Garantziotis S. Size Matters: Molecular Weight Specificity of Hyaluronan Effects in Cell Biology. Int J Cell Biol. 2015;2015:563818.
10. Cicero AFG, Girolimetto N, Bentivenga C, Grandi E, Fogacci F, Borghi C. Short-Term Effect of a New Oral Sodium Hyaluronate Formulation on Knee Osteoarthritis: A Double-Blind, Randomized, Placebo-Controlled Clinical Trial. Diseases. 2020;8(3):26.
11. Liu L, Liu Y, Li J, Du G, Chen J. Microbial production of hyaluronic acid: current state, challenges, and perspectives. Microb Cell Fact. 2011;10:99.
12. Sun Q, Wu J, Qian G, Cheng H. Effectiveness of Dietary Supplement for Skin Moisturizing in Healthy Adults: A Systematic Review and Meta-Analysis of Randomized Controlled Trials. Front Nutr. 2022;9:895192.
13. Oe M, Sakai S, Yoshida H, Okado N, Kaneda H, Masuda Y, et al. Oral hyaluronan relieves wrinkles: a double-blinded, placebo-controlled study over a 12-week period. Clin Cosmet Investig Dermatol. 2017;10:267-73.
14. Kawada C, Yoshida T, Yoshida H, Sakamoto W, Odanaka W, Sato T, et al. Ingestion of hyaluronans (molecular weights 800 k and 300 k) improves dry skin conditions: a randomized, double blind, controlled study. J Clin Biochem Nutr. 2015;56(1):66-73.
15. Kalman DS, Hewlings S. The effect of oral hydrolyzed eggshell membrane on the appearance of hair, skin, and nails in healthy middle-aged adults: A randomized double-blind placebo-controlled clinical trial. J Cosmet Dermatol. 2020;19(6):1463-72.
16. Guaitolini E, Cavezzi A, Cocchi S, Colucci R, Urso SU, Quinzi V. Randomized, Placebo-controlled Study of a Nutraceutical Based on Hyaluronic Acid, L-carnosine, and Methylsulfonylmethane in Facial Skin Aesthetics and Well-being. J Clin Aesthet Dermatol. 2019;12(4):40-5.
17. Michelotti A, Cestone E, De Ponti I, Pisati M, Sparta E, Tursi F. Oral intake of a new full-spectrum hyaluronan improves skin profilometry and ageing: a randomized, double-blind, placebo-controlled clinical trial. Eur J Dermatol. 2021;31(6):798-805.
18. Pechová V, Gajdziok J. [Possibilities of using sodium hyaluronate in pharmaceutical and medical fields]. Ceska Slov Farm. 2017;66(4):154-9.
19. Tashiro T, Seino S, Sato T, Matsuoka R, Masuda Y, Fukui N. Oral Administration of Polymer Hyaluronic Acid Alleviates Symptoms of Knee Osteoarthritis: A Double-Blind, Placebo-Controlled Study over a 12-Month Period. ScientificWorldJournal. 2012;2012:167928.
20. Simone P, Alberto M. Caution should be used in long-term treatment with oral compounds of hyaluronic acid in patients with a history of cancer. Clin Drug Investig. 2015;35(11):689-92.
21. Balogh L, Polyak A, Mathe D, Kiraly R, Thuroczy J, Terez M, et al. Absorption, uptake and tissue affinity of high-molecular-weight hyaluronan after oral administration in rats and dogs. J Agric Food Chem. 2008 Nov 26;56(22):10582-93.

22. Sato Y, Joumura T, Takekuma Y, Sugawara M. Transfer of orally administered hyaluronan to the lymph. Eur J Pharm Biopharm. 2020;154:210-3.
23. Oe M, Mitsugi K, Odanaka W, Yoshida H, Matsuoka R, Seino S, et al. Dietary hyaluronic acid migrates into the skin of rats. ScientificWorldJournal. 2014;2014:378024.
24. Kimura M, Maeshima T, Kubota T, Kurihara H, Masuda Y, Nomura Y. Absorption of Orally Administered Hyaluronan. J Med Food. 2016;19(12):1172-9.
25. Marinho A, Nunes C, Reis S. Hyaluronic Acid: A Key Ingredient in the Therapy of Inflammation. Biomolecules. 2021;11(10):1518.
26. How KN, Yap WH, Lim CLH, Goh BH, Lai ZW. Hyaluronic Acid-Mediated Drug Delivery System Targeting for Inflammatory Skin Diseases: A Mini Review. Front Pharmacol. 2020;11.

20

Lactoferrin (LF)

Lactoferrin and Colostrum

✍ Aseem Sharma

CONTENTS

LACTOFERRIN AND COLOSTRUM: NUTRIENT SNAPSHOT

- ▸ REQUIREMENT IN THE INDIAN CONTEXT | **201**
- ▸ ACTIVE FORMS | **202**
- ▸ SAFETY AND DOSAGE | **202**
- ▸ CLINICAL CONDITIONS | **203**
- ▸ SUPPLEMENTATION | **207**

INTRODUCTION | **208**

DIGESTION, ABSORPTION AND STORAGE | **208**

MECHANISM OF ACTION | **208**

KEY TOPICS

- ACNE VULGARIS
- ATOPIC DERMATITIS
- HAIR GROWTH
- PSORIASIS
- SKIN MOISTURE
- SKIN TEXTURE
- SKIN WHITENING/ PIGMENTATION
- TINEA PEDIS (ATHLETE'S FOOT)
- WOUND HEALING

Nutrient Snapshot

▶ **REQUIREMENT IN THE INDIAN CONTEXT**

- Lactoferrin (LF), also known as lactotransferrin, an iron-binding multifunctional glycoprotein. It is present in most biological secretions and reaches particularly high concentrations in colostrum and breast milk.[1]

- LF belongs to the transferrin family of glycoproteins. As the name suggests (lacto + ferrin = milk + iron), is an iron binding milk protein, which helps to balance iron levels in the body.[1] A key function of LF is considered to be a mediator linking innate and adaptive immune responses.[2]

- As a component of whey protein from milk, LF can be acquired from our diet. A glass of cow's milk has an estimated 25–75 mg of LF, whereas clinical doses are upwards of 100 mg.

- A lot of research is based on dietary bovine LF, which is 70% similar to human LF.[3] Since many functions of LF (such as the ability to bind iron) are highly dependent on the integrity of the protein structure, boiling milk and its gastrointestinal digestion may cause a loss of some of its properties.[1,2]

- Having said that, there is encouraging evidence to suggest that LF supplementation, possibly through the peptides produced, may be beneficial in acne, psoriasis, and diabetic ulcerations.[4] Low levels of lactoferrin have been reported in chronic telogen effluvium as well.[5] Upcoming studies also suggest that colostrum, rich in LF, growth factors and other bioactive components may help reduce skin aging.[6]

▶ ACTIVE FORMS

ACTIVE FORMS	SUPPLEMENT SOURCES	SALIENT FEATURES
Lactoferrin[7]	Bovine milk and colostrum	Bovine LF is GRAS approved by US FDA for infant formula.[8]
	Recombinant human lactoferrin	According to a study, bovine LF appears to be more resistant to degradation in human adults than human lactoferrin, suggesting that human LF is "designed" to be ingested orally only during infancy.[9]
	Camel, goat, sheep milk	These are not easily available in the market.
Colostrum	Bovine milk	Other than LF, colostrum contains immunoglobulins and growth factors. Their heterogeneity may lead to varied effects, as their composition is not standadized.

▶ SAFETY AND DOSAGE

GENERAL REQUIREMENTS	
Indian recommendations	N/A
Global recommendations and limits	NOAEL (apo-recombinant human lactoferrin): >1,800 mg/kg/day.[10] NOAEL (holo-recombinant human lactoferrin): >1,000 mg/kg/day.[11] Another study suggested 2,000 mg/kg/day for both sexes at which no adverse effect of bovine LF was observed.[12]
Notes:	Bovine LF is well-tolerated and safe for consumption. LF has been shown to improve dermatosis such as tinea pedis, acne vulgaris, plaque psoriasis, and atopic dermatitis. It may also be useful for diabetic wound healing.[13,14] Colostrum can vary significantly in the amount of LF and immunoglobulins it contains, as their levels are affected by animal species, time of collection, and temperature amongst others. While commercial producers may differentiate their products on the basis of IgG content or by specifying the collection time for the colostrum, no specific standards exist. This heterogeneity may be responsible for conflicting data on its effects.[13,15]

▶ CLINICAL CONDITIONS

EVIDENCE LEVEL	CONDITION OR USE CASE	DOSAGE	BENEFIT OR MECHANISM OF ACTION
++	Hair growth	In vitro tissue culture incubated with biotin labelled bovine LF, followed by topical application on mice	The bovine LF promoted the proliferation of dermal papillae cells and enhanced the phosphorylation of Erk and Akt (two major controllers of cell proliferation). LF stimulated hair growth in both young and aged mice when applied topically. It also induced the expression of Wnt signaling-related proteins, including Wnt3a, Wnt7a, Lef1, and β-catenin (which play a critical role in normal hair follicle development and cycling).[16]
+++	Acne vulgaris	Fermented milk with/without 200 mg of LF daily for 12 weeks	Acne showed improvement in the LF group by decreasing inflammatory lesion count, total lesion count, and acne grade compared to placebo at week 12. The sebum content in the LF group was decreased compared to placebo. The amount of total skin surface lipids decreased in both groups. The amount of free fatty acids decreased in both the groups while triacylglycerol amounts were only decreased in LF group. The latter was correlated with decreases in serum content, acne lesion counts, and acne grade.[17]

▶ CLINICAL CONDITIONS (Continued)

EVIDENCE LEVEL	CONDITION OR USE CASE	DOSAGE	BENEFIT OR MECHANISM OF ACTION
+++	Acne vulgaris	A chewable tablet formulation of bovine LF twice daily for 8 weeks	There was a mean reduction in inflammatory lesion count, in non-inflammatory lesion count, and in total lesion count as compared with baseline.[18]
+++++	Acne vulgaris	Subjects either received a capsule containing 100 mg LF with 11 IU vitamin E and 5 mg zinc or a placebo twice a day for 3 months.	The LF group showed a reduction in total lesions as early as 2 weeks, with the maximum reduction occurring at week 10 compared to the placebo. Maximum reduction in comedones and inflammatory lesions was also seen at week 10 compared to the placebo. Sebum scores were improved by week 12.[19]
++	Acne vulgaris	Human keratinocytes were induced by heat-killed Propionibacterium acne and then was treated with LF in vitro, followed by injection of P. acnes in mice ears	The expression of proinflammatory cytokines IL-8 increased after induction of cells by heat-killed P. acnes, but it decreased significantly after LF treatment. The injection of active P. acnes into the ear skin of mice resulted in increased IL-8 expression in the acne model. The expression of IL-8, decreased with LF treatment. The levels of TLR2 (proinflammatory cytokines), nuclear factor kappa B (NFkB) and intercellular cell adhesion molecule 1 protein were induced by P. acnes in cells, and the results showed that the levels were inhibited by LF.[20]

▶ CLINICAL CONDITIONS (Continued)

EVIDENCE LEVEL	CONDITION OR USE CASE	DOSAGE	BENEFIT OR MECHANISM OF ACTION
+++++	Skin texture and moisture	Subjects received 6 tablets daily containing either a placebo, 200 mg or 600 mg of LF for 12 weeks	Changes in the scores of moisture were greater in the 200 mg and 600 mg groups, and of texture were greater in the 600 mg group than in the placebo group.[21]
+++	Tinea pedis (Athlete's foot)	Individuals predicted to have mild-to-moderate tinea pedis were given either 600 mg or 2,000 mg of LF, or a placebo daily for 8 weeks	The dermatological symptom scores in all groups decreased but the differences were not significant. For subjects with moderate vesicular or interdigital tinea pedis, dermatological symptom scores in the LF groups decreased in comparison with placebo. A mycological (fungal) cure was not seen in any of the subjects.[22]
++++	Atopic dermatitis	Patients consumed a tablet daily containing 250 mg bovine whey-derived LF +250 mg bovine whey-derived Ig-rich fraction or placebo for 56 days.	There were more cases of a reduction in the SCORAD (SCORing of Atopic Dermatitis) index from severe-to-moderate or mild or from moderate-to-mild in the LF+Ig group compared to placebo. Improvements were also seen in the Dermatology Life Quality Index (DLQI) score.[23]

▶ **CLINICAL CONDITIONS** (*Continued*)

EVIDENCE LEVEL	CONDITION OR USE CASE	DOSAGE	BENEFIT OR MECHANISM OF ACTION
++	Skin whitening/pigmentation	Bovine LF was studied on melanin-producing cell in vitro	There was a 20% reduction in pigmentation. There was dose-dependent suppression of melanin production. There was a downregulation of the microphthalmia-associated transcription factor (MITF), leading to the suppression of tyrosinase activity.[24]
+++	Psoriasis	5 g of oral XP-828L (nutraceutical compound obtained by the extraction of a growth factors-enriched protein fraction from bovine milk) twice daily for 56 days.	At day 28, 6 of the 11 patients showed a reduction in PASI score (psoriasis area-and-severity index). At 56 days, 7 subjects had a decrease in PASI score. 8 out of 11 patients agreed to participate in an additional 8-week extension treatment phase, during which the improvement of psoriasis was maintained.[25]
++	Wound healing	Human epidermal keratinocytes from neonatal foreskin were treated with rice-derived recombinant human LF (holo-rhLF) for 7 days	Holo-rhLF showed strong migration-promoting effects on keratinocytes. With cells under starvation or exposure to the tumor promoter called TPA, the addition of holo-rhLF greatly increased cell viability and inhibited cell apoptosis.[26]

▶ SUPPLEMENTATION

	BASIS	WHAT TO LOOK OUT FOR
Supplementation form	Apo-LF (without bound iron) Holo-LF (with bound iron)[27] Microparticles LF Liposomal LF As LF is susceptible to peptic digestion, the liposomal form has shown to improve stability.[28]	The form of LF may not be stated on the label but the information can be obtained from the product manufacturer.
Administration form	Capsules or tablets	N/A
Purity considerations	Purity may vary depending on the source.[29] This is especially true for colostrum.	The packaging normally states the amount of LF in the product.
Patient considerations	It is recommended to take bovine LF before meals so as to avoid its gastric degradation due to very low pH during digestion. Patients with an allergy to dairy can consider taking a recombinant human LF.[9] However, liposomal forms may be better absorbed with a meal. Those who are lactose intolerant may be able to tolerate LF, but not colostrum as the latter contains lactose.	The instructions for administration are usually be mentioned on the packaging. The manufacturer can often provide a test report for the quantification of lactose.
Safety considerations	Human studies did not record any adverse effects due to intake of bovine LF. Milk is considered an allergen (one of the big 8 allergens), and those allergic to it should avoid it.	Patients with an allergy to dairy should consult a doctor before taking LF supplement.

▶ **INTRODUCTION**

Belonging to the transferrin family of glycoproteins, LF has multifaceted effects on the body, not all mechanisms of which have been thoroughly investigated yet, which is why it is referred to as a multipotent protein. This is possible because LF can occur in many variants.

LF is produced by mucosal epithelial cells and is present in most biological fluids. The presence of LF has been confirmed in kidneys, lungs, gallbladder, pancreas, intestine, liver, prostate, saliva, tears, sperm, cerebrospinal fluid, urine, bronchial secretions, vaginal discharge, synovial fluid, umbilical cord blood, blood plasma, and cells of the immune system.[1]

LF is present in significant amounts in polymorphonuclear granules, and its net positive charge and distribution in various tissue allows it to play a role in several physiological processes. These include regulation of iron absorption in the bowel, immune response, as well as antimicrobial, antioxidant, anticarcinogenic, and anti-inflammatory processes.

Given its antibacterial and anti-inflammatory action, LF supplementation has beneficial effects on acne severity. However, the concern of whey protein worsening acne is often raised as any increase in IGF-1 levels attributable to milk ingestion may counteract the benefit.[30] While there is little evidence to back up the whey-acne connection, there is considerable evidence to suggest LF supplementation helps manage acne.

▶ **DIGESTION, ABSORPTION AND STORAGE**

Digestion and Absorption

- Similar to other proteins, lactoferrin is denatured and broken down by proteases in the stomach, followed by further breakdown and absorption in the small intestine.

- However, protein degradation also has positive aspects as some peptides produced by its digestion, such as lactoferricin and lactoferrampin, display potent anti-inflammatory and antimicrobial activity.[2,31]

- Some delivery mechanisms like microencapsulation, PEGylation and absorption enhancers are being used in order to for LF to pass through the stomach and reach the intestine without being degraded.[32]

Storage

- LF is normally secreted at epithelial-lining mucosal surfaces. It is also present in specific granules of neutrophils.[33]

- It is not clear whether dietary LF or its peptides form part of the LF pool in the human body. It is likely to undergo glomerular filtration and eliminated thereafter.[34]

▶ **MECHANISM OF ACTION**

01 | Iron Chelation

Excess iron can be toxic because it has the ability to donate electrons to oxygen, resulting in the formation of reactive oxygen species (ROS) such as superoxide anions and hydroxyl radicals. LF has the ability to strongly and reversibly bind iron ions, supporting the body in maintaining iron homeostasis. This antioxidant activity protects cells from DNA damage and mitochondrial dysfunction. Iron chelation also reduces its availability to pathogens that need it for their growth.[1]

02 | Immunoregulation

Its major functions are antioxidant, antimicrobial and anti-inflammatory. LF acts as a transcription factor, triggering the expression of a variety of genes, including genes related to the innate immune response.[3]

The interaction of LF with the surface of the immune cells induce an anti-inflammatory reaction.[35] Moreover, it regulates cytokine synthesis by activated B cells by blocking NF-kB (nuclear factor kappa-light-chain-enhancer). It decreases the production of some proinflammatory cytokines, such as tumor necrosis factor alpha (TNF-α), interleukin 1α (IL-1α), IL-6 and IL-8 and increases the levels of anti-inflammatory IL-10.[3]

Iron chelation by LF can deprive microbes of iron and restrict their growth. Other than that, LF interacts with variable hosts' and microbial molecules, such as cell receptors, glycosaminoglycans, lysozyme, nucleic acids, lipoteichoic acid (LTA), lipopolysaccharide (LPS) to confer its antimicrobial activities. For example, LF destroys bacterial cells by interacting with enterobacterial LPS and destabilizes the bacterial membrane.[36] LF can bind to some viral surface proteins or block receptors on host cells. Finally, it also increases the sensitivity of pathogens to drugs.[36]

03 | DNA Protection

The protective role of LF against human DNA damage resulting from environmental and physiological conditions is poorly documented. A proper balance between DNA repair, proliferation, and apoptosis prevents accumulation of mutations within the human genome. LF acts similarly to p53 protein, which is a known as the "guardian of the genome", which helps maintain the genetic integrity of the cell after DNA damage by acting as a sensor. When DNA damage is extensive and unrepairable, LF induces apoptosis, whereas when the DNA damage is repairable, it stops the cell in the G1 phase of the cell cycle to permit DNA repair mechanisms to work.[3]

04 | Wound Healing and Hair Growth

Further to the effects of LF on our immune system, LF promotes both, the formation of granulation tissue and re-epithelialization, important stages of wound healing. However, its positive effect on wound healing and hair growth is mainly based on its ability to promote fibroblast and keratinocyte migration, thereby helping with wound contraction and proliferation of dermal papilla cells (in the hair follicle). Early evidence suggests its benefits in diabetic wound healing,[14] and promoting hair growth **(Figure 1)**.[16]

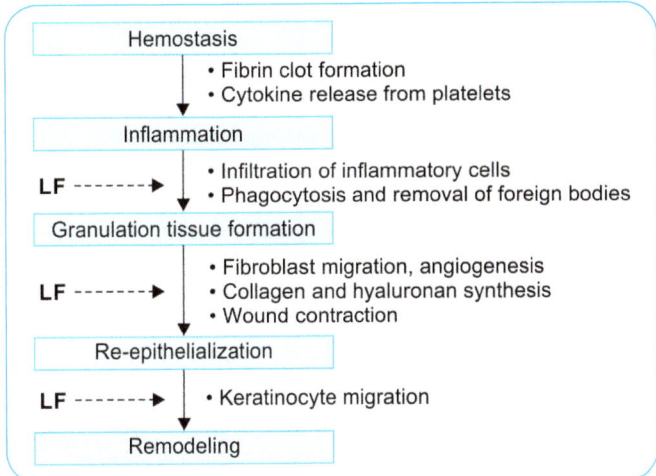

Figure 1: Schematic representation of normal wound healing. The sequential events in the wound-healing process, i.e., hemostasis, inflammation, granulation tissue formation, re-epithelialization, and tissue remodeling, are shown. Lactoferrin (LF) promotes wound healing in multiple ways.

▶ REFERENCES

1. Kowalczyk P, Kaczyńska K, Kleczkowska P, Bukowska-Ośko I, Kramkowski K, Sulejczak D. The Lactoferrin Phenomenon—A Miracle Molecule. Molecules. 2022;27(9):2941.
2. Superti F. Lactoferrin from Bovine Milk: A Protective Companion for Life. Nutrients. 2020;12(9):2562.
3. Bukowska-Ośko I, Sulejczak D, Kaczyńska K, Kleczkowska P, Kramkowski K, Popiel M, et al. Lactoferrin as a Human Genome "Guardian"—An Overall Point of View. Int J Mol Sci. 2022;23(9):5248.
4. Hassoun LA, Sivamani RK. A systematic review of lactoferrin use in dermatology. Crit Rev Food Sci Nutr. 2017;57(17):3632-9.
5. Milad GT, Diab HM, Elhusseiny RM. Role of Lactoferrin in Chronic Telgon Effluvium. QJM: An International Journal of Medicine. 2020;113(Suppl 1):hcaa046.011.
6. Jogi R, Tager MJ, Perez D, Tsapekosc M. Bovine Colostrum, Telomeres, and Skin Aging. Journal of Drugs in Dermatology. 2021;20(5).
7. Ashraf MF, Zubair D, Bashir MN, Alagawany M, Ahmed S, Shah QA, et al. Nutraceutical and Health-Promoting Potential of Lactoferrin, an Iron-Binding Protein in Human and Animal: Current Knowledge. Biol Trace Elem Res. 2023;1-17.
8. Superti F. Lactoferrin from Bovine Milk: A Protective Companion for Life. Nutrients. 2020;12(9):2562.
9. Cutone A, Rosa L, Ianiro G, Lepanto MS, Bonaccorsi di Patti MC, Valenti P, et al. Lactoferrin's Anti-Cancer Properties: Safety, Selectivity, and Wide Range of Action. Biomolecules. 2020;10(3):456.

10. Cerven D, DeGeorge G, Bethell D. 28-Day repeated dose oral toxicity of recombinant human apo-lactoferrin or recombinant human lysozyme in rats. Regul Toxicol Pharmacol. 2008;51(2):162-7.
11. Cerven D, DeGeorge G, Bethell D. 28-day repeated dose oral toxicity of recombinant human holo-lactoferrin in rats. Regul Toxicol Pharmacol. 2008;52(2):174-9.
12. Yamauchi K, Toida T, Nishimura S, Nagano E, Kusuoka O, Teraguchi S, et al. 13-Week oral repeated administration toxicity study of bovine lactoferrin in rats. Food Chem Toxicol. 2000;38(6):503-12.
13. Guberti M, Botti S, Capuzzo MT, Nardozi S, Fusco A, Cera A, et al. Bovine Colostrum Applications in Sick and Healthy People: A Systematic Review. Nutrients. 2021;13(7):2194.
14. Takayama Y, Aoki R. Roles of lactoferrin on skin wound healing. Biochem Cell Biol. 2012;90(3):497-503.
15. Guberti M, Botti S, Capuzzo MT, Nardozi S, Fusco A, Cera A, et al. Bovine Colostrum Applications in Sick and Healthy People: A Systematic Review. Nutrients. 2021;13(7):2194.
16. Huang HC, Lin H, Huang MC. Lactoferrin promotes hair growth in mice and increases dermal papilla cell proliferation through Erk/Akt and Wnt signaling pathways. Arch Dermatol Res. 2019;311(5):411-20.
17. Kim J, Ko Y, Park YK, Kim NI, Ha WK, Cho Y. Dietary effect of lactoferrin-enriched fermented milk on skin surface lipid and clinical improvement of acne vulgaris. Nutrition. 2010;26(9):902-9.
18. Mueller EA, Trapp S, Frentzel A, Kirch W, Brantl V. Efficacy and tolerability of oral lactoferrin supplementation in mild to moderate acne vulgaris: an exploratory study. Curr Med Res Opin. 2011;27(4):793-7.
19. Chan H, Chan G, Santos J, Dee K, Co JK. A randomized, double-blind, placebo-controlled trial to determine the efficacy and safety of lactoferrin with vitamin E and zinc as an oral therapy for mild to moderate acne vulgaris. Int J Dermatol. 2017;56(6):686-90.
20. Su Y, Cui W, Wei H. Influence of lactoferrin on Propionibacterium acnes-induced inflammation in vitro and in vivo. Dermatologic Therapy. 2020;33(6):e14483.
21. Oda H, Miyakawa M, Mizuki M, Misawa Y, Tsukahara T, Tanaka M, et al. Effects of Lactoferrin on Subjective Skin Conditions in Winter: A Preliminary, Randomized, Double-Blinded, Placebo-Controlled Trial. Clin Cosmet Investig Dermatol. 2019;12:875-80.
22. Yamauchi K, Hiruma M, Yamazaki N, Wakabayashi H, et al. Oral administration of bovine lactoferrin for treatment of tinea pedis. A placebo-controlled, double-blind study. Mycoses. 2000;43(5):197-202.
23. Tong PL, West NP, Cox AJ, Gebski VJ, Watts AM, Dodds A, et al. Oral supplementation with bovine whey-derived Ig-rich fraction and lactoferrin improves SCORAD and DLQI in atopic dermatitis. Journal of Dermatological Science. 2017;85(2):143-6.
24. Ishii N, Ryu M, Suzuki YA. Lactoferrin inhibits melanogenesis by down-regulating MITF in melanoma cells and normal melanocytes. Biochem Cell Biol. 2017;95(1):119-25.
25. Poulin Y, Pouliot Y, Lamiot E, Aattouri N, Gauthier SF. Safety and efficacy of a milk-derived extract in the treatment of plaque psoriasis: an open-label study. J Cutan Med Surg. 2005;9(6):271-5.
26. Tang L, Wu JJ, Ma Q, Cui T, Andreopoulos FM, Gil J, et al. Human lactoferrin stimulates skin keratinocyte function and wound re-epithelialization. British Journal of Dermatology. 2010;163(1):38-47.
27. Giansanti F, Panella G, Leboffe L, Antonini G. Lactoferrin from Milk: Nutraceutical and Pharmacological Properties. Pharmaceuticals (Basel). 2016;9(4):61.
28. Onishi H. Lactoferrin delivery systems: approaches for its more effective use. Expert Opin Drug Deliv. 2011;8(11):1469-79.
29. Cao X, Ren Y, Lu Q, Wang K, Wu Y, Wang Y, et al. Lactoferrin: A glycoprotein that plays an active role in human health. Front Nutr. 2023;9:1018336.
30. Simonart T. Acne and Whey Protein Supplementation among Bodybuilders. Dermatology. 2012;225(3):256-8.
31. Gruden Š, Poklar Ulrih N. Diverse Mechanisms of Antimicrobial Activities of Lactoferrins, Lactoferricins, and Other Lactoferrin-Derived Peptides. Int J Mol Sci. 2021;22(20):11264.
32. Yao X, Bunt C, Cornish J, Quek SY, Wen J. Oral Delivery of Lactoferrin: A Review. International Journal of Peptide Research and Therapeutics. 2012;19:1-10.
33. Ramos OL, Pereira RN, Rodrigues RM, Teixeira JA. Whey and Whey Powders: Production and Uses. In: Benjamin Caballero, et al. (Eds). Encyclopedia of Food and Health. Academic Press, 2016, pp. 498-505.
34. Diao L, Meibohm B. Pharmacokinetics and pharmacokinetic-pharmacodynamic correlations of therapeutic peptides. Clin Pharmacokinet. 2013;52(10):855-68.
35. Legrand D. Overview of Lactoferrin as a Natural Immune Modulator. J Pediatr. 2016;173:S10-15.
36. Drago-Serrano ME, de la Garza-Amaya M, Luna JS, Campos-Rodríguez R. Lactoferrin-lipopolysaccharide (LPS) binding as key to antibacterial and antiendotoxic effects. Int Immunopharmacol. 2012;12(1):1-9.

SECTION 04

Fatty Acids

21. Omega-3 Fatty Acids — *Madhulika Mhatre*
22. Omega-6 Fatty Acids — *Madhulika Mhatre*
23. Phytoceramides — *Madhulika Mhatre*

21

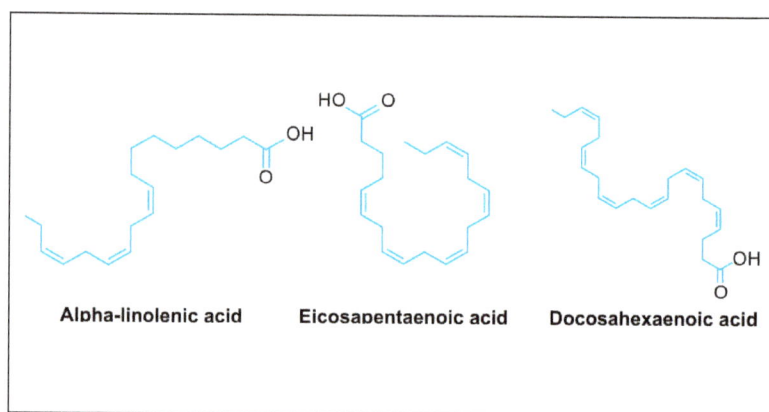

Omega-3 fatty acids (ALA, EPA, and DHA)

Omega-3 Fatty Acids

✍ Madhulika Mhatre

CONTENTS

OMEGA-3 FATTY ACIDS: NUTRIENT SNAPSHOT

▸ REQUIREMENT IN THE INDIAN CONTEXT | 213

▸ ACTIVE FORMS | 214

▸ SAFETY AND DOSAGE | 214

▸ CLINICAL CONDITIONS | 215

▸ SUPPLEMENTATION | 216

INTRODUCTION | 217

DIGESTION, ABSORPTION AND STORAGE | 217

MECHANISM OF ACTION | 218

KEY TOPICS

- ACNE VULGARIS
- DERMATITIS
- DRY SKIN
- HAIR GROWTH
- ISOTRETINOIN TREATMENT FOR ACNE VULGARIS
- PSORIASIS (ALONGSIDE MEDICATION)
- WOUND HEALING

Nutrient Snapshot

▶ **REQUIREMENT IN THE INDIAN CONTEXT**

- Omega-3 (ω3) and omega-6 (ω6) fatty acids are polyunsaturated fatty acids (PUFAs), and known as essential fats as they cannot be synthesized in the body.

- They are structural components of cells and tissue, and are involved in regulating various biological processes, mainly the inflammatory response, where ω6 fats give rise to inflammatory molecules while ω3 fats give rise to anti-inflammatory molecules. This is why the ω6: ω3 ratio is of importance to our long-term health.

- The ideal ratio is 1:1 to 3:1. However, in India, ratios in urban areas range between 38:1 and 50:1, whereas in rural areas from 5:1 to 6.1:1.[1,2] The lower ability to resolve inflammation is thought to be responsible for the rise in lifestyle diseases.[3]

- In the dermatological context, ω3 fats contribute to epidermal lipids, and its local inflammation. Lowering inflammation in skin can help manage inflammation-mediated pathologies, like acne, dermatitis and psoriasis.

- α-linolenic acid (ALA) is converted to its longer forms, eicosapentaenoic acid (EPA) and docosahexaenoic acid (DHA), in the body. This conversion, however, is very inefficient. Preformed EPA and DHA are therefore often supplemented.

ACTIVE FORMS

ACTIVE FORMS	SUPPLEMENT SOURCES	SALIENT FEATURES
α-linolenic acid (ALA)	Algae oil Flaxseed oil	This is the parent compound of the ω3 series, which can be converted to anti-inflammatory actives, EPA and DHA, however this conversion is very poor in the modern diet.[4–6]
Eicosapentaenoic acid (EPA)	Fish oil Krill oil	These provide preformed EPA but their purity needs to be checked on the label. The amount of fish oil or krill oil does not equal to the amount of the omega-3 fats. Krill oil normally has a lower purity than fish oil.
Docosahexaenoic acid (DHA)	Fish oil Krill oil Marine algae	Fish and krill oil provide preformed DHA, and their purity needs to be checked from the label. Marine algae is the only vegan source of DHA.[7]

SAFETY AND DOSAGE

GENERAL REQUIREMENTS	
Indian recommendations	ICMR-NIN (acceptable minimum dietary range): 250–2,000 mg/day ω3 fats.[8]
Global recommendations and limits	FDA: Daily intake should not exceed 3 g/day of EPA and DHA combined, with no more than 2 g/day derived from supplements.[9]
	EFSA: EPA and DHA combined at doses up to 5 g/day, and supplemental intakes of EPA alone up to 1.8 g/day.
	The WHO and FAO recommended an intake of 0.25–2 g EPA + DHA per day.
	EFSA set a daily intake of 250 mg of omega-3 fatty acids for adults in order to reduce the risk of heart disease.[10]
	Global Organization for EPA and DHA (GOED): 500 mg for general adult population inorder to lower to lower the risk coronary heart disease.[11] 2.1 g EPA + 1.1 g DHA/day do not perturb immune homeostasis or suppress immune responses.
Notes:	Those who have a known allergy toward fish may want to opt for the vegan sources of ω3 fats. Ideally, a preformed source of EPA and DHA from marine algae should be taken.

▶ CLINICAL CONDITIONS

EVIDENCE LEVEL	CONDITION OR USE CASE	DOSAGE	BENEFIT OR MECHANISM OF ACTION
++++	Dry skin	2.2 g flaxseed oil (approximately 50% ALA) for 12 weeks, versus a placebo of medium-chain fatty acids	There was a reduction in TEWL by 10% by week 6, with a further reduction after 12 weeks (compared to placebo). There was an improvement in roughness and scaling of the skin too.[12]
++++	Acne vulgaris	2 g EPA + DHA/day for 10 weeks in mild-to-moderate acne patients versus placebo	There was an anti-inflammatory effect of ω3 fats and reduction in interleukin-8 intensity in acne lesions, which is stimulated by IGF-1.[13]
+++	Alongside isotretinoin for acne vulgaris	1 g EPA + DHA/day for 16 weeks	There was a reduction in cheilitis, xerosis, and dryness of nose and eyes, compared to the group that received isotretinoin alone.[14]
+++	Dermatitis	5.4 g DHA/day for 8 weeks compared to placebo	The active group saw a significant clinical improvement of atopic eczema (SCORAD) compared to placebo. There was a reduction of anti-CD40/interleukin 4-mediated IgE synthesis of peripheral blood mononuclear cells.[15]
+++	Hair growth	Ex vivo hair follicles were cultured in mackerel-derived fermented fish oil (FFO) extract, alongside a positive control of minoxidil.	The fish oil markedly increased the length of hair-fiber comparable to minoxidil. EPA and DHA promote hair growth through anagen-activating pathways in dermal papilla cells.[16]
+	Psoriasis (alongside medication)	N/A (scientific review)	An ω3 rich diet and a reduction in ω6 intake has shown an improvement in clinical symptoms.[17]
+++	Chronic wound healing	1.6 g of EPA and 1.2 g of DHA per day for 28 days versus placebo	There was an increase in plasma levels of EPA and DHA, compared to the placebo group. There was a reduction in wound fluid levels of two 15-lipoxygenase products of ω6 PUFAs at 24 hours postwounding. The active group also had lower levels of myeloperoxidase, a leukocyte marker, at 12 hours and more reepithelialization on day 5 postwounding.[18]

▶ **SUPPLEMENTATION**

	BASIS OR MORE INFORMATION	**WHAT TO LOOK OUT FOR**
Supplementation form	Fish oil comes in phospholipid, triglyceride or ethyl ester forms. There is no clinical difference between these forms with long-term use. Krill oil generally has lower amounts of ω3 fats than fish oil. Flaxseed oil only provides ALA,[19] the conversion of which is not efficient in the body.[4–6] Marine algae is the only vegan source of DHA. It comes commonly in an oil form but some brands do offer powder form as well.	The respective amounts of ALA, EPA and DHA should be mentioned in the nutrition table or ingredients section of the product packaging.
Administration form	Capsules, gummies or syrup	Softgel capsules are often made of gelatin (non-vegetarian) unless stated otherwise. When using ω3 syrups, the bottle must be refrigerated (once opened) to avoid oxidation.
Purity considerations	Oils are a mixture of different fatty acids. The quantity of ω3 fatty acids in the oil may vary considerably.	This is stated on the packaging. However, companies can provide a gas chromatography report to show their purity at time points throughout the shelf-life of the product. Limits established by the FSSAI.
Patient considerations	'Fishy burps' after consumption	Enteric-coated or burp-free capsules are available in the market, or certain ω3 products are also flavored.
Safety considerations	Heavy metals can accumulate in marine species.	A heavy metal test report can be provided by the manufacturer. There are acceptable limits of heavy metals established by the FSSAI.
Other considerations	ω3 fats are very prone to oxidation.	Manufacturers can provide oxidation tests of their products over time. These include acid, peroxide value, anisidine and totox values. Authorities like GOED and CODEX Alimentarius have upper limits for assessment.
	Fish is a common allergen Contraindicated during warfarin treatments[20]	Patients with known fish allergies must avoid fish oils. Individuals with known medical conditions such as epilepsy or on any medications such as blood thinners should consult their doctors before taking ω3 supplements.

INTRODUCTION

ω3 and ω6 fats are polyunsaturated fatty acids (PUFAs) and are essential for normal development and health. Mammals cannot synthesize the parent compound in the ω3 series, α-linolenic acid (ALA), and the parent compound in the 6 series, linoleic acid (LA), de novo because they lack the enzymes to produce double bonds at the ω3 and ω6 position. Therefore, we must obtain these fats from the diet.[21-23]

As shown in **Figure 1**, PUFAs are converted from one another in the body via enzymes known as desaturases and elongases.[21,22] Humans can synthesize the long-chain ω3 fatty acids, eicosapentaenoic acid (EPA) and docosahexaenoic acid (DHA) from ALA.[23] EPA and DHA, which are not found in vegetarian foods, give rise to anti-inflammatory eicosanoids in the body and are therefore, important for resolving inflammation. DHA also contributes to lipids of the retina and nervous system. Both EPA and DHA are incorporated in the cell membranes, providing fluidity to the membrane on account of the kink caused by the double bonds in their structure, which limits close packing of the lipid bilayer.[24,25]

The enzyme known as Δ6 desaturase is the rate-limiting step for producing DHA in the body, and supplementation of DHA tends to circumvent this rate limit. Studies of ALA metabolism in healthy individuals indicated that approximately 5–10% of dietary ALA was converted to EPA and 0–4% was converted to docosahexaenoic acid (DHA). This is due to the high intake of ω6 fats, which give rise to inflammatory compounds, in our diet (rich in vegetable and seed oils) competing for Δ6 desaturase. This is why the ω6 to ω6 ratio is of significance to our health.

▶ DIGESTION, ABSORPTION AND STORAGE

Digestion and Absorption

- EPA and DHA are digested and taken up as normal dietary fats, by getting packaged into micelles in the intestines.[26]

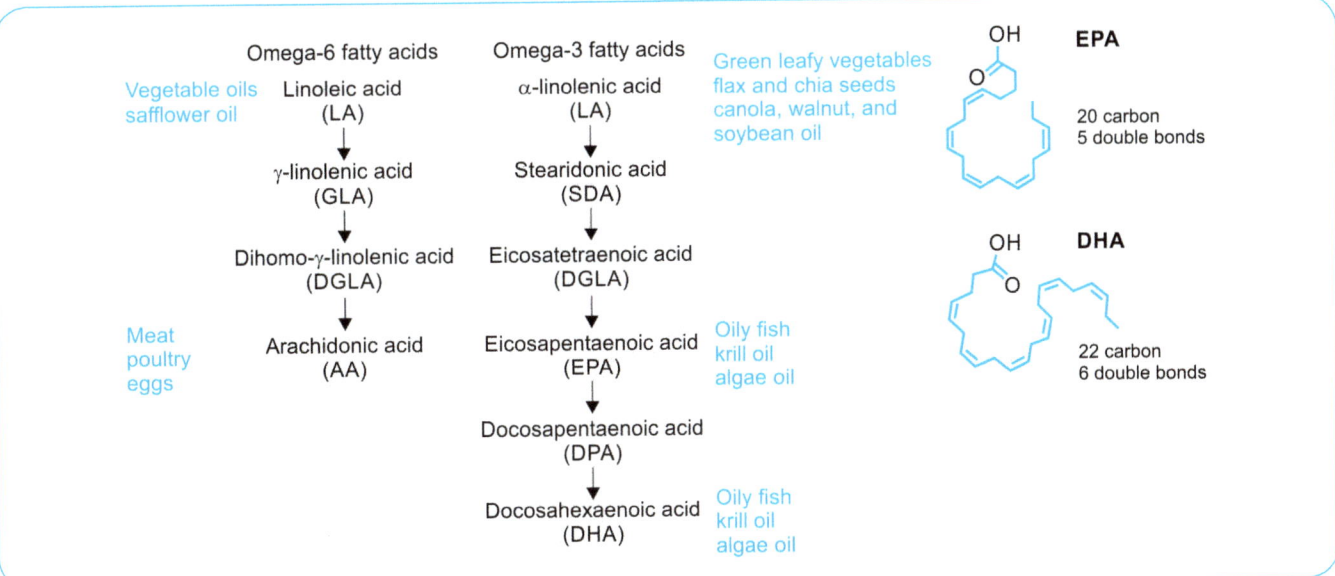

Figure 1: *The parent compound of each, ω3 and ω6 fatty acids, linoleic acid (LA) and α-linolenic acid (ALA), respectively, give rise to longer chain derivatives inside the body. Due to the poor conversion of ALA to the long-chain ω6 fats, EPA and DHA, it is recommended to obtain them from additional dietary sources.*
Source: *Linus Pauling website.*

- Digestion begins in the stomach with gastric lipases that break down triacylglycerols into diacylglycerol and fatty acids.[26]

- Once broken down, they form fat globules that are subsequently broken down by pancreatic lipases and bile salts in the small intestines.[26]

Storage

ω3 fats are incorporated into membrane phospholipids. It has been proposed that once incorporated into phospholipids,[24] they could alter the structure and functionality of membranes. i.e., fluidity, flexibility and thickness.[25]

▶ MECHANISM OF ACTION

01 | Anti-inflammatory Action and Photoprotection

ω3 and ω6 fats give rise to eicosanoids, a large class of signaling molecules that includes prostaglandins (PGs), thromboxanes, leukotrienes, mono-and poly-hydroxy fatty acids, and lipoxins. This occurs by the action of enzymes known as cyclooxygenases (COX) and lipoxygenases (LOX) **(Figure 2)**.

Long-chain ω3 fats have three major molecular targets:

MOLECULAR TARGETS	MODE OF ACTION
The peroxisome proliferator-activated receptor **(PPAR)** system, a class of receptors (PPARα, PPARβ/δ, and PPARγ)[26-29]	These inhibit the nuclear factor kappa B **(NF-κB)** pathway
GRP120, is a G-protein coupled receptor (rhodopsin-like)[30]	NF-κB acts to up-regulate inflammatory gene expression, which exists as in inactive form in the cytosol of cells, until the presence of an inflammatory trigger or stimulus.
Adenosine monophosphate kinase **(AMPK)** is a nutrient signalling molecule that also inhibits **NF-κB**.[31,32]	It is antagonistic of mTOR and activated in periods of nutrient deprivation; it is the molecular target of various drugs like Metformin – ω3 is used for diabetes and weight management.

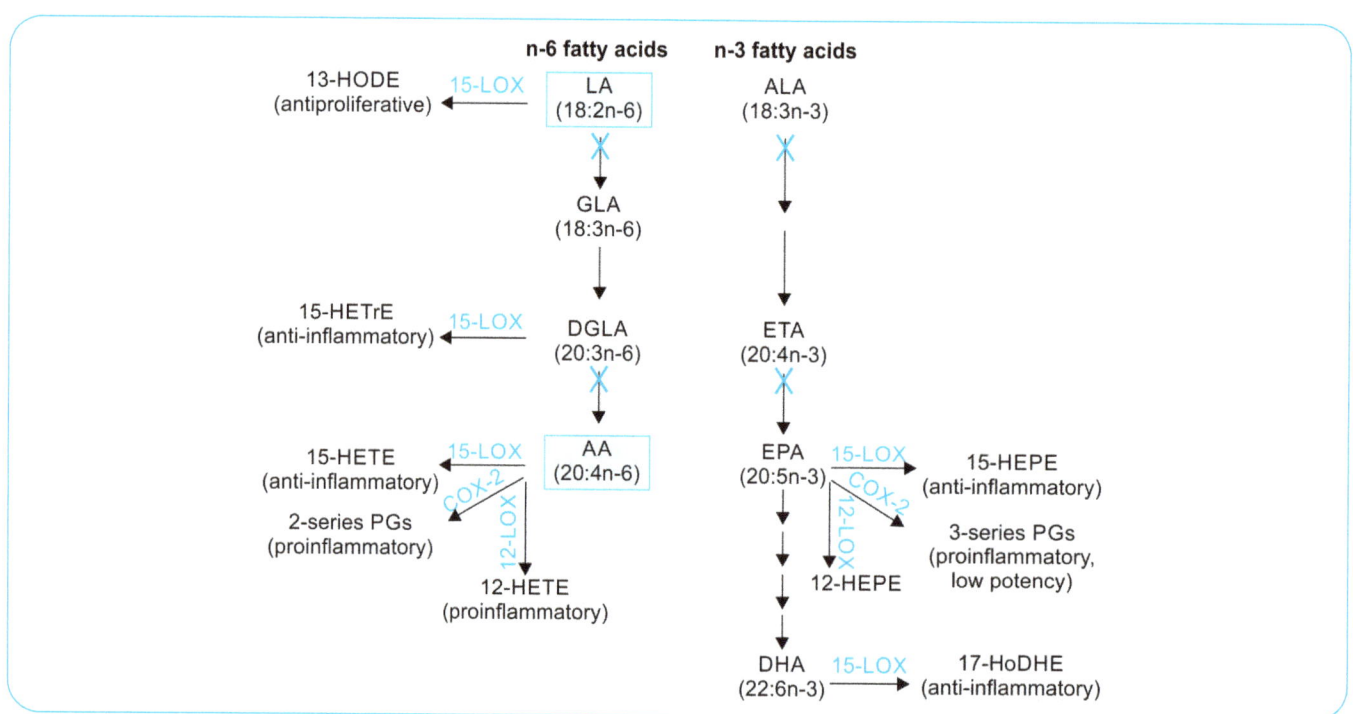

Figure 2: ω3 and ω6 fats give rise to eicosanoids by enzymes known as cyclooxygenases (COX) and lipoxygenases (LOX).
Source: Adapted from Linus Pauling website.

The skin expresses two cyclooxygenase isoforms: COX-1 and COX-2. COX-2 is induced in response to ROS and UV radiation leading to an increased production of prostaglandins from AA and EPA substrates.[33-35]

- AA is converted to PGE2, a major contributor to UV-induced inflammation and immunosuppression. UVR induced inflammation gives rise to three matrix metalloproteinases (MMPs): MMP-1, MMP-3, and MMP-9, that cleave and degrade skin's matrix.[36]

- EPA is converted to PGE3, a less potent inflammatory eicosanoid.

Mammalian skin expresses 5-, 12-, and 15-LOX enzyme isoforms.[33,37,38]

- 5- and 12-LOX produce monohydroxy fatty acids with potent chemoattractant and proinflammatory effects.

- 15-LOX products display antiproliferative and anti-inflammatory effects in skin.

The enzyme phospholipase A2 releases stored PUFAs in response to stress, including inflammation and oxidation.[35]

- The cellular membrane ratio of ω6 to ω3 fatty acids is important as phospholipase A2 is not discriminatory as to which PUFA it releases.[35,39-41]

- The eicosanoids that are produced when a cell is stressed therefore correlate directly with the PUFAs that make up its membrane.

- EPA and eicosatrienoic acid, an ω3 fat in the epidermis block the expression of matrix metalloproteinases (MMP1 and MMP9), enzymes causing collagen layer damage, thus offering photoprotection.[42-44]

Increasing the availability of ω3 fats shifts the eicosanoid content of the skin to an ω3 profile, thereby attenuating the negative effects of UV exposure. This is why the ω6 to ω3 ratio is important for skin health.

02 | Promoting Barrier Properties

Transepidermal water loss (TEWL) is directly related to the essential fatty acid composition of structural lipids in the stratum corneum. ω6 fats are the main component of epidermal lipids, whilst ω3 fats are predominantly immunomodulatory. Barrier damage, dry skin and itch are intricately linked and form the basis of many common skin diseases, management of which can be supported by these fats.[45] Skin barrier dynamics seem to be positively influenced by a decrease in skin's ω6/ω3 ratio.[46]

▶ REFERENCES

1. Pella D, Dubnov G, Singh RB, Sharma R, Berry EM, Manor O, et al. Effects of an Indo-Mediterranean Diet on the Omega-6/Omega-3 Ratio in Patients at High Risk of Coronary Artery Disease: The Indian Paradox. World Rev Nutr Diet. 2003:92:74-80.

2. Udipi SA, Karandikar S, Mukherjee R, Agarwal S, Ghugre PS. Variations in fat and fatty acid intakes of adult males from three regions of India. Indian J Public Health. 2006;50(3):179-86.

3. Simopoulos AP. Importance of the Ratio of Omega-6/Omega-3 Essential Fatty Acids: Evolutionary Aspects. World Review of Nutrition and Dietetics. 2003;92: 1-22.

4. Burdge GC, Jones AE, Wootton SA. Eicosapentaenoic and docosapentaenoic acids are the principal products of alpha-linolenic acid metabolism in young men*. Br J Nutr. 2002;88(4):355-63.

5. Burdge GC, Wootton SA. Conversion of alpha-linolenic acid to eicosapentaenoic, docosapentaenoic and docosahexaenoic acids in young women. Br J Nutr. 2002;88(4):411-20.

6. Burdge G. Alpha-linolenic acid metabolism in men and women: nutritional and biological implications. Curr Opin Clin Nutr Metab Care. 2004;7(2):137-44.

7. Senanayake J, Fichtali J. Single-Cell Oils as Sources of Nutraceutical and Specialty Lipids: Processing Technologies and Applications. 2006:265-94.

8. National Institute of Nutrition Indian Council of Medical Research. Recommended Dietary Allowances and Estimated Average Requirements for Indians - 2020. RDA Full Report 2020.

9. Bradberry JC, Hilleman DE. Overview of Omega-3 Fatty Acid Therapies. 2013;38(11):681-91.

10. Pasini F, Gómez-Caravaca AM, Blasco T, Cvejić J, Caboni MF, Verardo V. Assessment of Lipid Quality in Commercial Omega-3 Supplements Sold in the French Market. Biomolecules. 2022;12(10):1361.

11. GOED. Omega 3. EPA+DHA daily intake recommendations.

12. Spirt SD, Stahl W, Tronnier H, Sies H, Bejot M, Maurette JM, Heinrich U. Intervention with flaxseed and borage oil supplements modulates skin condition in women. Br J Nutr. 2009;101(3):440-5.

13. Jung JY, Kwon HH, Hong JS, Yoon JY, Park MS, Jang MY, et al. Effect of dietary supplementation with omega-3 fatty acid and gamma-linolenic acid on acne vulgaris: a randomised, double-blind, controlled trial. Acta Derm Venereol. 2014p;94(5):521-5.

14. Mirnezami M, Hoda R. Is Oral Omega-3 Effective in Reducing Mucocutaneous Side Effects of Isotretinoin in Patients with Acne Vulgaris? Dermatol Res Pract. 2018:2018:6974045.
15. Koch C, Dölle S, Metzger M, Rasche C, Jungclas H, Rühl R, et al. Docosahexaenoic acid (DHA) supplementation in atopic eczema: a randomized, double-blind, controlled trial. Br J Dermatol. 2008;158(4):786-92.
16. Kang JII, Hoon-Seok Y, Min KS, Park JE, Hyun YJ, Ko A, et al. Mackerel-Derived Fermented Fish Oil Promotes Hair Growth by Anagen-Stimulating Pathways. Int J Mol Sci. 2018;19(9):2770.
17. Balić A, Vlašić D, Žužul K, Marinović B, Zrinka BM. Omega-3 Versus Omega-6 Polyunsaturated Fatty Acids in the Prevention and Treatment of Inflammatory Skin Diseases. Int J Mol Sci. 2020;21(3):741.
18. McDaniel JC, Massey K, Nicolaou A. Fish oil supplementation alters levels of lipid mediators of inflammation in microenvironment of acute human wounds. Wound Repair Regen. 2011;19(2):189-200.
19. Shahidi F, Ambigaipalan P. Omega-3 Fatty Acids. Encyclopedia of Food Chemistry. 2022:465-71.
20. Fact Sheet for Health Professionals. Omega-3 Fatty Acids [Online]. Available from: https://ods.od.nih.gov/factsheets/Omega3FattyAcids-HealthProfessional/
21. Leonard AE, Pereira SL, Sprecher H, Huang YS. Elongation of long-chain fatty acids. Prog Lipid Res. 2004;43(1):36-54.
22. Zhuang XY, Zhang YH, Xiao AF, Zhang AH, Fang, BS. Key Enzymes in Fatty Acid Synthesis Pathway for Bioactive Lipids Biosynthesis. Front Nutr. 2022:9:851402.
23. Nakamura MT, Nara TY. Structure, function, and dietary regulation of delta6, delta5, and delta9 desaturases. Annu Rev Nutr. 2004:24:345-76.
24. Leng X, Kinnun JJ, Cavazos AT, Canner SW, Shaikh SR, Feller SE, et al. All n-3 PUFA are not the same: MD simulations reveal differences in membrane organization for EPA, DHA and DPA. Biochim Biophys Acta Biomembr. 2018;1860(5):1125-34.
25. Hishikawa D, Valentine WJ, Iizuka-Hishikawa Y, Shindou H, Shimizu T. Metabolism and functions of docosahexaenoic acidcontaining membrane glycerophospholipids. doi:10.1002/1873-3468.12825.
26. Omega-3 Fatty Acids - StatPearls - NCBI Bookshelf. https://www.ncbi.nlm.nih.gov/books/NBK564314/.
27. Yu K, Bayona W, Kallen CB, Harding HP, Ravera CP, McMahon G, et al. Differential activation of peroxisome proliferator-activated receptors by eicosanoids. J Biol Chem. 1995;270(41):23975-83.
28. Issemann I, Prince RA, Tugwood JD, Green S. The peroxisome proliferator-activated receptor:retinoid X receptor heterodimer is activated by fatty acids and fibrate hypolipidaemic drugs. J Mol Endocrinol. 1993;11(1):37-47.
29. Hertz R, Berman I, Keppler D, Bar-Tana J. Activation of gene transcription by prostacyclin analogues is mediated by the peroxisome-proliferators-activated receptor (PPAR). Eur J Biochem . 1996;235:242-7.
30. Oh, DY, Talukdar S, Bae EJ, Imamura T, Morinaga H, Fan W, et al. GPR120 is an omega-3 fatty acid receptor mediating potent anti-inflammatory and insulin-sensitizing effects. Cell. 2010;142(5):687-98.
31. Lorrente-Cabrián S, Bustos M, Marti A, Martinez JA, Moreno-Aliaga MJ. Eicosapentaenoic acid stimulates AM P-activated protein kinase and increases visfatin secretion in cultured murine adipocytes. Clin Sci (Lond). 2009;117:243-9.
32. Xue B, Yang Z, Wang X, Shi H. Omega-3 polyunsaturated fatty acids antagonize macrophage inflammation via activation of AM PK/SIRT1 pathway. PLoS One. 2012;7(10):e45990.
33. Lands WE. Biochemistry and physiology of n-3 fatty acids. FASEB J. 1992;6(8):2530-6.
34. Tripp CS, Blomme EAG, Chinn KS, Hardy MM, LaCelle P, Pentland AP. Epidermal COX-2 Induction Following Ultraviolet Irradiation: Suggested Mechanism for the Role of COX-2 Inhibition in Photoprotection. J Invest Dermatol. 2003;121(4):853-61.
35. Rhodes LE, Gledhill K, Masoodi M, Haylett AK, Brownrigg M, Thody AJ, et al. The sunburn response in human skin is characterized by sequential eicosanoid profiles that may mediate its early and late phases. FASEB J. 2009;23(11):3947-56.
36. Fisher GJ, Kang S, Varani J, Bata-Csorgo Z, Wan Y, Datta S, et al. Mechanisms of photoaging and chronological skin aging. Arch Dermatol. 2002;138(11):1462-70.
37. Ziboh VA, Cho Y, Mani I, Xi S. Biological significance of essential fatty acids/prostanoids/lipoxygenase- derived monohydroxy fatty acids in the skin. Arch Pharm Res. 2002;25(6):747-58.
38. Ziboh VA. Prostaglandins, Leukotrienes, and Hydroxy Fatty Acids in Epidermis. Seminars in Dermatology. 1992;11(2): 114-20.
39. Pilkington SM, Watson REB, Nicolaou A, Rhodes LE. Omega-3 polyunsaturated fatty acids: photoprotective macronutrients. Exp Dermatol. 2011;20(7):537-43.
40. Norris PC, Dennis EA, Karin M. Omega-3 fatty acids cause dramatic changes in TLR4 and purinergic eicosanoid signaling. Proc Natl Acad Sci U S A. 2012;109(22):8517-22.
41. Hruza LL, Pentland AP. Mechanisms of UV-induced inflammation. J Invest Dermatol. 1993;100(1):35S-41S.
42. Ju KE, Min-Kyoung K, Xing-Ji J, Jang-Hee OH, Kim JE, Chung JH. Skin Aging and Photoaging Alter Fatty Acids Composition, Including 11,14,17-eicosatrienoic Acid, in the Epidermis of Human Skin. J Korean Med Sci. 2010;25(6):980-3.
43. Kim HH, Cho S, Lee S, Kim KH, Kwang HC, Eun HC, Chung JH. Photoprotective and anti-skin-aging effects of eicosapentaenoic acid in human skin in vivo. J Lipid Res. 2006;47(5):921-30.
44. Pilkington SM, Watson REB, Nicolaou A, Rhodes LE. Omega-3 polyunsaturated fatty acids: photoprotective macronutrients. Exp Dermatol. 2011;20(7):537-43.
45. Yosipovitch G, Misery L, Proksch E, Metz M, Ständer S, Schmelz M. Skin Barrier Damage and Itch: Review of Mechanisms, Topical Management and Future Directions. Acta Derm Venereol. 2019;99(13):1201-9.
46. Barcelos RCS, Mello-Sampayo CD, Antoniazzi CTD, Segat HJ, Silva H, Veit JC, et al. Oral supplementation with fish oil reduces dryness and pruritus in the acetone-induced dry skin rat model. J Dermatol Sci. 2015;79(3):298-304.

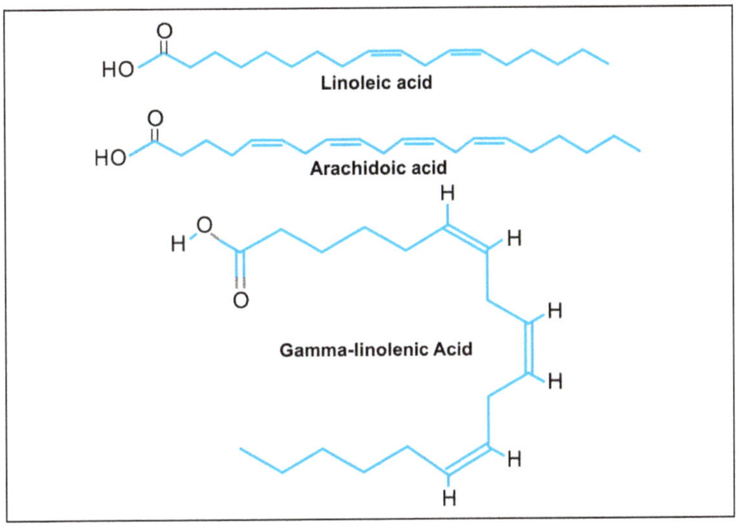

Linoleic Acid (LA), Arachidonic Acid (AA), Gamma-linolenic Acid (GLA)

Omega-6 Fatty Acids

✍ Madhulika Mhatre

CONTENTS

OMEGA-6 FATTY ACIDS: NUTRIENT SNAPSHOT

▶ REQUIREMENT IN THE INDIAN CONTEXT | 222

▶ ACTIVE FORMS | 223

▶ SAFETY AND DOSAGE | 223

▶ CLINICAL CONDITIONS | 223

▶ SUPPLEMENTATION | 224

INTRODUCTION | 225

DIGESTION, ABSORPTION AND STORAGE | 225

MECHANISM OF ACTION | 226

KEY TOPICS

- ACNE VULGARIS
- ATOPIC DERMATITIS
- DRY SKIN
- FEMALE PATTERN HAIR LOSS
- ISOTRETINOIN TREATMENT RELATED FOR ACNE VULGARIS

Nutrient Snapshot

▶ **REQUIREMENT IN THE INDIAN CONTEXT**

- Omega-3 (ω3) and omega-6 (ω6) fatty acids are polyunsaturated fatty acids (PUFAs), and are known as essential fats as they cannot be synthesized in the body.

- They are structural components of cells and tissue, and are involved in regulating various biological processes, mainly the inflammatory response, where ω6 fats give rise to inflammatory molecules while ω3 fats give rise to anti-inflammatory molecules. This is why the ω6: ω3 ratio is of importance to our long-term health.

- Linoleic acid (LA), the parent compound of ω6 fats, and its derivatives play a central role in the lipid barrier of the skin. Normally, ω6 fats are ubiquitous in the Indian diet, with very little ω3 fats. However, an anti-inflammatory derivative of LA, gamma-linolenic acid (GLA), can be conditionally essential i.e., in physiologically stressful conditions, its biosynthesis from LA may be inadequate.

- Activity of the enzyme that catalyses the reaction of LA to GLA decreases with age, and in people suffering from various diseases including arthritis, diabetes, hypertension, eczema, psoriasis, etc. Lifestyle factors (like stress, smoking and excessive consumption of alcohol, LA, saturated and trans-fatty acids) and nutritional deficiencies of vitamin B6, zinc, and magnesium also inhibit this enzyme.[1] Due to limitations in the in vivo production of GLA, supplementation with preformed GLA is becoming important, which appears to improve skin barrier function in subjects with dry skin conditions and atopic dermatitis.[2]

Nutrition in Dermatology

▶ ACTIVE FORMS

ACTIVE FORMS	SUPPLEMENT SOURCES	SALIENT FEATURES
Linoleic acid (LA)	Excessive in the Indian diet and often not supplemented	The body converts LA to its long-chain derivatives based on the requirement.
Gamma linolenic acid (GLA)	Evening primrose oil Borage oil Blackcurrant oil	Anti-inflammatory precursor. Blackcurrant oil is not approved by FSSAI
Dihomo-gamma linolenic acid (DGLA)	It is synthesized from GLA	Anti-inflammatory precursor.
Arachidonic acid (AA)	It is synthesized from LA	Pro-inflammatory precursor.

▶ SAFETY AND DOSAGE

GENERAL REQUIREMENTS	
Indian recommendations	ICMR-NIN: Adequate intake (AI) of 2–3% of total energy intake[3] Accepted macronutrient dietary range (AMDR): 2.5–9% of total energy intake
Global recommendations and limits	IOC's Food and Nutrition Board: AI (19–50 years of age) of LA is 17 g/day for male and 12 g/day for female (5–6% of energy)[4]
	EFSA recommendations of GLA for promoting and maintaining healthy skin: 33–720 mg/day[5]
Notes:	Side effects are rare. The most common side effects of GLA are temporary gastrointestinal symptoms such as abdominal pain, fullness, or nausea.

▶ CLINICAL CONDITIONS

EVIDENCE LEVEL	CONDITION OR USE CASE	DOSAGE	BENEFIT OR MECHANISM OF ACTION
+++++	Dry skin and atopic dermatitis	200 mg GLA-rich food for 12 weeks	There was an improvement in skin barrier function and a reduction in transepidermal water loss (TEWL).[2]
++++	Acne vulgaris	GLA (400 mg) for 10 weeks vs placebo	Acne lesions decreased. Mechanism: Reductions in inflammation and IL-8.[6]

▶ CLINICAL CONDITIONS (Continued)

EVIDENCE LEVEL	CONDITION OR USE CASE	DOSAGE	BENEFIT OR MECHANISM OF ACTION
++++	Female pattern hair loss	Blackcurrant seed oil (460 mg GLA) for 6 months	A reduction in hair loss, and an improvement in hair diameter and hair density was seen.[7]
+++	Acne vulgaris	LA: 694 mg, GLA: 84.8 mg for 9 months	Evening primrose oil with isotretinoin increased skin hydration.[8]
+++	Xerotic cheilitis (side effect of Isotretinoin treatment in acne)	Subjects received oral isotretinoin with or without 240 mg GLA for 8 weeks	No increase in TEWL in patients receiving combination as compared to patients receiving just isotretinoin treatment.[9]

▶ SUPPLEMENTATION

	BASIS	WHAT TO LOOK OUT FOR
Supplementation form	LA, GLA, DHLA	The form and source of ω6 fat is often stated on the product packaging, if not can be obtained from the product company.
Administration form	Soft gel capsules, chewable capsules, syrups, powders	N/A
Purity considerations	The type and purity of ω6 fats as per the source: Evening primrose oil: Over 70% LA and approximately 9% GLA Borage oil: Approximately 21% GLA Blackcurrant oil: Approximately 17% GLA[10] Borage oil has the highest GLA	The content of ω6 fats is often stated in the nutritional information but gas chromatography report from the product company can be obtained to know the purity of the product.
Patient considerations	GLA should be taken with the meal or after the meal. Some softgel capsule coatings can be made of gelatin (non-vegetarian).	N/A
Safety considerations	Evening primrose oil is generally well tolerated, with minor adverse effects, including abdominal pain, indigestion, nausea, softening of stools and headaches.[11] According to literature, GLA is generally safe for supplementation.	N/A
Other considerations	PUFAs are prone to oxidation and must be protected from heat, light and air exposure.	Storage conditions given on the packaging should be strictly considered. Product manufacturers should be able to provide laboratory reports of oxidation parameters.

INTRODUCTION

ω3 and ω6 fats are PUFAs and are essential for normal development and health. Mammals cannot synthesize the parent compound in the ω3 series, α-linolenic acid (ALA), and the parent compound in the ω6 series, LA, de novo because they lack the enzymes to produce double bonds at the ω3 and ω6 position. Therefore, these fats must be obtained from the diet.[12-14]

As shown in **Figure 1**, PUFAs are converted from one another in the body via an enzymes known as desaturases and elongases.[12,13] LA is converted to GLA, DGLA and AA. LA and AA give rise to proinflammatory eicosanoids while GLA, which is converted to DGLA, gives rise to anti-inflammatory eicosanoids. The delta-6 (Δ6) desaturase lacks in the skin and thus the body relies on the liver for the conversion of LA into GLA.[15]

DIGESTION, ABSORPTION AND STORAGE

Digestion and Absorption

- ω6 fats are digested and taken up as normal dietary fats, by getting packaged into micelles in the intestines.

- Digestion begins in the stomach with gastric lipases that break down triacylglycerols into diacylglycerol and fatty acids.

- Once broken down, they form fat globules that are subsequently broken down by pancreatic lipases and bile salts in the small intestines

After consumption, LA can be desaturated and elongated to form other ω6 PUFAs such as GLA and DGLA. The DGLA is converted to the metabolically important ω6 PUFA, AA, the substrate for a wide array of reactive oxygenated metabolites.

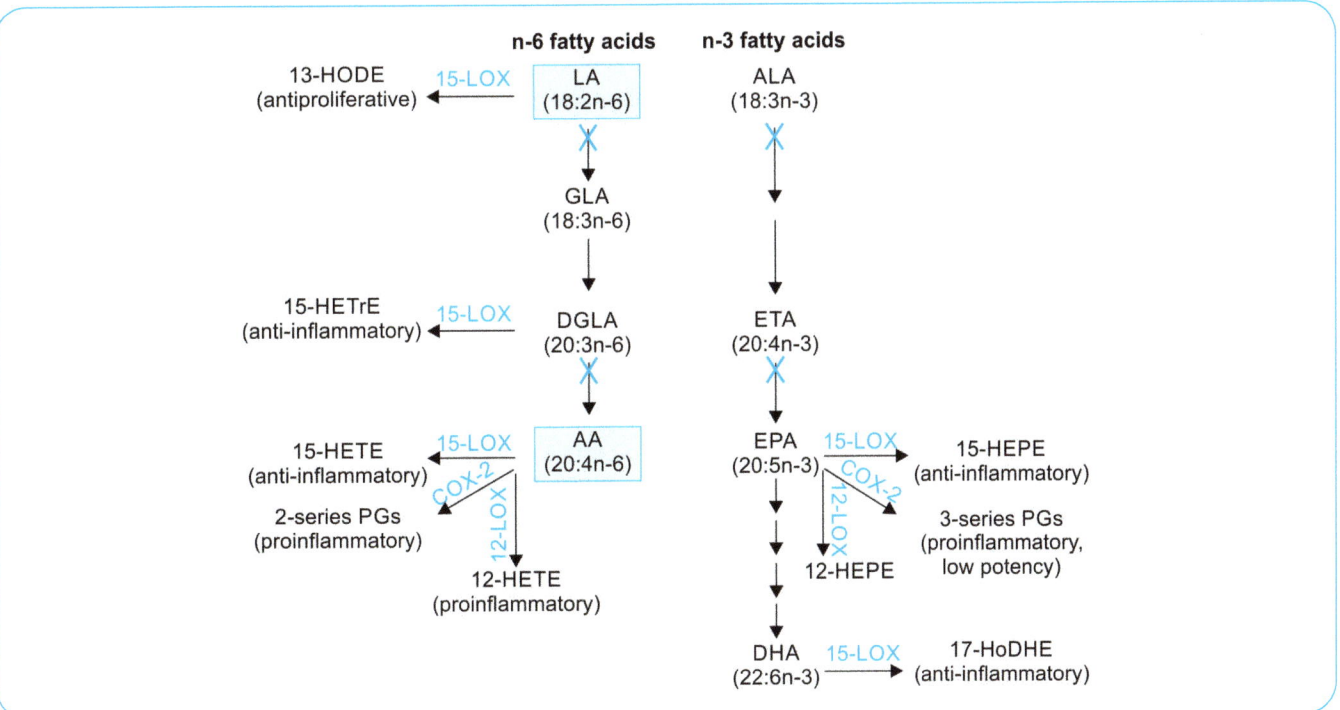

Figure 1: *ω3 and ω6 fats give rise to eicosanoids by enzymes known as cyclooxygenases (COX) and lipoxygenases (LOX).*

(LA: linoleic acid; GLA: gamma-linolenic acid; DGLA: dihomo-gamma linolenic acid; AA: arachidonic acid; HETE: hydroxyeicosatetraenoic acids; PGs: prostaglandins; ALA: alpha-linolenic acid; ETA: eicosatetraenoic acid; EPA: eicosapentaenoic acid; DHA: docosahexaenoic acid)

Source: *Adapted from Linus Pauling.*

Storage

The essential fatty acids which are assimilated into phospholipids are particularly important in the body as phospholipids maintain both the structural integrity and functioning of cellular membranes throughout the body.

▶ MECHANISM OF ACTION

01 | Skin Lipid Barrier

LA is the most abundant PUFA present in the epidermis, and it has a specific and unique role in the structural integrity of the skin and in barrier function because it is as an essential constituent of ceramides.[16]

The fluidity of the lipid barrier function is dependent on the content of LA. Its presence in the stratum corneum ceramides directly correlates with the permeability of the barrier function of the skin,[17] therefore affecting TEWL. The major and early deficiency symptoms of ω6 fatty acids are growth defects, scaly skin, and increased TEWL.

02 | Anti-inflammatory Property

ω3 and ω6 fats give rise to eicosanoids, a large class of signaling molecules that includes prostaglandins (PGs), thromboxanes, leukotrienes, mono-and polyhydroxy fatty acids, and lipoxins. This occurs by the action of enzymes known as cyclooxygenases (COX) and lipoxygenases (LOX) **(Figure 1)**.

AA is the second most abundant PUFA in the epidermis (approximately 9%). It is a structural component of phospholipids found in the membranes of epidermal keratinocytes.

The skin expresses two COX isoforms: COX-1 and COX-2. COX-2 is induced in response to reactive oxygen species (ROS) and UV radiation leading to an increased production of prostaglandins from AA and EPA substrates.[18-20] AA is released from phospholipids by the enzyme phospholipase A2 (PLA2) and is converted to prostaglandins E2 (PGE2), a major contributor to UV radiation-induced inflammation and immunosuppression. UV-radiation induced inflammation gives rise to three matrix metalloproteinases (MMPs): MMP-1, MMP-3, and MMP-9, that cleave and degrade skin's matrix.[21-23]

GLA is rapidly converted to DGLA that gives rise to anti-inflammatory prostaglandins. GLA supplementation in humans has shown an increase in GLA and DGLA with little change in AA levels.[1] Prevention of active inflammation and the improvement of epidermal barrier function with different PUFAs may be an excellent therapeutic approach for patients with inflammatory skin disorders e.g., atopic dermatitis, eczema and psoriasis, most likely through changes in the ratio of pro-and anti-inflammatory eicosanoids. For example, combined ω6 PUFAs (LA and GLA) and long-chain ω3 PUFAs (EPA and DHA) has the potential to ameliorate inflammatory processes in the skin, helping with disease management.[16]

03 | Cellular Activity

AA is not only involved in inflammation; It triggers multiple intracellular signal transduction pathways and affects a variety of cellular functions. For example, AA affects the signal transduction cascades that mediate cell proliferation via the expression of fibroblast growth factor-7 (FGF-7), FGF-10, and hepatocyte growth factor (HGF) in human dermal papillae cells and hair follicle cells.[24]

GLA and DGLA also affect the expression of various genes that regulate the levels of matrix proteins.[1]

▶ REFERENCES

1. Kapoor R, Huang YS. Gamma linolenic acid: an antiinflammatory omega-6 fatty acid. Curr Pharm Biotechnol. 2006;7(6):531-4.
2. Kawamura A, Ooyama K, Kojima K, Kachi H, Abe T, Amano K, et al. Dietary Supplementation of Gamma-Linolenic Acid Improves Skin Parameters in Subjects with Dry Skin and Mild Atopic Dermatitis. Journal of Oleo Science. 2011;60(12):597-607.
3. National Institute of Nutrition Indian Council of Medical Research. Recommended Dietary Allowances and Estimated Average Requirements for Indians – 2020. RDA Full Report 2020.
4. Harris WS, Dariush M, Eric R, Penny KE, Rudel LL, Appel LJ, et al. Omega-6 Fatty Acids and Risk for Cardiovascular Disease: A Science Advisory From the American Heart Association Nutrition Subcommittee of the Council on Nutrition, Physical Activity, and Metabolism; Council on Cardiovascular Nursing; and Council on Epidemiology and Prevention. 2009;119(6):902-7.

5. EFSA Panel on Dietetic Products, Nutrition and Allergies (NDA). Scientific Opinion on the substantiation of health claims related to gamma linolenic acid (GLA) and maintenance of normal blood LDL cholesterol concentrations (ID 2661, 4452, 4453), maintenance of normal blood pressure (ID 2662), reduction of menstrual discomfort (ID 495, 640, 1773, 1775), contribution to normal cognitive function (ID 1770), maintenance of the barrier function of the skin (ID 499, 591, 639, 676, 1554, 2003, 2065), "function of the cell membrane" (ID 1769), maintenance of normal structure, elasticity and appearance of the skin (ID 2660, 4296), and "anti-inflammatory properties" (ID 4454) pursuant to Article 13(1) of Regulation (EC) No 1924/2006. EFSA Journal. 2011;9(4):2059.

6. Jung JY, Kwon HH, Hong JS, Yoon JY, Park MS, Jang MY, et al. Effect of dietary supplementation with omega-3 fatty acid and gamma-linolenic acid on acne vulgaris: a randomised, double-blind, controlled trial. Acta Derm Venereol. 2014;94(5):521-5.

7. Le Floc'h C, Cheniti A, Connétable S, Piccardi N, Vincenzi C, Tosti A. Effect of a nutritional supplement on hair loss in women. J Cosmet Dermatol. 2015;14(1):76-82.

8. Kaźmierska A, Bolesławska I, Polańska A, Dańczak-Pazdrowska A, Jagielski P, Drzymała-Czyż S, et al. Effect of Evening Primrose Oil Supplementation on Selected Parameters of Skin Condition in a Group of Patients Treated with Isotretinoin—A Randomized Double-Blind Trial. Nutrients. 2022;14(14):2980.

9. Young PK, Jung KE, Su KI, Kapsok L, Kim BJ, Seoet SJ, et al. The Effect of Evening Primrose Oil for the Prevention of Xerotic Cheilitis in Acne Patients Being Treated with Isotretinoin: A Pilot Study. Ann Dermatol. 2014;26(6):706-12.

10. Sergeant S, Rahbar E, Chilton FH. Gamma-linolenic acid, Dihommo-gamma linolenic, Eicosanoids and Inflammatory Processes. Eur J Pharmacol. 2016;785:77-86.

11. Bayles B, Usatine R. Evening Primrose Oil. afp. 2009;80(12):1405-8.

12. Leonard AE, Pereira SL, Sprecher H, Huang YS. Elongation of long-chain fatty acids. Progress in Lipid Research. 2004;43(1):36-54.

13. Zhuang XY, Zhang YH, Xiao AF, Zhang AH, Fang BS. Key Enzymes in Fatty Acid Synthesis Pathway for Bioactive Lipids Biosynthesis. Frontiers in Nutrition. 2022;9:175.

14. Nakamura MT, Nara TY. Structure, function, and dietary regulation of delta6, delta5, and delta9 desaturases. Annu Rev Nutr. 2004;24:345-76.

15. Chapkin RS, Ziboh VA. Inability of skin enzyme preparations to biosynthesize arachidonic acid from linoleic acid. Biochem Biophys Res Commun. 1984;124(3):784-92.

16. Djuricic I, Calder PC. Beneficial Outcomes of Omega-6 and Omega-3 Polyunsaturated Fatty Acids on Human Health: An Update for 2021. Nutrients. 2021;13(7):2421.

17. Hansen HS, Jensen B. Essential function of linoleic acid esterified in acylglucosylceramide and acylceramide in maintaining the epidermal water permeability barrier. Evidence from feeding studies with oleate, linoleate, arachidonate, columbinate and alpha-linolenate. Biochim Biophys Acta. 1985;834(3):357-63.

18. Lands WE. Biochemistry and physiology of n-3 fatty acids. FASEB J. 1992;6(8):2530-6.

19. Tripp CS, Blomme EAG, Chinn KS, Hardy MM, LaCelle P, Pentland AP, et al. Epidermal COX-2 Induction Following Ultraviolet Irradiation: Suggested Mechanism for the Role of COX-2 Inhibition in Photoprotection. Journal of Investigative Dermatology. 2003;121:853-61.

20. Rhodes LE, Gledhill K, Masoodi M, Haylett AK, Brownrigg M, Thody AJ, et al. The sunburn response in human skin is characterized by sequential eicosanoid profiles that may mediate its early and late phases. FASEB J. 2009;23:3947-56.

21. Fisher GJ, Kang S, Varani J, Bata-Csorgo Z, Wan Y, Datta S, et al. Mechanisms of photoaging and chronological skin aging. Arch Dermatol. 2002;138:1462-70.

22. Wertz PW. Epidermal lipids. Semin Dermatol. 1992;11:106-113.

23. Chapkin RS, Ziboh VA, McCullough JL. Dietary influences of evening primrose and fish oil on the skin of essential fatty acid-deficient guinea pigs. J Nutr. 1987;117:1360-70.

24. Munkhbayar S, Jang S, Cho AR, Choi SJ, Shin CY, Eun HC, et al. Role of Arachidonic Acid in Promoting Hair Growth. Ann Dermatol. 2016;28(1):55-64.

23

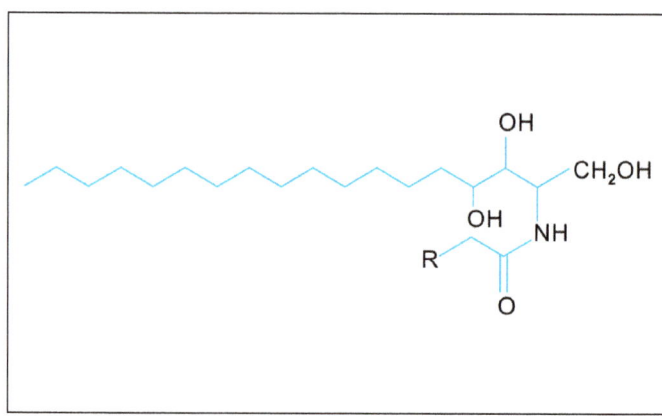

Phytocermide

Phytoceramides

✍ Madhulika Mhatre

CONTENTS

PHYTOCERAMIDES: NUTRIENT SNAPSHOT

- ▸ REQUIREMENT IN THE INDIAN CONTEXT | 229
- ▸ ACTIVE FORMS | 230
- ▸ SAFETY AND DOSAGE | 230
- ▸ CLINICAL CONDITIONS | 230
- ▸ SUPPLEMENTATION | 232

INTRODUCTION | 233

DIGESTION, ABSORPTION AND STORAGE | 233

MECHANISM OF ACTION | 233

KEY TOPICS

- ANTI-AGING
- ATOPIC DERMATITIS
- CERAMIDES AND GLUCOSYLCERAMIDE CONTENT IN THE SKIN
- DRY SKIN
- HYPERPIGMENTATION/ DEPIGMENTATION
- SKIN BARRIER FUNCTION
- SKIN HYDRATION

Nutrient Snapshot

▶ **REQUIREMENT IN THE INDIAN CONTEXT**

- Ceramides are a group of naturally occurring, long-chain fatty acids that makes up about 50% of the epidermis.[1] Ceramides are important elements of the skin barrier and are involved in limiting transepidermal water loss (TEWL). In addition, ceramides regulate processes such as proliferation, differentiation and apoptosis of keratinocytes.[1]

- Although the skin naturally makes ceramides, environmental factors like cold weather, air pollution, UV rays, and low humidity can reduce their concentration. Ceramide production in the skin reduces with age, which is one of the reasons for an increase in skin's TEWL, irritation and structural damage.

- Phytoceramides refer to plant-derived ceramides and are similar in structure to ceramides found in the skin. The bioactivity of ceramides varies considerably with the physical properties, so phytoceramides are being explored for a range of health outcomes. In dermatology, their research has been limited to utilizing their role in epidermal barrier function and related conditions like psoriasis and atopic dermatitis. While these conditions are prominent not only in India, but world over, the use of phytoceramides for its bioactive abilities in the long run is likely.

- Although ceramide-containing foods like rice and wheat are frequent in the Indian diet, they may not naturally occur in sufficient quantities to have a clinical impact.[2] While not essential, phytoceramides can be a useful tool to manage dry skin and skin conditions like psoriasis and atopic dermatitis, where barrier function is compromised.

▶ ACTIVE FORMS

ACTIVE FORMS	SUPPLEMENT SOURCES	SALIENT FEATURES
Ceramides	Plant (wheat, rice, spinach) derived in the form of glucosylceramide extracts, gram negative bacteria derived ceramides, yeast derived ceramides	Due to the sheer variation in sphingolipids as well as the development of synthetic varieties, their bioavailability and mechanism of action may vary considerably.

▶ SAFETY AND DOSAGE

GENERAL REQUIREMENTS	
Indian recommendations	There are no recommendations for phytoceramides. They are produced from dietary lipids. Phytoceramides or ceramides are not approved by the FSSAI.
Global recommendations and limits	There are no recommendations for phytoceramides.
Notes:	As per human clinical trials, ceramides are well tolerated. Phytoceramides or ceramides are not approved by the FSSAI. Thus, phytoceramide supplements are not manufactured in India and are not available on Indian e-commerce platforms.
	Those who have gluten sensitivities may want to ensure that they purchase supplements that do not contain gluten.

▶ CLINICAL CONDITIONS

EVIDENCE LEVEL	CONDITION OR USE CASE	DOSAGE	BENEFIT OR MECHANISM OF ACTION
+++++	Dry skin	Food with acetic acid bacteria containing 0.8 mg of dihydroceramide for 12 weeks	There was an improvement in stratum corneum hydration.[3]
+++	Ceramides and glucosylceramide content in the skin	Rice-derived glucosylceramides 3 or 10 mg/kg body weight/day were fed to mice for 12 days	Oral dosing of glucosylceramides improved TEWL. In the skin, epidermal ceramide 1 was increased along with enhancing glucosylceramide synthase and glucocerebrosidase (enzyme that breaks glucosylceramide into ceramides).[4]

▶ **CLINICAL CONDITIONS** (*Continued*)

EVIDENCE LEVEL	CONDITION OR USE CASE	DOSAGE	BENEFIT OR MECHANISM OF ACTION
+++++	Skin moisturizing	N/A (meta-analysis)	As per this meta-analysis, oral ceramides are effective in skin moisturizing and reducing TEWL.[5]
+++++	Anti-aging and skin hydration	Placebo or wheat polar lipid complex containing 1.6 or 1.7 mg/day, with 11.5 mg of digalactosyl diglycerides (DGDG); measured after 15, 30 and 60 days.	Supplementation increased skin hydration, elasticity, and smoothness, and decreased TEWL, roughness, and wrinkles in both the dosage groups compared to placebo.[2]
+++	Dry skin, hyperpigmentation, itchiness and skin hydration	5 mg of glucosylceramide using amorphophallus konjac extract for 6 weeks.	Oral intake of extract decreased skin dryness, hyperpigmentation, redness, itching and oiliness.[6]
+++	Skin barrier function and depigmentation	40 mg of rice ceramides for 12 weeks	There was an improvement in skin hydration, an increase in sebum production and composition, firmness and elasticity, and wrinkle severity. It also reduced TEWL, levels of melanin index and erythema index.[7]
+++	Atopic dermatitis (AD)	Glucosylceramides from yeast and maize was added in the diet of mice at 0.1%, fed for 7 weeks	The ceramide-containing diet led to a decrease in Ceramide-containing diet led to decrease in plasma IgE levels and an increase in interleukin (IL)-12, which induces cellular immunity, in the AD mice compared to the control. Glucosylceramide can prevent AD like symptoms in AD model mice via regulation of Th1/Th2 (T helper cells) balance.[8]

▶ SUPPLEMENTATION

	BASIS	WHAT TO LOOK OUT FOR
Supplementation form	Glucosylceramide, glycosylceramides, dihydroceramide, and sphingosine are obtained from plant extract, yeast extract or gram negative bacteria. There are no studies recommending the best form or source of ceramides.	The source of the product is mentioned on the product packaging.
Administration form	Capsules, tablets	N/A
Purity considerations	Some manufacturers suggest that the wheat extract powder has a higher amount of phytoceramide compared to the oil form.	The purity of phytoceramides is stated in the nutritional label, if not can be obtained from the product company.
Patient considerations	Plant-based ceramides are vegan.	Vegetarian products will have a vegetarian logo (green dot) on the supplement.
Safety considerations	A dose of 9.06 mg of ceramide a day for 4 weeks did not show any adverse effects.[9] Much higher doses are used in several supplements. Caution must be exercised for people with cardiovascular concerns as ceramides play an important role in heart disease.[10]	Safety and tolerability data must be provided by the company.
Other considerations	Wheat extract may contain gluten, so caution must be exercised for those who are intolerant.	A gluten ELIZA report showing < 20 ppm or mg/kg gluten shows the product is gluten-free. The manufacturer should be able to provide this laboratory report.

▶ INTRODUCTION

Ceramides are a heterogeneous class of lipids present in the stratum corneum of the skin epidermis. They constitute the backbone structure of all sphingolipids, as well as being a minor component of cellular membranes.[11] Along with other lipids present in stratum corneum, ceramides form a highly ordered lamellar structure which is involved in skin barrier function. Therefore, they are involved in regulating TEWL through skin as well as biological activities.

Ceramides are involved in a variety of cellular processes and in diseases. Their biological functions are dependent on their unique biophysical properties, which promote strong alterations to the cell membrane and the consequent triggering of signaling events.[12]

Phytoceramides, or broadly speaking, plant sphingolipids are structurally diverse, and therefore have a range of bioactivities.[13] Phytoceramides, or even those produced by other means, are mostly employed in topical concoctions; more recently its oral supplementation has been explored.[2]

▶ DIGESTION, ABSORPTION AND STORAGE

Digestion and Absorption

- The fate of ingested sphingolipids in humans is hypothesized to follow a similar track of metabolism as described in animal studies. Some components of sphingolipids (like sphingosine) reach systemic circulation following transport through the mucosa.[16]

- After reaching the skin, they may activate the ceramide synthesis in the skin, rather than direct reutilization.[14]

- Animal studies have shown that radiolabeled ingested ceramides are delivered to the skin.[15]

Storage

Components of phytoceramides are used to synthesize ceramides in the skin. Animal studies also suggest a large proportion of ingested sphingolipids are excreted in the feces.[6,15]

▶ MECHANISM OF ACTION

01 | Barrier Function

Dermatological diseases, including psoriasis, atopic dermatitis and ichthyosis, are associated with altered composition and metabolism of epidermal sphingolipids. Oral intake of phytoceramides helps restore the ceramide content of skin. They are hypothesized to do so by assimilating its components into epidermal ceramides. Whether the bioactivity of ceramides increases de novo ceramide synthesis or not remains to be clarified further.[1,16,16]

An in vitro study shows that treatment of phytosphingosine to the cultured keratinocyte increased its ceramide content. There was an increase in expression of the three genes [SPT, ceramide synthase 3 (CERS3), and ELOVL4] and their proteins. The expression of the dihydroceramide C4-desaturase (DES2), an enzyme which converts dihydroceramide into ceramide NP was also enhanced by phytosphingosine treatment.[16]

02 | Cell Signaling

Within the cell membrane, there are tightly-packed, ordered regions called lipid rafts that are enriched with cholesterol and sphingolipids. Ceramides greatly stabilize these lipid rafts and displace cholesterol from them. Recently, ceramide-platforms also emerged as an important class of membrane domains.[17] Together they affect the cell's physical properties like lipid-protein interactions and attract signaling molecules.[18]

By virtue of this, sphingolipids also play an important role in epidermal signaling. As a chief mediator of the sphingolipid metabolic pathway, ceramides and its metabolites regulate processes such as proliferation, differentiation, and apoptosis **(Figure 1)**. Ceramides have also been shown to induce apoptosis in cultured human keratinocytes triggered by UVB radiation.[1]

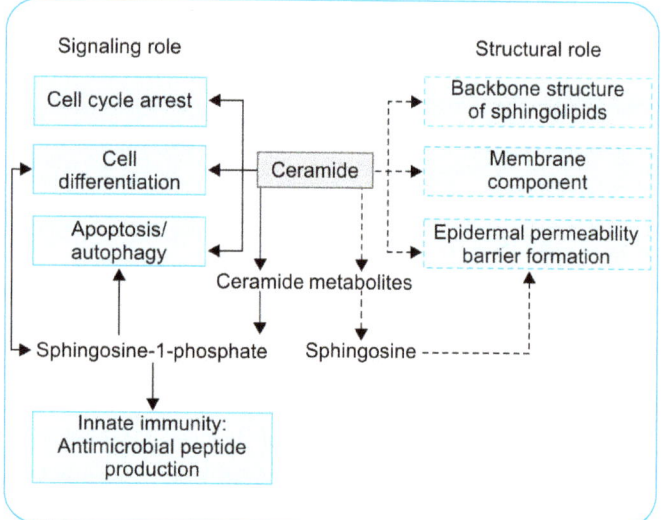

Figure 1: *The role of ceramides and their metabolites in the epidermis.*
Source: *Adapted from Uchida (2014).[11]*

Recent studies have further demonstrated that a ceramide metabolite, sphingosine-1-phosphate, modulates innate immunity against infecting pathogens.[18] It does so by stimulating cathelicidin antimicrobial peptide expression, which exhibits a broad spectrum of antimicrobial activity, and can also trigger specific defence responses in the host.

► REFERENCES

1. Borodzicz S, Rudnicka L, Mirowska-Guzel D, Cudnoch-Jedrzejewska A. The role of epidermal sphingolipids in dermatologic diseases. Lipids Health Dis. 2016;15(1):13.
2. Bizot V, Cestone E, Michelotti A, Nobile V. Improving Skin Hydration and Age-related Symptoms by Oral Administration of Wheat Glucosylceramides and Digalactosyl Diglycerides: A Human Clinical Study. Cosmetics. 2017;4(4):37.
3. Tsuchiya Y, Ban M, Kishi M, Ono T, Masaki H. Safety and Efficacy of Oral Intake of Ceramide-Containing Acetic Acid Bacteria for Improving the Stratum Corneum Hydration: A Randomized, Double-Blind, Placebo-Controlled Study over 12 Weeks. J Oleo Sci. 2020;69(11):1497-508.
4. Shimoda H, Terazawa S, Hitoe S, Tanaka J, Nakamura S, Matsuda H, et al. Changes in ceramides and glucosylceramides in mouse skin and human epidermal equivalents by rice-derived glucosylceramide. J Med Food. 2012;15(12):1064-72.
5. Sun Q, Wu J, Qian G, Cheng H. Effectiveness of Dietary Supplement for Skin Moisturizing in Healthy Adults: A Systematic Review and Meta-Analysis of Randomized Controlled Trials. Front Nutr. 2022;9:895192.
6. Venkataramana SH, Puttaswamy N, Kodimule S. Potential benefits of oral administration of AMORPHOPHALLUS KONJAC glycosylceramides on skin health – a randomized clinical study. BMC Complement Med Ther. 2020;20:26.
7. Leo TK, Tan ESS, Amini F, Rehman N, Ng ESC, Tan CK. Effect of Rice (Oryza sativa L.) Ceramides Supplementation on Improving Skin Barrier Functions and Depigmentation: An Open-Label Prospective Study. Nutrients. 2022;14(13):2737.
8. Ono J, Kinoshita M, Aida K, Tamura M, Ohnishi M. Effects of dietary glucosylceramide on dermatitis in atopic dermatitis model mice. European Journal of Lipid Science and Technology. 2010;112(7):708-11.
9. Tsuchiya Y, Ban M, Kishi M, Ono T. Safety Evaluation of the Excessive Intake of Ceramide-Containing Acetic Acid Bacteria – A Randomized, Double-Blind, Placebo-Controlled Study Over a 4-week Period. J Oleo Sci. 2021;70(3):417-30.
10. Zietzer A, Düsing P, Reese L, Nickenig G, Jansen F. Ceramide Metabolism in Cardiovascular Disease: A Network With High Therapeutic Potential. Arterioscler Thromb Vasc Biol. 2022;42(10):1220-8.
11. Uchida Y. Ceramide signaling in mammalian epidermis. Biochim Biophys Acta. 2014;1841(3):453-62.
12. Castro BM, Prieto M, Silva LC. Ceramide: a simple sphingolipid with unique biophysical properties. Prog Lipid Res. 2014;54:53-67.
13. Markham JE, Lynch DV, Napier JA, Dunn TM, Cahoon EB. Plant sphingolipids: function follows form. Curr Opin Plant Biol. 2013;16(3):350-7.
14. Duan J, Sugawara T, Hirose M, Aida K, Sakai S, Fujii A, et al. Dietary sphingolipids improve skin barrier functions via the upregulation of ceramide synthases in the epidermis. Exp Dermatol. 2012;21(6):448-52.
15. Ueda O, Hasegawa M, Kitamura S. Distribution in Skin of Ceramide after Oral Administration to Rats. Drug Metab Pharmacokinet. 2009;24(2):180-4.
16. Choi HK, Kim HJ, Liu KH, Park CS. Phytosphingosine Increases Biosynthesis of Phytoceramide by Uniquely Stimulating the Expression of Dihydroceramide C4-desaturase (DES2) in Cultured Human Keratinocytes. Lipids. 2018;53(9):909-18.
17. Megha, Sawatzki P, Kolter T, Bittman R, London E. Effect of ceramide N-acyl chain and polar headgroup structure on the properties of ordered lipid domains (lipid rafts). Biochim Biophys Acta. 2007;1768(9):2205-12.
18. Huang FC. The Role of Sphingolipids on Innate Immunity to Intestinal Salmonella Infection. Int J Mol Sci. 2017;18(8):1720.

SECTION 05

Antioxidants and Enzymes

24. Non-provitamin A Carotenoids — *Rajat Kandhari*
25. Glutathione — *Geetanjali Shetty*
26. Coenzyme Q10 — *Geetanjali Shetty*
27. Alpha Lipoic Acid — *Geetanjali Shetty*
28. Polyphenols — *Rajesh Mikkilineni*
29. Phytoestrogens — *Rajesh Mikkilineni*

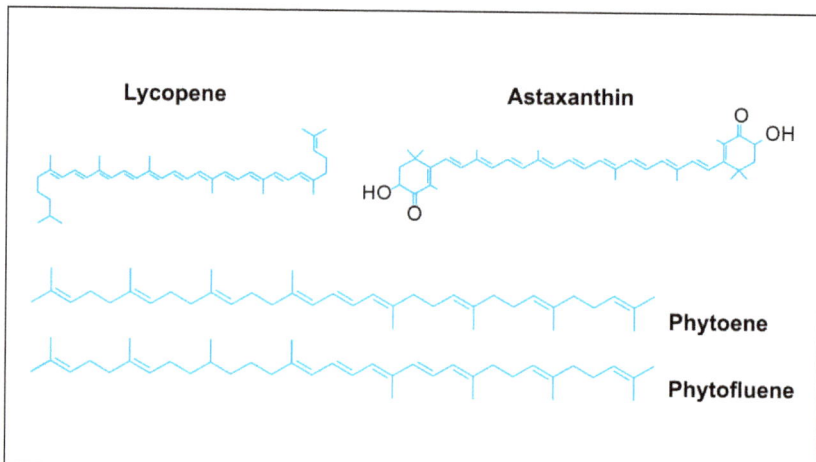

Non-provitamin A Carotenoids (Lycopene, Astaxanthin, Phytoene, Phytofluene)

Non-provitamin A Carotenoids

✍ Rajat Kandhari

CONTENTS

NON-PROVITAMIN A CAROTENOIDS: NUTRIENT SNAPSHOT

- ▸ REQUIREMENT IN THE INDIAN CONTEXT | **237**
- ▸ ACTIVE FORMS | **238**
- ▸ SAFETY AND DOSAGE | **238**
- ▸ CLINICAL CONDITIONS | **240**
- ▸ SUPPLEMENTATION | **245**

INTRODUCTION | **247**

DIGESTION, ABSORPTION AND STORAGE | **247**

MECHANISM OF ACTION | **247**

KEY TOPICS

- ACNE VULGARIS
- ANTI-AGING
- ANTI-INFLAMMATION
- ATOPIC DERMATITIS
- COLLAGEN DEPOSITION
- ERYTHEMA
- ERYTHEMA-INDUCED MMP-1 PRODUCTION
- OXIDATIVE DAMAGE
- PHOTOAGING
- POLYMORPHIC LIGHT ERUPTION (PLE) PHOTODERMATOSIS
- UNDEREYE DARK CIRCLES
- UV-INDUCED ERYTHEMA

Nutrient Snapshot

▶ **REQUIREMENT IN THE INDIAN CONTEXT**

- Carotenoids are a class of natural pigments that can be classified as provitamin A or non-provitamin A. Provitamin A carotenoids, like α-carotene, β-carotene, and α-cryptoxanthin, can be metabolized into retinal and retinol, and therefore contribute to vitamin A intake. Conversely, non-provitamin A carotenoids, including lycopene, lutein, zeaxanthin, and astaxanthin, have been associated with a variety of health benefits unrelated to vitamin A function.

- Although no intake recommendations are currently proposed for carotenoids, existing recommendations for increased consumption of carotenoid-rich fruits and vegetables are supported. Given that too much supplemental vitamin A can cause hypervitaminosis, non-provitamin A carotenoids offer a safer option to increase carotenoid intake through supplements.

- In dermatology, carotenoids are deposited in the skin, where they absorb UV radiation and neutralize free radicals. Carotenoid coloration in the skin, increases its yellowness, making it appear healthier. There are also reports of carotenoids and some other phytonutrients to be effective blockers of dihydrotestosterone (DHT) production, thereby promoting hair health.

- Most of the lycopene consumption in our diet comes from tomatoes. Astaxanthin is found in algae, yeast, certain fish and crustaceans. However, these sources may not provide appreciable amounts for a clinical benefit.

▶ ACTIVE FORMS

ACTIVE FORMS	SUPPLEMENT SOURCES	SALIENT FEATURES
Lycopene	Synthetic	As per research, the natural form has the benefit of additional carotenoids such as phytoene and phytofluene that absorb light in the UV and work synergistically with lycopene.[1,2]
	Tomatoes, red guava, grapefruit, papaya, watermelon, fungus (Blakeslea trispora)	
Astaxanthin (ASX)	Microalgae, fungi, lichen and bacteria or redfish and crustaceans.	It is not known whether natural or synthetic astaxanthin works better.[3] Astaxanthin derived from microalgae *Haematococcus pluvialis* is GRAS approved.[3]
	Synthetic	As per FSSAI guidelines, (2022) synthetic astaxanthin is not allowed to be used in nutraceuticals.
Lutein and zeaxanthin	Flower marigold	They are normally used in supplements for eye health.
Phytoene and phytofluene	Tomato	These two have maximum absorption in the UV range.[4,5]

▶ SAFETY AND DOSAGE

GENERAL REQUIREMENTS	
Indian recommendations	Lycopene: Permitted range not available. Astaxanthin: FSSAI permitted range of natural astaxanthin that can be used for products is 2–12 mg/day

▶ SAFETY AND DOSAGE (Continued)

GENERAL REQUIREMENTS	
Global recommendations and limits	Lycopene: - GRAS* approved by the FDA - The daily lycopene intake for its benefits is suggested to be 2–20 mg.[6] - EFSA acceptable daily intake(ADI): 0.5 mg/kg body weight per day - NOAEL: 500 mg/kg body weight per day Astaxanthin: - GRAS* approved by the FDA for astaxanthin from H. pluvialis for dosages up to 12 mg/day and up to 24 mg/ day for no more than 30 days[7-9] Studies suggest that 3–6 mg/day has shown benefits on skin health.[10] - EFSA ADI: 0.2 mg/day - EFSA: 8 mg/day from food supplements is safe for adults.[11] - NOAEL: 3 g/kg body weight per day.[12] - Phytoene and phytofluene: ADIs not established.[13]
Notes:	Lycopene: There are no known adverse effects from low (12 mg/day) to very high (150 mg/day) intake of lycopene in a healthy population.[14] Astaxanthin: No significant side effects have been reported so far in published human studies.[3]

▶ **CLINICAL CONDITIONS**

EVIDENCE LEVEL	CONDITION OR USE CASE	DOSAGE	BENEFIT OR MECHANISM OF ACTION
++++	Acne vulgaris (lycopene)	50 g ice cream containing 7 mg of lycopene (and one group without lycopene) daily in the evening for 4 weeks	Control ice cream increased corneocyte desquamation and bacterial presence in the residual skin surface components (RSSC) analysis, which remained unchanged in the lycopene group. Lycopene also decreased systemic oxidative stress biomarkers (IOD and LDL-px) compared to control.[15]
+++++	UV-induced erythema (lycopene)	N/A (meta-analysis)	In this analysis of 21 studies, supplementation of tomato and lycopene were associated with reductions in Δa*, MMP-1, ICAM-1 and skin pigmentation. Their supplementation was also associated with an increase in minimal erythema dose, skin thickness and skin density.[16]
+++++	Erythema (tomato carotenoids)	Carotenoid-rich tomato nutrient complex containing 15 mg lycopene, 5.8 mg phytoene and phytofluene, 0.8 mg β-carotene, 5.6 mg tocopherols, and 4 mg carnosic acid (from rosemary extract) daily or placebo daily for 12 weeks	The carotenoid-containing supplement protected against UVB-induced erythema formation as compared to the placebo. The supplement protected against UVB-induced upregulation of IL-6 and TNF-α as compared with the intake of placebo.[17]
+++	UV-induced erythema (tomato paste)	Tomato paste (40 g), providing approximately 16 mg/day of lycopene, was ingested with 10 g of olive oil vs placebo for 10 weeks	Serum levels of lycopene increased in subjects; the other carotenoids did not change significantly. At week 10, skin erythema formation was 40% lower in the tomato paste group compared with controls.[18,19]

▶ CLINICAL CONDITIONS (Continued)

EVIDENCE LEVEL	CONDITION OR USE CASE	DOSAGE	BENEFIT OR MECHANISM OF ACTION
+++	UV-induced erythema (mixed carotenoids)	Subjects were divided into 3 groups: synthetic lycopene (10.2 mg), natural tomato extract of 9.8 mg lycopene, 0.8 mg phytofluene, 1 mg phytoene, and 0.4 mg β-carotene; and the third group consumed a drink containing 8.2 mg lycopene, 3.2 mg phytofluene, 4.6 mg phytoene, and 0.4 mg β-carotene, for 12 weeks.	The a-values (which indicates the redness of the skin) before irradiation were similar in all groups at all time points. The treatment with synthetic lycopene, a slight decrease in the Δ a-value was observed between weeks 0 and 12. In the lycopene with other carotenoids groups, there was a significant reduction in a-values.[20]
+++	Erythema (phytoene and phytofluene)	Subjects ingested an oral supplement with 5 mg total of phytoene and phytofluene daily for 12 weeks.	There was an average increase of the minimal erythema dose (MED) in all subjects. Erythema after exposure to 1.25 MED was also measured, showing no increase in skin color. Skin quality was reportedly improved in 55–95% of the subjects by clinical and subjective assessment.[21]
+++++	Polymorphic light eruption (PLE): Photodermatosis (mix carotenoids)	One capsule containing 2.5 mg lycopene, 4.7 mg of β-carotene, and 5.108 cfu of the probiotic *L. johnsonii* or placebo for 12 weeks.	The intake of the supplement reduced the PLE score after one exposure of UV radiation as compared to placebo. After two exposures of UV light, these differences were no longer significant. The development of skin lesions was associated with an increased expression of intercellular adhesion molecule 1 (ICAM-1) mRNA, which was reduced after supplementation, unlike placebo.[22]

▶ **CLINICAL CONDITIONS** (*Continued*)

EVIDENCE LEVEL	CONDITION OR USE CASE	DOSAGE	BENEFIT OR MECHANISM OF ACTION
+++++	Anti-aging and undereye dark circles (natural lycopene)	Women were first given a placebo daily for 30 days to establish a baseline, followed by a product containing hydrolyzed collagen peptide (5.5 g), lycopene (5 mg), grape seed extract, green tea extract, taurine, vitamin C and E for 60 days.	On day 30, skin hydration, firmness, elasticity and barrier function improved from baseline. The product reduced wrinkle width, pore size, skin roughness, and the color of hyperpigmented blemishes at day 60 from baseline. Clinical evaluation showed that periorbital hyperpigmentation and wrinkles also reduced after 60 days.[23]
+++	Skin aging, dermal density and skin pH (tomato extract)	Oral supplement containing 210 mg marine protein, 54 mg vitamin C, 27.5 mg grape seed extract, 4 mg zinc, and 28.8 mg tomato extract for 180 days	Clinical improvements on both investigator- and subject-rated outcomes were found for the following parameters: Erythema, hydration, radiance, and overall appearance. Improvements from baseline were also seen in skin hydration, dermal ultrasound density, and reduction of skin pH.[24]
+++	Collagen deposition and MMP-1 production caused by erythema (tomato paste)	Subjects ingested 55 g tomato paste (16 mg lycopene) in olive oil daily for 12 weeks	Mean erythemal D(30) was higher following tomato paste versus control. Post supplementation, UVR-induced MMP-1 was reduced, while procollagen I deposition was increased in the tomato paste group compared to control. mtDNA 3895-bp deletion (highly sensitive biomarker of UV radiation) following UVR was also reduced.[25]
+++++	UV radiation induced photoprotection (tomato extract and lutein)	Subjected received softgels of either 5 mg tomato nutrient rich complex (TNC) or 10 mg of lutein or placebo for 12 weeks (2 times)	TNC completely inhibited UVA/B induced upregulation of HO-1, ICAM-1 and MMP1 mRNA (genes known to cause UV radiation induced damage). TNC was more effective than lutein.[26]

▶ CLINICAL CONDITIONS (Continued)

EVIDENCE LEVEL	CONDITION OR USE CASE	DOSAGE	BENEFIT OR MECHANISM OF ACTION
+++	UV radiation induced skin deterioration (astaxanthin)	Placebo or capsule containing 4 mg of natural astaxanthin derived from *H. pluvialis* for 10 weeks	The astaxanthin group showed increased MED compared to placebo. The astaxanthin group had more moisture in the irradiated area compared to placebo. Subjective skin conditions for "improvement of rough skin" and "texture" in non-irradiated areas were improved by astaxanthin.[27]
+++	Photoaging and undereye dark circles (phytofluene and phytoene)	1 softgel containing a mix of tomato carotenes predominantly phytoene and phytofluene, zeta-carotene, daily for 12 weeks (dose not available)	After 12 weeks, the score of different skin parameters was improved, including skin elasticity, firmness, brightness, skin tone, reduction in dark spots and periorbital dark circles, skin hydration, texture and fine lines and wrinkles. These improvements persisted even after treatment was stopped.[28]
++++	Oxidative damage (lycopene)	Healthy women ingested a single large dose of β-carotene (120 mg). Lycopene wasn't supplemented.	When skin was subjected to UV light stress, more skin lycopene was destroyed compared with β-carotene, suggesting a role of lycopene in mitigating oxidative damage in tissues.
++++	Skin aging (astaxanthin)	Oral supplementation containing AstaReal® Oil 50F, astaxanthin, either 12 mg or 6 mg or a placebo for 16 weeks.	The level of an inflammatory cytokine, IL-1α, in the stratum corneum increased in the placebo and low-dose groups but not in the high-dose group from baseline. The skin moisture content and wrinkles did not change in the astaxanthin-supplemented groups, whereas these parameters worsened in the placebo group.[29]
+++	Skin aging (astaxanthin)	4 mg of astaxanthin daily for 4 weeks	The analysis of residual skin surface components (RSSC) samples revealed decreased levels of corneocyte desquamation and microbial presence at the end of the study. The described RSSC changes correspond to a shift toward characteristics of younger skin.[30]
++++	Skin aging (astaxanthin)	2 mg of astaxanthin or placebo daily for 6 weeks	Improvements of moisture, wrinkles, fine lines and elasticity were observed at 6 weeks in the astaxanthin group compared to placebo. Over 50% of the subjects in the treated group showed subjective improvement of all parameters (skin dryness, moisture content, roughness, elasticity and fine lines/wrinkles).[31]

▶ CLINICAL CONDITIONS (Continued)

EVIDENCE LEVEL	CONDITION OR USE CASE	DOSAGE	BENEFIT OR MECHANISM OF ACTION
+++	Anti-aging (astaxanthin)	Study 1: 6 mg of astaxanthin along with 2 mL topical application of astaxanthin for 8 weeks. Study 2: Supplement containing 6 mg of astaxanthin for 6 weeks	Study 1: Improvements were seen in skin wrinkle, dark spot size, elasticity, skin texture, and the moisture content of the corneocyte layer. Study 2: Crow's feet wrinkle and elasticity and TEWL were improved after daily astaxanthin supplementation. Moisture content and sebum oil level improved.
+++	UV irradiated skin changes (lutein and zeaxanthin)	Subjects were divided into 4 groups: Group A: Placebo for both oral and topical treatments, group B: Oral placebo while lutein + zeaxanthin topical application twice daily, group C: lutein 5 mg + zeaxanthin 0.3 mg twice daily and topical placebo and group 4: Oral lutein 5 mg + zeaxanthin 0.3 mg twice daily and topical lutein + zeaxanthin twice daily for 12 weeks.	The oral administration of lutein provided better UV protection than that topical application as measured by changes in lipid peroxidation and photoprotective activity following UV irradiation.[32]
++	Anti-inflammatory property (phytofluene and phytoene)	Human dermal fibroblasts cell culture was first exposed to UV radiation or IL-1 and then incubated with either CoQ10 or phytoene + phytofluene or with combination of both for 24 hours in vitro.	There was an increase in the production of various inflammatory mediators including PGE-2, IL-1, and IL-6 and proteases such as MMP-1 by human fibroblasts due to exposure to UV radiation or IL-1. Treatment of fibroblasts with CoQ10 suppressed the UVR- or IL-1-induced increase in PGE-2, IL-6, and MMP-1. The combination of carotenoids and CoQ10 produced an enhanced inhibition of these inflammatory mediators. The colorless carotenoids, phytoene and phytofluene, protected CoQ10 from degradation by ROS.[33]

▶ CLINICAL CONDITIONS (Continued)

EVIDENCE LEVEL	CONDITION OR USE CASE	DOSAGE	BENEFIT OR MECHANISM OF ACTION
+++	Atopic dermatitis (astaxanthin)	Rodents received astaxanthin (100 mg/kg) or placebo (olive oil) once a day and 3 times a week for 26 days.	The astaxanthin group showed a reduction in the clinical skin severity score compared to placebo. The spontaneous scratching in AD model mice was reduced in the treatment group. Serum IgE level, and the number of eosinophils and total and degranulated mast cells was decreased by astaxanthin. The mRNA and protein levels of eotaxin, MIF, IL-4, IL-5 and L-histidine decarboxylase were decreased in the skin of mice in the astaxanthin group.[34]
++	DHT inhibition	The DHT blocking ability of botanical extracts (like curcumin, lycopene, astaxanthin and β-carotene) was tested on prostate cancer cells that grow in response to DHT.	Prostate cancer cells that grow in response to DHT, were inhibited most effectively by lycopene. The combinations of several carotenoids (lycopene, phytoene and phytofluene), or carotenoids and polyphenols (like carnosic acid and curcumin) and/or other compounds (e.g., vitamin E) synergistically inhibited DHT, even at low, noneffective concentrations.[35]

▶ SUPPLEMENTATION

	BASIS	WHAT TO LOOK OUT FOR
Supplementation form	Cis and trans lycopene All foods contain predominantly all-trans lycopene while human tissue contain cis lycopene. As per studies, the cis isomer is easily absorbed and has more bioavailability as compared to the trans form.[36] Phytoene and phytofluene has higher bioavailability and bioaccessibility due to its cis form and molecular flexibility.[37,38]	The form of lycopene is normally not given on the label but mostly it will be the trans form. Synthetic lycopene is nature-identical. However, the natural extract have phytofluene and phytoene, which promote its benefits.
Administration form	Capsule, softgel, powder, liquid	N/A

▶ SUPPLEMENTATION (Continued)

	BASIS	WHAT TO LOOK OUT FOR
Purity considerations	Lycopene: Beadlets and powders have a 5% concentration. Oil format has higher concentrations. Astaxanthin: Oil format (10%) has higher concentration as compared to powders (4%).	Normally the amount of lycopene-containing extract is given on the label, of which the purity is 5%. The concentration of pure lycopene in a product must be inquired from the manufacturer.
Patient considerations	As these are fat soluble antioxidants, they should be taken with or after a meal for better absorption.	N/A
Safety considerations	Lycopene has a very good safety profile. No known side effects recorded with a 150 mg dose.[14] Astaxanthin is safe, with no side effects when it is consumed with food.[39] However, FSSAI's permitted range of natural astaxanthin is 2–12 mg/day. Several phytoene and phytofluene-rich products, notably tomato-derived, have been regarded as safe for human consumption by different competent bodies, such as the US FDA or the EFSA.[4,40]	The dose per serving is stated in the nutritional table of the product packaging.
	Individuals on blood thinners should exercise caution while taking any phytonutrients and supplements.[41,42] Astaxanthin is not recommended for individuals with diabetes. While lycopene is generally recommended to promote cardiac health, it is not recommended for low blood pressure, and pregnant and lactating women.	Patients with chronic disorders or on medication should seek their doctor's advice prior to consuming any supplements

▶ INTRODUCTION

Carotenoids function in plants and in photosynthetic bacteria as accessory pigments in photosynthesis and protect against photosensitization in animals, plants, and bacteria. Blood concentrations of carotenoids are the best biological markers for consumption of fruits and vegetables. A large body of observational epidemiological evidence suggests that higher blood concentrations of carotenoids obtained from foods are associated with lower risk of several chronic diseases.[43]

By virtue of their vitamin A activity, provitamin A carotenoids are involved in skin turnover and immune function directly. However, there has been great interest in the potential role of non provitamin A carotenoids in enhancement of skin and hair. Astaxanthin, lycopene, phytofluene and phytoene are amongst the most popular, due to their ability to neutralize ROS, prevent lipid peroxidation, reduce inflammation and promote UV protection.[44] Natural extracts with combinations of these carotenoids have been thought to work synergistically to promote their benefits.[35]

▶ DIGESTION, ABSORPTION AND STORAGE

Digestion and Absorption

- The intestinal absorption of dietary carotenoids is facilitated by the formation of bile acid micelles.[43]

- The carotenoids are transported in blood exclusively by lipoproteins. Their delivery to extrahepatic tissue is accomplished through lipoprotein interaction with receptors and the degradation of lipoproteins by enzymes.[43]

- Encapsulation with materials is being used to improve the bioavailability of carotenoids and shield them from the harsh environment of the stomach.

- Carotenoid absorption requires the presence of fat in a meal. While this may vary within carotenoids, as little as 3–5 g of fat (approximately 1 teaspoon) appears sufficient to ensure absorption.[45]

Storage

They are mostly stored in the liver, adrenals, and prostate. They can be found in other body parts (e.g., brain and skin) in lower concentrations.[6]

▶ MECHANISM OF ACTION

01 | Antioxidant Activity and Photoprotection

Non-provitamin A carotenoids can protect DNA, proteins, and lipids against oxidation. Lycopene is one of the most potent dietary antioxidants. Its long, acyclic polyene chain gives it a singlet oxygen quenching capacity higher than that of β-carotene and α-tocopherol (vitamin E).[6,46] While astaxanthin is believed to be a stronger antioxidant than lycopene, limited safety data and dosage constraints can limit its long-term use.

The concentration of carotenoids in skin, especially lycopene, have been associated with reducing the level of skin damage caused by UV light exposure (e.g., roughness), and increasing the minimum amount of UV exposure required to cause sunburn (minimum erythema dose).[18,19,25,47] Furthermore, a lycopene-rich supplement has shown to reduce UVR-induced MMP-1, abrogate UVR-induced reduction in fibrillin-1, and increase procollagen I deposition in skin.[25] Similarly, astaxanthin has been shown to reduce MMP production in certain cells.[7]

Carotenoids are thought to synergistically improve photoprotection too. For example, the combination of lycopene with colorless carotenoids like phytofluene and phytoene, is more effective at photoprotection than lycopene alone.[1,25] This is possibly because it covers the UV spectra more efficiently.[48]

Finally, reduction in ROS caused by lycopene or other antioxidants found in tomatoes regulate immune function and lower inflammation by multiple mechanisms, which is possibly the reason for its use for psoriasis.[49]

02 | Enhancing Skin Appearance

Skin color is mostly determined by melanin concentration, but also by blood and the carotenoids in skin. Human skin color is described using the L*a*b* colorimetric model defined by the Commission Internationale del'Eclairage (CIE L*a*b*), which expresses color as three values: L* for perceptual lightness and a* (green-red) and b* (blue-yellow), modeled on the human visual system. Carotenoids increase skin's b* value (yellowness), which is thought to provide a perceptible cue to health and play a role in attraction. The photoprotection may also be responsible for improving skin's appearance.[47,50]

03 | Preventing DHT Activity

Testosterone is converted to DHT by 5-α-reductase. DHT can bind to androgen receptors longer, and miniaturize hair follicles as well as shorten anagen and lengthen telogen, causing hair to thin and stunts hair growth. While the mechanism of androgenic alopecia is highly complex, this is accepted as the main cause based on our current understanding.[51] By virtue of downregulating DHT activity and production, phytonutrients, especially carotenoids, can be a dietary intervention for DHT-mediated hair loss. Lycopene may be exerting this effect by downregulating IGF-1.[52,53] This is also the reason why lycopene is becoming an important candidate for not only acne vulgaris treatment, but also human prostate cancer prevention.[54,55] In fact, one study stated that lycopene, especially in combination with phytofluene, and phytoene, can inhibit DHT, even at low non-effective concentrations.[35]

▶ **REFERENCES**

1. Aust O, Stahl W, Sies H, Tronnier H, Heinrich U. Supplementation with tomato-based products increases lycopene, phytofluene, and phytoene levels in human serum and protects against UV-light-induced erythema. Int J Vitam Nutr Res. 2005;75(1):54-60.
2. Meléndez-Martínez AJ, Stinco CM, Mapelli-Brahm P. Skin Carotenoids in Public Health and Nutricosmetics: The Emerging Roles and Applications of the UV Radiation-Absorbing Colourless Carotenoids Phytoene and Phytofluene. Nutrients. 2019;11(5):1093.
3. Fassett RG, Coombes JS. Astaxanthin: A Potential Therapeutic Agent in Cardiovascular Disease. Mar Drugs. 2011;9(3):447-65.
4. So B, Kwon KH. Nutritional Approaches of the Changing Consumer after the Pandemic: Sustainable Potential of Phytoene and Phytofluene for Photoprotection and Skin Health. Sustainability. 2023;15(5):4416.
5. Engelmann NJ, Clinton SK, Erdman JW. Nutritional Aspects of Phytoene and Phytofluene, Carotenoid Precursors to Lycopene12. Adv Nutr. 2011;2(1):51-61.
6. Imran M, Ghorat F, Ul-Haq I, Ur-Rehman H, Aslam F, Heydari M, et al. Lycopene as a Natural Antioxidant Used to Prevent Human Health Disorders. Antioxidants (Basel). 2020;9(8):706.
7. Davinelli S, Nielsen ME, Scapagnini G. Astaxanthin in Skin Health, Repair, and Disease: A Comprehensive Review. Nutrients. 2018;10(4):522.
8. Visioli F, Artaria C. Astaxanthin in cardiovascular health and disease: mechanisms of action, therapeutic merits, and knowledge gaps. Food Funct. 2017;8(1):39-63.
9. Sztretye M, Dienes B, Gönczi M, Czirják T, Csernoch L, Dux L, et al. Astaxanthin: A Potential Mitochondrial-Targeted Antioxidant Treatment in Diseases and with Aging. Oxid Med Cell Longev. 2019;2019:3849692.
10. Ng QX, De Deyn MLZQ, Loke W, Foo NX, Chan HW, Yeo WS. Effects of Astaxanthin Supplementation on Skin Health: A Systematic Review of Clinical Studies. J Diet Suppl. 2021;18(2):169-82.
11. EFSA Panel on Nutrition, Novel Foods and Food Allergens (NDA). Safety of astaxanthin for its use as a novel food in food supplements. EFSA Journal 2020;18(2):5993.
12. Trumbo PR. Are there Adverse Effects of Lycopene Exposure?1. The Journal of Nutrition. 2005;135(8):2060S-1S.
13. Havas F, Krispin S, Meléndez-Martínez AJ, von Oppen-Bezalel L. Preliminary Data on the Safety of Phytoene- and Phytofluene-Rich Products for Human Use including Topical Application. Journal of Toxicology. 2018;2018(1):5475784.
14. Saini RK, Rengasamy KRR, Mahomoodally FM, Keum YS. Protective effects of lycopene in cancer, cardiovascular, and neurodegenerative diseases: An update on epidemiological and mechanistic perspectives. Pharmacol Res. 2020;155:104730.
15. Chernyshova MP, Pristenskiy DV, Lozbiakova MV, Chalyk NE, Bandaletova TY, Petyaev IM. Systemic and skin-targeting beneficial effects of lycopene-enriched ice cream: A pilot study. Journal of Dairy Science. 2019;102(1):14-25.
16. Zhang X, Zhou Q, Qi Y, Chen X, Deng J, Zhang Y, et al. The effect of tomato and lycopene on clinical characteristics and molecular markers of UV-induced skin deterioration: A systematic review and meta-analysis of intervention trials. Crit Rev Food Sci Nutr. 2023;1-20.
17. Groten K, Marini A, Grether-Beck S, Jaenicke T, Ibbotson SH, Moseley H, et al. Tomato Phytonutrients Balance UV Response: Results from a Double-Blind, Randomized, Placebo-Controlled Study. Skin Pharmacol Physiol. 2019;32(2):101-8.
18. Stahl W, Heinrich U, Aust O, Tronnier H, Sies H. Lycopene-rich products and dietary photoprotection. Photochem Photobiol Sci. 2006;5(2):238-42.
19. Stahl W, Heinrich U, Wiseman S, Eichler O, Sies H, Tronnier H. Dietary tomato paste protects against ultraviolet light-induced erythema in humans. J Nutr. 2001;131(5):1449-51.

20. Aust O, Stahl W, Sies H, Tronnier H, Heinrich U. Supplementation with tomato-based products increases lycopene, phytofluene, and phytoene levels in human serum and protects against UV-light-induced erythema. Int J Vitam Nutr Res. 2005;75(1):54-60.
21. Bezalel Liki VO, Fishbein D, Havas F, Ben-Chitrit O, Khaiat A. The photoprotective effects of a food supplement tomato powder rich in phytoene and phytofluene, the colorless carotenoids, a preliminary study. Glob Dermatol. 2015;2(4).
22. Marini A, Jaenicke T, Grether-Beck S, Le Floc'h C, Cheniti A, Piccardi N, et al. Prevention of polymorphic light eruption by oral administration of a nutritional supplement containing lycopene, β-carotene, and Lactobacillus johnsonii: results from a randomized, placebo-controlled, double-blinded study. Photodermatol Photoimmunol Photomed. 2014;30(4):189-94.
23. Motwani MS, Khan K, Pai A, Joshi R. Efficacy of a collagen hydrolysate and antioxidants-containing nutraceutical on metrics of skin health in Indian women. Journal of Cosmetic Dermatology. 2020;19(12):3371-82.
24. Costa A, Pegas Pereira ES, Assumpção EC, Calixto dos Santos FB, Ota FS, de Oliveira Pereira M, et al. Assessment of clinical effects and safety of an oral supplement based on marine protein, vitamin C, grape seed extract, zinc, and tomato extract in the improvement of visible signs of skin aging in men. Clin Cosmet Investig Dermatol. 2015;8:319-28.
25. Rizwan M, Rodriguez-Blanco I, Harbottle A, Birch-Machin MA, Watson REB, Rhodes LE. Tomato paste rich in lycopene protects against cutaneous photodamage in humans in vivo: a randomized controlled trial. Br J Dermatol. 2011;164(1):154-62.
26. Grether-Beck S, Marini A, Jaenicke T, Stahl W, Krutmann J. Molecular evidence that oral supplementation with lycopene or lutein protects human skin against ultraviolet radiation: results from a double-blinded, placebo-controlled, crossover study. Br J Dermatol. 2017;176(5):1231-40.
27. Ito N, Seki S, Ueda F. The Protective Role of Astaxanthin for UV-Induced Skin Deterioration in Healthy People—A Randomized, Double-Blind, Placebo-Controlled Trial. Nutrients. 2018;10(7):817.
28. Tarshish E, Hermoni K, Sharoni Y, Muizzuddin N. Effect of Lumenato oral supplementation on plasma carotenoid levels and improvement of visual and experiential skin attributes. Journal of Cosmetic Dermatology. 2022;21(9):4042-52.
29. Tominaga K, Hongo N, Fujishita M, Takahashi Y, Adachi Y. Protective effects of astaxanthin on skin deterioration. J Clin Biochem Nutr. 2017;61(1):33-9.
30. Chalyk NE, Klochkov VA, Bandaletova TY, Kyle NH, Petyaev IM. Continuous astaxanthin intake reduces oxidative stress and reverses age-related morphological changes of residual skin surface components in middle-aged volunteers. Nutr Res. 2017;48:40-8.
31. Yamashita E. The Effects of a Dietary Supplement Containing Astaxanthin on Skin Condition. Carotenoid Science. 2006;10.
32. Palombo P, Fabrizi G, Ruocco V, Ruocco E, Fluhr J, Roberts R, et al. Beneficial long-term effects of combined oral/topical antioxidant treatment with the carotenoids lutein and zeaxanthin on human skin: a double-blind, placebo-controlled study. Skin Pharmacol Physiol. 2007;20(4):199-210.
33. Fuller B, Smith D, Howerton A, Kern D. Anti-inflammatory effects of CoQ10 and colorless carotenoids. J Cosmet Dermatol. 2006;5(1):30-8.
34. Yoshihisa Y, Andoh T, Matsunaga K, Rehman MU, Maoka T, and Shimizu T. Efficacy of Astaxanthin for the Treatment of Atopic Dermatitis in a Murine Model. PLoS One. 2016;11(3):e0152288.
35. Linnewiel-Hermoni K, Khanin M, Danilenko M, Zango G, Amosi Y, Levy J, et al. The anti-cancer effects of carotenoids and other phytonutrients resides in their combined activity. Arch Biochem Biophys. 2015;572:28-35.
36. Boileau T, Boileau A, Erdman Jr J. Bioavailability of all-trans and cis–Isomers of Lycopene. Experimental biology and medicine (Maywood, NJ). 2002;227:914-9.
37. Mapelli-Brahm P, Margier M, Desmarchelier C, Halimi C, Nowicki M, Borel P, et al. Comparison of the bioavailability and intestinal absorption sites of phytoene, phytofluene, lycopene and β-carotene. Food Chem. 2019;300:125232.
38. Mapelli-Brahm P, Desmarchelier C, Margier M, Reboul E, Meléndez Martínez AJ, Borel P. Phytoene and Phytofluene Isolated from a Tomato Extract are Readily Incorporated in Mixed Micelles and Absorbed by Caco-2 Cells, as Compared to Lycopene, and SR-BI is Involved in their Cellular Uptake. Mol Nutr Food Res. 2018;62(22):e1800703.
39. Ambati RR, Siew Moi P, Ravi S, Aswathanarayana RG. Astaxanthin: Sources, Extraction, Stability, Biological Activities and Its Commercial Applications—A Review. Mar Drugs. 2014;12(1):128-52.
40. Meléndez-Martínez AJ, Stinco CM, Mapelli-Brahm P. Skin Carotenoids in Public Health and Nutricosmetics: The Emerging Roles and Applications of the UV Radiation-Absorbing Colourless Carotenoids Phytoene and Phytofluene. Nutrients. 2019;11(5):1093.
41. Santiyanon N, Yeephu S. Interaction between warfarin and astaxanthin: A case report. J Cardiol Cases. 2019;19(5):173-5.
42. Sawardekar SB, Patel TC, Uchil D. Comparative evaluation of antiplatelet effect of lycopene with aspirin and the effect of their combination on platelet aggregation: An in vitro study. Indian J Pharmacol. 2016;48(1):26-31.
43. Institute of Medicine (US) Panel on Dietary Antioxidants and Related Compounds. Dietary Reference Intakes for Vitamin C, Vitamin E, Selenium, and Carotenoids. National Academies Press (US), 2000.
44. Milani A, Basirnejad M, Shahbazi S, Bolhassani A. Carotenoids: biochemistry, pharmacology and treatment. Br J Pharmacol. 2017;174(11):1290-324.
45. van Het Hof KH, West CE, Weststrate JA, Hautvast JG. Dietary factors that affect the bioavailability of carotenoids. J Nutr. 2000;130(3):503-6.
46. Przybylska S. Lycopene – a bioactive carotenoid offering multiple health benefits: a review. International Journal of Food Science & Technology. 2020;55(1):11-32.
47. Ian DS, Coetzee V, David IP. Carotenoid and melanin pigment coloration affect perceived human health. Evolution and Human Behavior. 2011;32:216-27.
48. Hermoni KL, Yoav S. Carotenoids and Polyphenols Synergistically Balance Skin Response to UV(P02-007-19). Current Developments in Nutrition. 2019;3(Suppl 1):nzz029.P02-007-19.
49. Shih CM, Hsieh CK, Huang CY, Huang CY, Wang KH, Fong TH, et al. Lycopene Inhibit IMQ-Induced Psoriasis-Like Inflammation by Inhibiting ICAM-1 Production in Mice. Polymers (Basel). 2020;12(7):1521.
50. Perrett DI, Talamas SN, Cairns P, Henderson AJ. Skin Color Cues to Human Health: Carotenoids, Aerobic Fitness, and Body Fat. Front Psychol. 2020:11:392.

51. Ustuner ET. Cause of Androgenic Alopecia: Crux of the Matter. Plast Reconstr Surg Glob Open. 2013;1(7):e64.
52. Xie Z, Yang F. The effects of lycopene supplementation on serum insulin-like growth factor 1 (IGF-1) levels and cardiovascular disease: A dose-response meta-analysis of clinical trials. Complement Ther Med. 2021;56:102632.
53. Liu X, Allen JD, Arnold JT, Blackman MR. Lycopene inhibits IGF-I signal transduction and growth in normal prostate epithelial cells by decreasing DHT-modulated IGF-I production in co-cultured reactive stromal cells. Carcinogenesis. 2008;29(4):816-23.
54. Wan L, Tan HL, Thomas-Ahner JM, Pearl DK, Erdman JW, Moran NE, et al. Dietary tomato and lycopene impact androgen signaling- and carcinogenesis-related gene expression during early TRAMP prostate carcinogenesis. Cancer Prev Res (Phila). 2014;7(12):1228-39.
55. Chernyshova MP, Pristenskiy DV, Lozbiakova MV, Chalyk NE, Bandaletova TY, Petyaev IM. Systemic and skin-targeting beneficial effects of lycopene-enriched ice cream: A pilot study. Journal of Dairy Science. 2019;102(1):14-25.

25

Glutathione (GSH)

Glutathione

✍ **Geetanjali Shetty**

CONTENTS

GLUTATHIONE: NUTRIENT SNAPSHOT

- ▶ REQUIREMENT IN THE INDIAN CONTEXT | 252
- ▶ ACTIVE FORMS | 253
- ▶ SAFETY AND DOSAGE | 253
- ▶ CLINICAL CONDITIONS | 254
- ▶ SUPPLEMENTATION | 255

INTRODUCTION | 256

DIGESTION, ABSORPTION AND STORAGE | 256

MECHANISM OF ACTION | 256

KEY TOPICS

- ANTI-AGING
- SKIN COLOR
- SKIN WHITENING

Nutrient Snapshot

▶ REQUIREMENT IN THE INDIAN CONTEXT

- Glutathione, a tripeptide of cysteine, glutamic acid, and glycine, is found in all forms of life. Glutathione is the main nonprotein thiol in cells and prevents cellular damage by reacting with free radicals, peroxides, and heavy metals.

- Glutathione levels decrease as a result of aging, stress, and toxin exposure. Insufficient supply of amino acids due to a low protein diet, which is typical in India, may also impact its levels. Chronic inflammation, or low omega 3 fatty acid status, can contribute to oxidative stress and deplete glutathione supply. Increasing glutathione levels may be beneficial as it is involved in the reduction of oxidative stress, detoxification and promotes the maintenance of disulphide bonds in proteins.[1] However, in dermatology, its use seems to be limited to skin lightening, the effect of which is temporary.[2]

- Research suggests that nutritional interventions, including amino acids, vitamins, minerals, phytochemicals, and foods can have important effects on circulating glutathione levels. Furthermore, there is a degree of genetic variability in an individual's capacity to produce glutathione. With upregulated oxidative stress, malnutrition or increased toxic burden due to exposure to environmental contaminants, a case can be made for preformed glutathione.[1] However, in a well-rounded diet, and when cost is a constraint, increasing glutathione levels may be possible by using cysteine (its rate limiter) and other antioxidants.

- Orally administered glutathione is thought to be degraded by digestive peptidases. That's why protein-bound glutathione has been produced to increase circulating levels.[3]

▶ ACTIVE FORMS

ACTIVE FORMS	SUPPLEMENT SOURCES	SALIENT FEATURES
Oxidized glutathione (GSSG)	Synthetically manufactured	According to a study, oxidized glutathione has the same efficacy as the reduced one.[4]
Reduced glutathione (GSH)	Sourced from yeast or synthetically manufactured	Reduced glutathione supplementation leads to increase in body stores of glutathione.[5] Studies show that the GSH form has a role in skin lightening.[6]
Gamma-glutamylcysteine (γ-GC)	Synthetically manufactured	This precursor compound bypasses the cellular regulation of glutathione synthesis and it has been proven to increase intracellular glutathione production above homeostasis.[7]

▶ SAFETY AND DOSAGE

GENERAL REQUIREMENTS	
Indian recommendations	FSSAI permitted range: 50–600 mg/day
Global recommendations and limits	There are no guidelines for glutathione supplementation and dose is based on the research.
Notes:	Glutathione is well tolerated. Glutathione is believed to be degraded in the body, and may simply serve as a source of sulfur. It is important to look at clinical studies of the ingredient in question to ensure whether it increases cellular glutathione levels (and the dose for the same). Another strategy to increase glutathione levels is to supplement N-acetylcysteine (NAC), a cysteine precursor. Cysteine is the main factor limiting the synthesis of GSH. However, this technique relies upon the body's ability to synthesize glutathione, which may be diminished in some circumstances.[8]

▶ **CLINICAL CONDITIONS**

EVIDENCE LEVEL	CONDITION OR USE CASE	DOSAGE	BENEFIT OR MECHANISM OF ACTION
++++	Aging and skin color	GSSG or GSH 250 mg/day or placebo for 12 weeks	There was a reduction in the melanin index of dark spots and an increase in skin elasticity for both GSH and GSSH, compared to placebo. Subjects receiving GSH showed a significant reduction in wrinkles too.[4]
+++	Skin whitening	250 mg L-glutathione + 500 mg L-cysteine, a combination of both or placebo for for 12 weeks	The combination showed skin lightening and significant reduction in the size of dark spots after 6 and 12 weeks, compared to placebo and either nutrient alone.[9]
+++	Skin whitening	Topical GSH + vitamin C and 600 mg oral GSH along with 50 mg alpha lipoic acid, and 4 mg or placebo for 8 weeks	There was a reduction in melanin indices and L* score (lightness) with the combination, compared to placebo and either topical or oral treatment alone.[10]
++++	Skin whitening	500 mg GSH (divided into 2 doses) or placebo for 4 weeks	There was a reduction in melanin indices at various sites on the skin along with changes in the number of dark spots compared to placebo.[11]
++	Skin lightening	500 mg GSH lozenges for 8 weeks through the buccal route	There was a reduction in melanin indices compared to baseline.[12]
+++++	Skin lightening	250–500 mg GSH	Glutathione was effective as a skin-whitening agent in some parts of the body.[2]

▶ SUPPLEMENTATION

	BASIS	WHAT TO LOOK OUT FOR
Supplementation form	Oxidized form (GSSG) Reduced form (L-GSH) Liposomal glutathione is the best form as it helps to increase body stores and is highly tolerable.[13] S-acetyl glutathione Gamma-glutamylcysteine (γ-GC)	Clinical studies on whether the specific form of glutathione helps raise glutathione levels in blood.
Administration form	Tablet, capsule, effervescent tablet, lozenges. Sublingual form of GSH is superior in terms of bioavailability and efficacy over oral form.[8]	This is mentioned on the packaging.
Purity considerations	N/A	
Patient considerations	Glutathione needs to be taken after food	N/A
Safety considerations	Glutathione is well-tolerated	Dose per serving is given on the label.
Other considerations	Other nutrients that can promote its benefits, e.g., antioxidants like vitamin C and B-vitamins help recycle GSH. Zinc can help with detoxification by glutathione.	Product label

INTRODUCTION

Glutathione is a tripeptide that comprises of three amino acids–cysteine, glutamic acid, and glycine. It is the most important low molecular weight antioxidant synthesized in cells.[14] Glutathione exists in cells in two states: Reduced (GSH) and oxidized (GSSG). GSH is a critical cofactor for several antioxidant pathways, including thiol-disulfide exchange reactions and glutathione peroxidase.[15]

The ratio of GSH to GSSG determines cell redox status of cells. Healthy cells at rest have a GSH/GSSG ratio >100 while the ratio drops to 1 to 10 in cells exposed to oxidative stress. GSH is made available in cells in three ways: de novo synthesis (requires ATP), regeneration of oxidized GSSG to reduced GSH (requires NADPH) and recycling of cysteine from conjugated glutathione (requires NADPH). Considering the high level of metabolic activity required to produce glutathione, at a high level, underlines its importance.[15]

DIGESTION, ABSORPTION AND STORAGE

Digestion and Absorption

- Glutathione is poorly absorbed orally. It is likely broken down by digestive peptidases into amino acids.

- Liposomal or protein-bound glutathione has been shown to increase plasma levels.

Storage

- Most cells have a high concentration of glutathione i.e., 5 millimolar. Adequate levels of glutathione are essential in mitochondria, where ROS are constantly being formed as a minor by-product of oxidative respiration.[16]

- Hepatocytes have a 5–10 millimolar concentration.[16]

MECHANISM OF ACTION

Glutathione participates in many cellular reactions—it acts as an antioxidant, a detoxifying agent, and promotes the maintenance of disulphide bonds in proteins. However, it is most frequently used for its activity on melanogenesis.

01 | Antioxidant Activity

As a substrate for glutathione S-transferase, glutathione reacts with a number of harmful chemical species, such as halides, epoxides and free radicals, to form harmless inactive products. In erythrocytes, these reactions prevent oxidative damage through the reduction of methemoglobin and peroxides.[17]

Defence against oxidative stress is primarily dependent upon an orchestrated synergism between several endogenous and exogenous antioxidants. For example, vitamins C and E help recycle glutathione, while glutathione is recycled by these antioxidants as well. Glutathione is thought to play a central role in the antioxidant network (**Figure 1**).[17]

Glutathione may increase intracellular magnesium levels, depletion of which renders cells more sensitive to oxidative damage. This is thought to be one of the reasons for its effects on improving insulin resistance.[18]

02 | Antimelanogenic Activity

Melanin is produced from L-tyrosine that is converted to dopaquinone by the enzymatic activity of tyrosinase. UV radiation is the major extrinsic factor in the regulation of melanogenesis, through the generation of ROS. Antioxidants or antioxidant systems, namely the thioredoxin and glutathione systems, with the ability to scavenge ROS, and regulate melanogenesis. GSH acts as an antimelanogenic agent by promoting the reddish-yellow pheomelanin synthesis over the brownish-black eumelanin.[19] Its effectiveness in sun-exposed areas of the body suggests it may be more efficient on preventing new melanogenesis than to reduce existing pigments.[2]

03 | Detoxification

Glutathione conjugation (facilitated by a family of glutathione transferase enzymes) helps contribute to detoxification by binding electrophiles that could otherwise bind to proteins or nucleic acids, resulting in cellular damage and genetic mutations.[20]

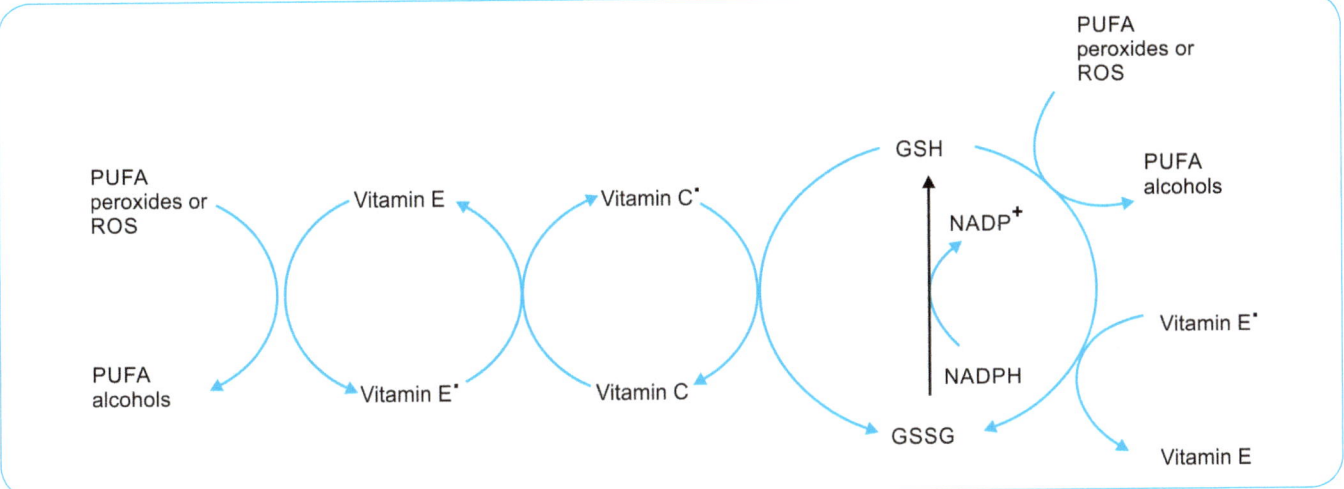

Figure 1: Glutathione plays a central role in the cellular antioxidant network.
(PUFA: polyunsaturated fatty acids; ROS: reactive oxygen species.)
Superscript dot represents radical form.

04 | Cell Metabolism

Glutathione plays important roles in the regulation of cellular events including gene expression, DNA and protein synthesis, cell proliferation and apoptosis, signal transduction, cytokine production and the immune response.[21] That's why glutathione is important for all tissue in the body.

Glutathione is involved in the uptake of amino acids from the intestinal lumen to the cytosol of intestinal mucosa cells. Glutathione is also involved in the formation and maintenance of disulfide bonds in proteins (like keratin). Low levels of glutathione within the cell can result in incorrect protein folding.[22] The amount of GSH in hair follicle keratinocytes reduces with age, causing structural changes in hair as well as becoming the limiting factor for cells to protect themselves from harm.[23]

▶ REFERENCES

1. Minich DM, Brown BI. A Review of Dietary (Phyto)Nutrients for Glutathione Support. Nutrients. 2019;11(9):2073.
2. Sitohang IBS, Ninditya S. Systemic Glutathione as a Skin-Whitening Agent in Adult. Dermatol Res Pract. 2020;2020:8547960.
3. Park EY, Shimura N, Konishi T, Sauchi Y, Wada S, Aoi W, et al. Increase in the protein-bound form of glutathione in human blood after the oral administration of glutathione. J Agric Food Chem. 2014;62(26):6183-9.
4. Weschawalit S, Thongthip S, Phutrakool P, Asawanonda P. Glutathione and its antiaging and antimelanogenic effects. Clin Cosmet Investig Dermatol. 2017;10:147-53.
5. Richie JP, Nichenametla S, Neidig W, Calcagnotto A, Haley JS, Schell TD, et al. Randomized controlled trial of oral glutathione supplementation on body stores of glutathione. Eur J Nutr. 2015;54(2):251-63.
6. Gandhi G, Malhotra SK, Kaur T, Tyagi S, Bassan RL. Glutathione: The master antioxidant – Beyond skin lightening agent. Pigment International. 2021;8(3):144.
7. Zarka MH, Bridge WJ. Oral administration of γ-glutamylcysteine increases intracellular glutathione levels above homeostasis in a randomised human trial pilot study. Redox Biol. 2017;11:631-6.
8. Effects of N-acetylcysteine, oral glutathione (GSH) and a novel sublingual form of GSH on oxidative stress markers: A comparative crossover study. Redox Biology. 2015;6:198-205.
9. Duperray J, Sergheraert R, Chalothorn K, Tachalerdmanee P, Perin F. The effects of the oral supplementation of L-Cystine associated with reduced L-Glutathione-GSH on human skin pigmentation: a randomized, double-blinded, benchmark- and placebo-controlled clinical trial. J Cosmet Dermatol. 2022;21(2):802-13.
10. Wahab S, Anwar AI, Zainuddin AN, Hutabarat EN, Anwar AA, Kurniadi I. Combination of topical and oral glutathione as a skin-whitening agent: a double-blind randomized controlled clinical trial. Int J Dermatol. 2021;60(8):1013-8.
11. Arjinpathana N, Asawanonda P. Glutathione as an oral whitening agent: a randomized, double-blind, placebo-controlled study. J Dermatolog Treat. 2012;23(2):97-102.
12. Handog EB, Datuin MSL, Singzon IA. An open-label, single-arm trial of the safety and efficacy of a novel preparation of glutathione as a skin-lightening agent in Filipino women. Int J Dermatol. 2016;55(2):153-7.

13. Sinha R, Sinha I, Calcagnotto A, Trushin N, Haley JS, Schell TD, et al. Oral supplementation with liposomal glutathione elevates body stores of glutathione and markers of immune function. Eur J Clin Nutr. 2018;72(1):105-11.
14. Forman HJ, Zhang H, Rinna A. Glutathione: Overview of its protective roles, measurement, and biosynthesis. Mol Aspects Med. 2009;30(1–2):1-12.
15. Pizzorno J. Glutathione! Integr Med (Encinitas). 2014;13(1):8-12.
16. Finsterer J. Treatment of Mitochondrial Disorders. European Journal of Paediatric Neurology. 2010;14(1):29-44.
17. Gul M, Kutay FZ, Temocin S, Hanninen O. Cellular and clinical implications of glutathione. Indian J Exp Biol. 2000;38(7):625-34.
18. Barbagallo M, Dominguez LJ, Tagliamonte MR, Resnick LM, Paolisso G. Effects of Glutathione on Red Blood Cell Intracellular Magnesium. Hypertension. 1999;34(1):76-82.
19. Lu Y, Tonissen KF, Trapani GD. Modulating skin colour: role of the thioredoxin and glutathione systems in regulating melanogenesis. Biosci Rep. 2021;41(5):BSR20210427.
20. SC Gad. Glutathione. Encyclopedia of Toxicology (3rd Edition) 2014. doi.org/10.1016/B978-0-12-386454-3.00850-2.
21. Wu G, Fang YZ, Yang S, Lupton JR, Turner ND. Glutathione metabolism and its implications for health. J Nutr. 2004;134(3):489-92.
22. Chakravarthi S, Bulleid NJ. Glutathione Is Required to Regulate the Formation of Native Disulfide Bonds within Proteins Entering the Secretory Pathway. J Biol Chem. 2004;279(38):39872-9.
23. Pruche F, Kermici M, Prunieras M. Changes in glutathione content in human hair follicle keratinocytes as a function of age of donor: relation with glutathione dependent enzymes. Int J Cosmet Sci. 1991;13(3):117-24.

26

Coenzyme Q10 (Ubiquinone)

Coenzyme Q10

Geetanjali Shetty

CONTENTS

COENZYME Q10: NUTRIENT SNAPSHOT

- REQUIREMENT IN THE INDIAN CONTEXT | 260
- ACTIVE FORMS | 261
- SAFETY AND DOSAGE | 261
- CLINICAL CONDITIONS | 261
- SUPPLEMENTATION | 263

INTRODUCTION | 264

DIGESTION, ABSORPTION AND STORAGE | 264

MECHANISM OF ACTION | 264

KEY TOPICS

- ANTI-AGING
- HAIR AGING
- PHOTOPROTECTION

Nutrient Snapshot

▶ REQUIREMENT IN THE INDIAN CONTEXT

- Coenzyme Q10 (ubiquinone, ubiquinol, CoQ10) is a fat-soluble quinone with a structure similar to that of vitamin K. The primary biochemical action of CoQ10 is as a cofactor in the electron-transport chain, in the series of redox reactions that are involved in the synthesis of adenosine triphosphate (ATP). As most cellular functions are dependent on an adequate supply of ATP, CoQ10 is essential for the health of virtually all human tissues and organs.[1,2] In fact, the 'mitochondrial theory of aging' suggests that damage to the mitochondria is a major cause of cellular aging, tissue dysfunction, and degeneration.[3]

- CoQ10 is an important antioxidant for protection of mitochondrial DNA during cellular stress. It is no surprise that CoQ10 has been shown to be a beneficial therapeutic agent in various degenerative conditions such as neurodegeneration, macular degeneration, and cardiovascular diseases.[4]

- The skin is a high turnover organ, and its constant renewal depends on the rapid proliferation of its progenitor cells, the metabolic activities of which are met by mitochondrial respiration.[2] In dermatology, CoQ10 can be used to counteract the slowing cellular metabolism in skin and hair follicles, a hallmark of aging and the cause or effect of conditions like female pattern hair loss.[5]

- While CoQ10 is made endogenously, its synthesis decreases with age, and can be compromised in certain disease states. Primary dietary sources of CoQ10 include oily fish, organ meats (such as liver), and whole grains, all of which are low in the Indian diet, especially for vegetarians. Unsurprisingly, a study found that the reduced form of coenzyme Q10, CoQ10H2, and total Q10 concentrations in plasma were significantly lower in Indian males than Chinese males.[6]

ACTIVE FORMS

ACTIVE FORMS	SUPPLEMENT SOURCES	SALIENT FEATURES
Ubiquinol (reduced)	Synthetic	In vitro and small-size human studies suggest that the ubiquinol form has higher bioavailability as compared to the ubiquinone form.[7-9]
Ubiquinone (oxidized)	Synthetic or natural (extracted from yeast)[10,11]	Ubiquinone supplementation is equally effective as ubiquinol.[10,11] Its lower bioavailability can be improved using carriers, as this is more stable.

SAFETY AND DOSAGE

GENERAL REQUIREMENTS	
Indian recommendations	ICMR-NIN: There is no established RDA.
Global recommendations and limits	NOAEL: 1200 mg/kg body weight/day[12] Dietary consumption is estimated to contribute to about 25% of plasma coenzyme Q10, but there are currently no specific dietary intake recommendations. 30–100 mg/day are normally given to healthy individuals.[13] According to the observed safe level (OSL) risk assessment method, evidence of safety is strong with doses up to 1,200 mg/day of coenzyme Q10. Much higher levels have been tested without adverse effects, but the data is not sufficient for a confident conclusion of safety.[14]
Notes:	Smokers and vegans should consider CoQ10 supplementation. People taking statins should consider supplementing CoQ10 as statins may interfere with its endogenous synthesis.

CLINICAL CONDITIONS

EVIDENCE LEVEL	CONDITION OR USE CASE	DOSAGE	BENEFIT OR MECHANISM OF ACTION
+++	Signs of skin aging	50 and 150 mg CoQ10 or placebo daily for 12 weeks	Supplementation limited seasonal deterioration of viscoelasticity and reduced some visible signs of aging like wrinkles and microrelief lines, compared to placebo, and improved skin smoothness for both doses tested. There was no change in skin hydration, the minimal erythema dose (MED), dermis thickness and density.[15]

▶ **CLINICAL CONDITIONS** (*Continued*)

EVIDENCE LEVEL	CONDITION OR USE CASE	DOSAGE	BENEFIT OR MECHANISM OF ACTION
++	UVA protection	Human dermal fibroblasts and keratinocytes were treated with CoQ10 in vitro	CoQ10 was effective against UVA mediated oxidative stress in keratinocytes in terms of thiol depletion, activation of specific phosphotyrosine kinases and prevention of oxidative DNA damage. CoQ10 was also able to significantly suppress the expression of collagenase in fibroblasts following UVA irradiation.[16]
++	UVB protection	Human dermal fibroblast were exposed to either UVR or to IL-1 and then incubated with CoQ10, or CoQ10 with phytoene and phytofluene in vitro	Human fibroblasts cultured with CoQ10, suppressed the UVR-induced increase in PGE-2 and IL-6, and of the matrix-degrading enzyme, MMP-1. The combination of carotenoids and CoQ10 produced an enhanced inhibition of these three inflammatory mediators.[17] Another in vitro study similarly showed a reduction in IL-6 and MMP-1 by fibroblasts in vitro following UVB irradiation.[18]
++	Hair aging	Hair follicles were cultured with CoQ10 in vitro	In cultivated hair follicle keratinocytes, CoQ10 was identified as a potent bioactive that stimulates gene expression of different hair keratins, especially those which are reduced during aging processes in hair follicles.[3]

SUPPLEMENTATION

	BASIS	WHAT TO LOOK OUT FOR
Supplementation form	Ubiquinone (oxidized) Ubiquinol (reduced) No significant difference in the relative bioavailability of the two forms has been reported and may vary depending on individuals.[10,11,19] Ubiquinone with cyclodextrins (complex formed with cyclic oligosaccharides): Higher bioavailability as compared to other formulations.[20] Liposomal CoQ10: Shows better bioavailability than powdered form of CoQ10.[21-23] CoQ10 obtained from a natural source (yeast) is more bioavailable than the synthetic one.	If CoQ10 is in ubiquinol or liposomal form, it is generally mentioned on the back label of the products.
Administration form	Capsule, tablet, softgels	N/A
Purity considerations	N/A	N/A
Patient considerations	CoQ10 is fat-soluble and should be supplemented after a meal to aid absorption.	N/A
Safety considerations	CoQ10 is generally well tolerated, with no serious adverse events reported in long-term use. Some people have experienced gastrointestinal symptoms, such as nausea, diarrhea, appetite suppression, heartburn, and abdominal discomfort with daily doses ≥ 200 mg. These adverse effects may be minimized if daily doses >100 mg are divided into two or three smaller doses.	The dose per serving is given on the packaging.
Other considerations:	Coq10 is sensitive to heat, light, and oxygen and thus needs to be stored in a dry place away from light.	Storage conditions are mentioned on the packaging and coloured capsules/packaging should be considered.
	CoQ10 supplements are relatively safe but may reduce the response of certain medications such as warfarin, theophylline, pro-oxidant chemotherapeutic agents and increase the effect of antihypertensive drugs.	N/A

INTRODUCTION

CoQ10 is a naturally occurring quinone that is found in most aerobic organisms from bacteria to mammals. CoQ10, is a part of cellular membranes, and appears to be highly localized in the mitochondria as well as other parts of the cell. It is one of the most significant lipid antioxidants, which prevents the generation of free radicals and modifications of proteins, lipids, and DNA. In many disease conditions connected with increased generation of reactive oxygen species (ROS), the concentration of coenzyme Q10 in the human body decreases.[1] Its deficiency has also been observed in persons with inadequate nutrition and in smokers.[24,25] The impairment of CoQ10 status can result in profound deficits to mitochondrial function, thereby impairing ATP synthesis and increasing free radical damage.[26]

The whole body content of CoQ10 is only about 500–2,000 mg and decreases with age. As estimate of 500 mg of CoQ10 needs to be replaced daily by a combination of endogenous synthesis and dietary intake based on the average tissue turnover time of 4 days.[27] The average intake appears to be around 3–6 mg/day (European and Asian data) perhaps because of low intake of organ meats, fatty fish and whole grains in the Indian diet.

Plasma concentrations of CoQ10 in vegans and vegetarians has shown to be lower than omnivores.[28] Certain medications can also lower CoQ10 levels. Lipid-lowering medications (statins) inhibit the activity of 3-hydroxy-3-methylglutaryl (HMG)-coenzyme A (CoA) reductase, a critical enzyme in both cholesterol and coenzyme Q10 biosynthesis, thereby decreasing plasma CoQ10 concentrations.[29]

DIGESTION, ABSORPTION AND STORAGE

Digestion and Absorption

Supplementary CoQ10 absorption depends on the form used. Because of the extreme hydrophobicity of the molecule, orally administered CoQ10 has a low bioavailability.

Following its transit through the stomach, CoQ10 is integrated into micelles in the duodenum, which facilitates CoQ10 transport to the intestinal villi prior to its absorption by enterocytes.

CoQ10 is absorbed into enterocytes via a process of passive facilitated diffusion, where the facilitator molecule is believed to be the cholesterol transporter NPC1L1 (Niemann-Pick C1 Like 1).[10,11]

CoQ10 is then incorporated into chylomicrons, which are released into the distal abdominal lymph duct, where they can then enter the systemic blood circulation via the subclavian vein. Chylomicrons in the circulation are taken up by the liver where CoQ10 is then re-packaged into lipoprotein particles, mainly LDL and VLDL, and a small amount in HDL cholesterol.[10,11]

Storage

Other than cell and mitochondrial membranes, CoQ10 is present in other subcellular organelles, including lysosomes, peroxisomes, Golgi apparatus and endoplasmic reticulum.

Typically, tissues with higher metabolic activity in the body (heart, brain, kidneys, liver, skeletal muscle) have higher levels of CoQ10.

In skin, CoQ10 levels are 10-fold higher in the epidermis than the dermis.

MECHANISM OF ACTION

The benefits of CoQ10 is attributable to its ability to drive cellular metabolism via mitochondrial function, its antioxidant properties for lipid membranes, and its anti-inflammatory function.

01 | Mitochondrial ATP Synthesis

The conversion of energy from carbohydrates and fats to ATP, the form of energy used by cells, requires the presence of coenzyme Q10 in the inner mitochondrial membrane. As part of the mitochondrial electron transport chain, coenzyme Q10 accepts electrons from reducing equivalents generated during fatty acid and glucose metabolism and then transfers them to electron acceptors.[30]

Coenzyme Q10 also contributes to transfer protons (H⁺) from the mitochondrial matrix to the intermembrane space, creating a proton gradient across the inner mitochondrial membrane, which is used to form ATP.[30] In addition to its role in ATP synthesis, mitochondrial coenzyme Q10 mediates the oxidation of dihydroorotate to orotate in the de novo pyrimidine synthesis. Studies have suggested that supplemental coenzyme Q10 could promote mitochondrial biogenesis and respiration, the decline of which is one of the hallmarks of aging.[31,32] For example, mitochondrial dysfunction has been implicated in conditions such as female pattern hair loss.[5]

02 | Antioxidant Properties

In its reduced form, CoQ10 is a powerful lipid-soluble antioxidant. It is present in the cell membrane and subcellular organelles, protecting them from free radical-induced oxidative damage.[33] When LDL is oxidized, CoQ10H2 is the first antioxidant consumed, highlighting its importance in overall health.

03 | Anti-inflammatory Action

CoQ10 has been shown to directly affect the expression of a number of genes. It decreases the production of the pro-inflammatory cytokines TNF-α and IL-6, by inhibiting *NF-κB* gene expression.[34]

While studies on oral CoQ10 for skin and hair remain scant, the innate role of the mitochondria in maintaining skin homeostasis and pigmentation, its therapeutic use in the dermatology—either via an ATP production boost or free radical scavenging—may be warranted.[2]

▶ REFERENCES

1. Saini R. Coenzyme Q10: The essential nutrient. J Pharm Bioallied Sci. 2011;3(3):466-7.
2. Sreedhar A, Aguilera-Aguirre L, Singh KK. Mitochondria in skin health, aging, and disease. Cell Death Dis. 2020;11(6):1-14.
3. Giesen M, Welß T, Zur Wiesche ES, Scheunemann V, Gruedl S, Oezkabakcioglu Y, et al. Coenzyme Q10 has anti-aging effects on human hair. International Journal of Cosmetic Science. 2009;31(2):154-5.
4. Schniertshauer D, Gebhard D, Bergemann J. Age-Dependent Loss of Mitochondrial Function in Epithelial Tissue Can Be Reversed by Coenzyme Q10. J Aging Res. 2018;2018(1):6354680.
5. Piccini I, Sousa M, Altendorf S, Jimenez F, Rossi A, Funk W, et al. Intermediate Hair Follicles from Patients with Female Pattern Hair Loss Are Associated with Nutrient Insufficiency and a Quiescent Metabolic Phenotype. Nutrients. 2022 Aug;14(16):3357.
6. Hughes K, Lee BL, Feng X, Lee J, Ong CN. Coenzyme Q10 and differences in coronary heart disease risk in Asian Indians and Chinese. Free Radic Biol Med. 2002;32(2):132-8.
7. Failla ML, Chitchumroonchokchai C, Aoki F. Increased bioavailability of ubiquinol compared to that of ubiquinone is due to more efficient micellarization during digestion and greater GSH-dependent uptake and basolateral secretion by Caco-2 cells. J Agric Food Chem. 2014;62(29):7174-82.
8. Langsjoen PH, Langsjoen AM. Comparison study of plasma coenzyme Q10 levels in healthy subjects supplemented with ubiquinol versus ubiquinone. Clin Pharmacol Drug Dev. 2014;3(1):13-7.
9. Miles MV, Horn P, Miles L, Tang P, Steele P, DeGrauw T. Bioequivalence of coenzyme Q10 from over-the-counter supplements. Nutrition Research. 2002;22(8):919-29.
10. Mantle D, Heaton RA, Hargreaves IP. Coenzyme Q10, Ageing and the Nervous System: An Overview. Antioxidants. 2022;11(1):2.
11. Mantle D, Dybring A. Bioavailability of Coenzyme Q10: An Overview of the Absorption Process and Subsequent Metabolism. Antioxidants (Basel). 2020;9(5):386.
12. Hidaka T, Fujii K, Funahashi I, Fukutomi N, Hosoe K. Safety assessment of coenzyme Q10 (CoQ10). Biofactors. 2008;32(1–4):199-208.
13. Raizner AE. Coenzyme Q10. Methodist Debakey Cardiovasc J. 2019;15(3):185-91.
14. Hathcock JN, Shao A. Risk assessment for coenzyme Q10 (Ubiquinone). Regul Toxicol Pharmacol. 2006;45(3):282-8.
15. Žmitek K, Pogačnik T, Mervic L, Žmitek J, Pravst I. The effect of dietary intake of coenzyme Q10 on skin parameters and condition: Results of a randomised, placebo-controlled, double-blind study. Biofactors. 2017;43(1):132-40.
16. Hoppe U, Bergemann J, Diembeck W, Ennen J, Gohla S, Harris I, et al. Coenzyme Q10, a cutaneous antioxidant and energizer. Biofactors. 1999;9(2–4):371–8.
17. Fuller B, Smith D, Howerton A, Kern D. Anti-inflammatory effects of CoQ10 and colorless carotenoids. J Cosmet Dermatol. 2006;5(1):30-8.
18. Inui M, Ooe M, Fujii K, Matsunaka H, Yoshida M, Ichihashi M. Mechanisms of inhibitory effects of CoQ10 on UVB-induced wrinkle formation in vitro and in vivo. Biofactors. 2008;32(1–4):237-43.
19. Pravst I, Rodríguez Aguilera JC, Cortes Rodriguez AB, Jazbar J, Locatelli I, Hristov H, et al. Comparative Bioavailability of Different Coenzyme Q10 Formulations in Healthy Elderly Individuals. Nutrients. 2020;12(3):784.
20. Enhancement of oral bioavailability of coenzyme Q10 by complexation with γ-cyclodextrin in healthy adults. Nutrition Research. 2006;26(10):503-8.
21. Beg S, Javed S, Kohli K. Bioavailability enhancement of coenzyme Q10: an extensive review of patents. Recent Pat Drug Deliv Formul. 2010;4(3):245-55.
22. Yamada Y, Burger L, Kawamura E, Harashima H. Packaging of the Coenzyme Q10 into a Liposome for Mitochondrial Delivery and the Intracellular Observation in Patient Derived Mitochondrial Disease Cells. Biological and Pharmaceutical Bulletin. 2017;40(12):2183-90.
23. Pastor-Maldonado CJ, Suárez-Rivero JM, Povea-Cabello S, Álvarez-Córdoba M, Villalón-García I, Munuera-Cabeza M, et al. Coenzyme Q10: Novel Formulations and Medical Trends. Int J Mol Sci. 2020;21(22):8432.

24. Quinzii CM, Hirano M, DiMauro S. CoQ10 deficiency diseases in adults. Mitochondrion. 2007;7(Suppl):S122.
25. Elsayed NM, Bendich A. Dietary antioxidants: potential effects on oxidative products in cigarette smoke. Nutrition Research. 2001;21(3):551-67.
26. Yubero D, Allen G, Artuch R, Montero R. The Value of Coenzyme Q10 Determination in Mitochondrial Patients. J Clin Med. 2017;6(4):37.
27. Weber C, Bysted A, Hılmer G. The coenzyme Q10 content of the average Danish diet. Int J Vitam Nutr Res. 1997;67(2):123-9.
28. Kazunori H, Takao Y, Iwao F. Lower plasma coenzyme Q10 concentrations in healthy vegetarians and vegans compared with omnivores. International Journal on Nutraceuticals, Functional Foods and Novel Foods. 2022. doi.org/10.17470/NF-022-0047
29. Deichmann R, Lavie C, Andrews S. Coenzyme Q10 and Statin-Induced Mitochondrial Dysfunction. The Ochsner Journal. 2010 Spring;10(1):16.
30. Acosta MJ, Vazquez Fonseca L, Desbats MA, Cerqua C, Zordan R, Trevisson E, et al. Coenzyme Q biosynthesis in health and disease. Biochim Biophys Acta. 2016;1857(8):1079-85.
31. Schmelzer C, Kubo H, Mori M, Sawashita J, Kitano M, Hosoe K, et al. Supplementation with the reduced form of Coenzyme Q10 decelerates phenotypic characteristics of senescence and induces a peroxisome proliferator-activated receptor-alpha gene expression signature in SAMP1 mice. Mol Nutr Food Res. 2010;54(6):805-15.
32. Tian G, Sawashita J, Kubo H, Nishio S ya, Hashimoto S, Suzuki N, et al. Ubiquinol-10 Supplementation Activates Mitochondria Functions to Decelerate Senescence in Senescence-Accelerated Mice. Antioxid Redox Signal. 2014;20(16):2606-20.
33. Crane FL. Biochemical functions of coenzyme Q10. J Am Coll Nutr. 2001;20(6):591-8.
34. Schmelzer C, Lindner I, Rimbach G, Niklowitz P, Menke T, Döring F. Functions of coenzyme Q10 in inflammation and gene expression. BioFactors. 2008;32(1–4):179-83.

27

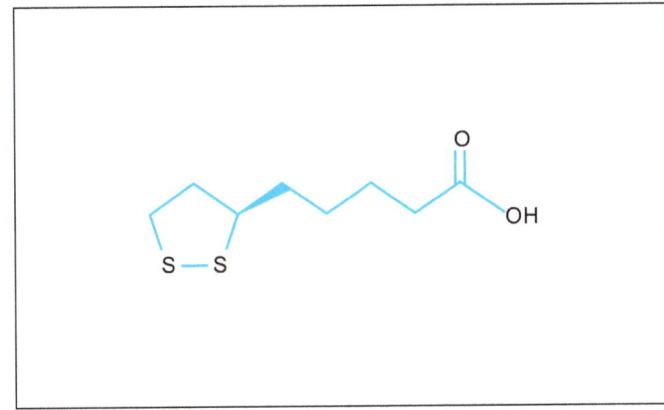

α-Lipoic Acid (or Lipoic Acid; LA)

Alpha Lipoic Acid

✎ Geetanjali Shetty

CONTENTS

ALPHA LIPOIC ACID: NUTRIENT SNAPSHOT

- ▶ REQUIREMENT IN THE INDIAN CONTEXT | 268
- ▶ ACTIVE FORMS | 269
- ▶ SAFETY AND DOSAGE | 269
- ▶ CLINICAL CONDITIONS | 269
- ▶ SUPPLEMENTATION | 270

INTRODUCTION | 271

DIGESTION, ABSORPTION AND STORAGE | 271

MECHANISM OF ACTION | 271

KEY TOPICS

- ANTI-AGEING
- NON-SEGMENTAL VITILIGO
- PIGMENTATION
- SKIN INFLAMMATION
- VITILIGO

Nutrient Snapshot

▶ REQUIREMENT IN THE INDIAN CONTEXT

α-Lipoic acid (or lipoic acid; LA), also known as 1,2-dithiolane-3-pentanoic acid or thioctic acid, is a sulfur-containing antioxidant that is involved in energy production in the mitochondria. It scavenges reactive oxygen species (ROS), and is produced in plants, animals, and humans from cysteine and fatty acids.[1]

Endogenously produced LA is covalently bound to certain proteins. However, there is increasing interest in the potential therapeutic uses of pharmacological doses of free (unbound) LA, which are likely as much as 1,000 times greater than the amounts that could be obtained from the diet. Typical dietary sources of LA are muscle meats, heart, kidney, and liver, and to a lesser degree, fruits and vegetables, all of which are not likely to provide appreciable amounts.[1]

Other than its use for glycemic control and diabetes which produce skin issues of their own, LA supplements are also added alongside glutathione and L-carnitine. They improve antioxidant status and age-related deterioration of cells and for skin pigmentation disorders.[2]

▶ ACTIVE FORMS

ACTIVE FORMS	SUPPLEMENT SOURCES	SALIENT FEATURES
α-lipoic acid (LA)	Synthetic	R isomer of LA is naturally synthesized in our body. In studies it is found that bioavailability of R-form is better than the mixture and also GI tolerability is better.

▶ SAFETY AND DOSAGE

GENERAL REQUIREMENTS	
Indian recommendations	N/A
Global recommendations and limits	EFSA Recommended intake 300 and 600 mg/day
	NOAEL: 60 mg/kg body weight/day
Side effects	LA is considered a safe supplement without any side effects.[3]
Notes:	LA has the capacity to regenerate and enhance the property of other antioxidants such as vitamin C, vitamin E and glutathione and reduces inflammation. Literature supports its role in case of diabetic neuropathy.[3,4]

▶ CLINICAL CONDITIONS

EVIDENCE LEVEL	CONDITION OR USE CASE	DOSAGE	BENEFIT OR MECHANISM OF ACTION
++++	Vitiligo	A supplement composed of 50 mg of LA plus vitamin C, vitamin E, PUFA and cysteine monohydrate along with narrow band UVB radiation therapy for 2 and 6 months	The supplement increased the therapeutic success of narrow band-UVB. It lead to an increase in catalase activity and a decrease in ROS level in peripheral blood mononuclear cells.[5]
++++	Nonsegmental vitiligo	Combination therapy-oral LA = 300 mg/day or placebo, betamethasone injection and narrow band UVB radiation for 6 months	In patients receiving the LA, there was significant improvement in the white patches. The treatment group achieved better efficacy than the control group at 3 months, while no difference was seen at 6 months. This suggests that LA could accelerate the initial response of repigmentation.[6]
++	Pigmentation	B16F10 melanoma cells were treated with LA bound to poly (ethylene) glycol (PEG) of molecular weight 2,000	LA suppressed the biosynthesis of melanin and reduced tyrosinase activity.[7]

▶ CLINICAL CONDITIONS (Continued)

EVIDENCE LEVEL	CONDITION OR USE CASE	DOSAGE	BENEFIT OR MECHANISM OF ACTION
++	Anti-aging	Skin-on-a-chip (SOC) technology of a single skin layer was used and treated with LA	There was an increase in *filaggrin* gene expression in the skin tissue layer.[7]
+++	Skin inflammation	Hairless mice were fed a diet containing 1.5 g/kg diet of R-LA or S-LA	Orally given R-LA significantly inhibited glucose oxidase-mediated skin inflammation, but S lipoate was marginally protective.[8]
+++	Aging	A supplement containing 200 mg of α-LA, marine protein complex, vitamins, minerals, lycopene, pine bark extract, red clover extract and soy extract or placebo was given for 6 months	There was a significant increase in skin thickness and elasticity of the treatment group, compared to placebo. Subjects also reported improvement in skin by self-evaluation method.[9]

▶ SUPPLEMENTATION

	BASIS	WHAT TO LOOK OUT FOR
Supplementation form	R-LA, S-LA[9] mixture of R and S-LA R-LA is more effective than S-LA.[8] Bioavailability of R-LA and mixture varies with age[10] but R-LA has higher gastrointestinal tolerability than the mixture.[11] Oxidized and reduced forms of LA show the same antioxidant activity.[12]	The form of LA is usually not mentioned on the packaging but most of the time it is a mixture of R and S-LA. The manufacturing company can provide information about the form of LA used in the formulation.
Administration form	Capsules or tablets	N/A
Purity considerations	N/A	N/A
Patient considerations	LA supplementation can be taken in a fasted state.	N/A
Safety considerations	LA is considered a safe supplement without any side effects. According to one study, adults can take up to 2,400 mg without experiencing any harmful side effects. However, high doses are not recommended as it does not provide any extra benefits.[13,14]	The Dose per serving is given on the packaging.
Other considerations	LA is heat and light sensitive and so should be protected accordingly.	Storage conditions are given on the package, and colored capsules/packaging should be considered.

INTRODUCTION

The biological roles of LA are quite diverse, due to its high permeability through the plasma membranes and its capacity to exert its numerous functions in both aqueous and lipid environments of the cell.[1,15] LA and its reduced counterpart, dihydrolipoic acid (DHLA), have been shown to combat oxidative stress by quenching a variety of reactive oxygen species (ROS) and acting as a metal chelator. In addition, LA has been shown to be involved in the recycling of other antioxidants in the body including vitamins C and E, glutathione and CoQ10. Supplementation has been found to provide protective benefits against oxidation, inflammation, diabetes, and cognitive decline.[1]

DIGESTION, ABSORPTION AND STORAGE

Digestion and Absorption

The bioavailability of LA supplementation is approximately 30%.[16,17]

It uses the monocarboxylic acid transporters transporter, and may not be absorbed as well if taken alongside medium-chained triglycerides.

Due to its partial similarity with biotin, the avidin from raw eggs can reduce its bioavailability.[18]

LA supplements are better absorbed on an empty stomach than with food.[19]

Storage

Unlike from food sources, high oral doses of free LA (≥ 50 mg) significantly, yet transiently, increase the concentration of free LA in plasma and cells.

Plasma concentrations generally peak within one hour or less and decline rapidly.[20-22]

In cells, LA is swiftly reduced to DHLA, and then rapidly exported from cells.[23]

MECHANISM OF ACTION

01 | Antioxidant Activity and Chelation of Metal Ions

The LA/DHLA constitutes a powerful endogenous antioxidant system that amplifies its chemical actions through the transfer of electrons, both, regenerating some endogenous antioxidant systems (glutathione, vitamin C, vitamin E, CoQ10) and chelating heavy metals (zinc, copper, lead, arsenic) to limit their toxicity and facilitate elimination.[24,25]

Lipoic acid might be able to increase glutathione synthesis in by up-regulating the expression of γ-glutamylcysteine ligase, the rate-limiting enzyme in glutathione synthesis, and by increasing cellular uptake of cysteine, which is required for glutathione synthesis. It does so by reducing hepatic expression of Nrf2, which mediates genes of the antioxidant response elements.[26] Unlike glutathione, for which only the reduced form is an antioxidant, both the oxidized and reduced forms of LA are powerful antioxidants.[27]

DHLA is a strong reductant that regenerates oxidized antioxidants such as vitamin C, vitamin E, glutathione and coenzyme Q10. Other than the direct reaction with tocopheroxyl radical, DHLA indirectly regenerates vitamin E by reducing the oxidized form of vitamin C and CoQ10, which in turn reduces alpha tocopherol and alpha-tocopheroxyl radical, respectively.[27] Animal studies also suggest that LA may improve endogenous vitamin C levels indirectly by inducing uptake from the blood.[1]

Because of the presence of two thiol groups, LA and DHLA both have metal chelating properties, which reduces the risk of oxidative stress. DHLA also regenerates vitamin C, which in turn reduces iron.[27]

02 | Inhibition of Melanogenesis

LA stimulates some signal transduction pathways that are sensitive to redox reactions due to its redox activity. The synthesis of melanin is modulated by LA decreasing levels of microphthalmia associated transcription factors (MITF) and subsequently those of melanogenic enzymes.

Because of its redox activity, LA also appears to stimulate certain signal transduction pathways and redox-sensitive gene expression. Furthermore, LA modulates melanin synthesis by decreasing levels of microphthalmia associated transcription factors (MITF), which has a downstream effect on tyrosinase, the main enzyme responsible for converting tyrosine into melanin, and other melanogenic enzymes.[28,29] UV-mediated pigmentation may also be reduced through the improvement of antioxidant defence capacity.

03 | Anti-inflammatory Action

Most anti-inflammatory effects of LA are mediated through its ability to inhibit NF-κB, a nuclear transcription factor that, upon its activation, induces an inflammatory cytokines, including interleukins (ILs) such as IL-1β and IL-6.[15] LA's anti-inflammatory effects are independent of TNF-α inhibition, which is the stage many antioxidants act on.[30]

The ability of LA to affect cellular signaling pathways is thought to account for its diverse biological roles far beyond its antioxidant and anti-inflammatory effects—as an insulin mimetic, a hypotriglyceridemic agent, a vasorelaxant/anti-hypertensive compound—which may have far reaching benefits on overall health.[1]

▶ REFERENCES

1. Shay KP, Moreau RF, Smith EJ, Smith AR, Hagen TM. Alpha-lipoic acid as a dietary supplement: Molecular mechanisms and therapeutic potential. Biochim Biophys Acta. 2009;1790(10):1149-60.
2. Sethumadhavan S, Chinnakannu P. L-Carnitine and α-Lipoic Acid Improve Age-Associated Decline in Mitochondrial Respiratory Chain Activity of Rat Heart Muscle. J Gerontol A Biol Sci Med Sci. 2006;61(7):650-9.
3. Nguyen H, Pellegrini MV, Gupta V. Alpha-Lipoic Acid. In: StatPearls. Treasure Island (FL): StatPearls Publishing; 2024.
4. Tutelyan VA, Makhova AA, Pogozheva AV, Shikh EV, Elizarova EV, Khotimchenko SA. [Lipoic acid: physiological role and prospects for clinical application]. Vopr Pitan. 2019;88(4):6-11.
5. Dell'Anna ML, Mastrofrancesco A, Sala R, Venturini M, Ottaviani M, Vidolin AP, et al. Antioxidants and narrow band-UVB in the treatment of vitiligo: a double-blind placebo controlled trial. Clin Exp Dermatol. 2007;32(6):631-6.
6. Li L, Lu L, Wu Y, Gao XH, Chen HD. Triple-combination treatment with oral α-lipoic acid, betamethasone injection, and NB-UVB for non-segmental progressive vitiligo. J Cosmet Laser Ther. 2016;18(3):182-5.
7. Kim JH, Sim GS, Bae JT, Oh JY, Lee GS, Lee DH, et al. Synthesis and anti-melanogenic effects of lipoic acid-polyethylene glycol ester. Journal of Pharmacy and Pharmacology. 2008;60(7):863-70.
8. Fuchs J, Milbradt R. Antioxidant inhibition of skin inflammation induced by reactive oxidants: evaluation of the redox couple dihydrolipoate/lipoate. Skin Pharmacol. 1994;7(5):278-84.
9. Thom E. A randomized, double-blind, placebo-controlled study on the clinical efficacy of oral treatment with DermaVite on ageing symptoms of the skin. J Int Med Res. 2005;33(3):267-72.
10. Keith DJ, Butler JA, Bemer B, Dixon B, Johnson S, Garrard M, et al. Age and gender dependent bioavailability of R- and R,S-α-lipoic acid: A pilot study. Pharmacol Res. 2012;66(3):199-206.
11. Cameron M, Taylor C, Lapidus J, Ramsey K, Koop D, Spain R. Gastrointestinal Tolerability and Absorption of R- Versus R,S-Lipoic Acid in Progressive Multiple Sclerosis: A Randomized Crossover Trial. J Clin Pharmacol. 2020;60(8):1099-106.
12. Rochette L, Ghibu S, Richard C, Zeller M, Cottin Y, Vergely C. Direct and indirect antioxidant properties of α-lipoic acid and therapeutic potential. Mol Nutr Food Res. 2013;57(1):114-25.
13. Cremer DR, Rabeler R, Roberts A, Lynch B. Safety evaluation of alpha-lipoic acid (ALA). Regul Toxicol Pharmacol. 2006;46(1):29-41.
14. Fogacci F, Rizzo M, Krogager C, Kennedy C, Georges CMG, Knežević T, et al. Safety Evaluation of α-Lipoic Acid Supplementation: A Systematic Review and Meta-Analysis of Randomized Placebo-Controlled Clinical Studies. Antioxidants (Basel). 2020;9(10):1011.
15. Packer L, Witt EH, Tritschler HJ. alpha-Lipoic acid as a biological antioxidant. Free Radic Biol Med. 1995;19(2):227-50.
16. Teichert J, Kern J, Tritschler HJ, Ulrich H, Preiss R. Investigations on the pharmacokinetics of alpha-lipoic acid in healthy volunteers. Int J Clin Pharmacol Ther. 1998;36(12):625-8.
17. Teichert J, Hermann R, Ruus P, Preiss R. Plasma kinetics, metabolism, and urinary excretion of alpha-lipoic acid following oral administration in healthy volunteers. J Clin Pharmacol. 2003;43(11):1257-67.
18. Hale G, Wallis NG, Perham RN. Interaction of avidin with the lipoyl domains in the pyruvate dehydrogenase multienzyme complex: three-dimensional location and similarity to biotinyl domains in carboxylases. Proc Biol Sci. 1992;248(1323):247-53.
19. Gleiter CH, Schug BS, Hermann R, Elze M, Blume HH, Gundert-Remy U. Influence of food intake on the bioavailability of thioctic acid enantiomers. Eur J Clin Pharmacol. 1996;50(6):513-4.
20. Teichert J, Hermann R, Ruus P, Preiss R. Plasma kinetics, metabolism, and urinary excretion of alpha-lipoic acid following oral administration in healthy volunteers. J Clin Pharmacol. 2003;43(11):1257-67.
21. Evans JL, Heymann CJ, Goldfine ID, Gavin LA. Pharmacokinetics, tolerability, and fructosamine-lowering effect of a novel, controlled-release formulation of alpha-lipoic acid. Endocr Pract. 2002;8(1):29-35.
22. Breithaupt-Grögler K, Niebch G, Schneider E, Erb K, Hermann R, Blume HH, et al. Dose-proportionality of oral thioctic acid--coincidence of assessments via pooled plasma and individual data. Eur J Pharm Sci. 1999;8(1):57-65.
23. Smith AR, Shenvi SV, Widlansky M, Suh JH, Hagen TM. Lipoic acid as a potential therapy for chronic diseases associated with oxidative stress. Curr Med Chem. 2004;11(9):1135-46.

24. Packer L. alpha-Lipoic acid: a metabolic antioxidant which regulates NF-kappa B signal transduction and protects against oxidative injury. Drug Metab Rev. 1998;30(2):245-75.
25. Ou P, Tritschler HJ, Wolff SP. Thioctic (lipoic) acid: a therapeutic metal-chelating antioxidant? Biochem Pharmacol. 1995;50(1):123-6.
26. Suh JH, Shenvi SV, Dixon BM, Liu H, Jaiswal AK, Liu RM, et al. Decline in transcriptional activity of Nrf2 causes age-related loss of glutathione synthesis, which is reversible with lipoic acid. Proc Natl Acad Sci U S A. 2004;101(10):3381-6.
27. Saeid G, Mohammad B, Ismail L. Diabetes and Alpha Lipoic Acid. Front Pharmacol. 2011;17:2:69
28. Lin CB, Babiarz L, Liebel F, Roydon Price E, Kizoulis M, Gendimenico GJ, et al. Modulation of microphthalmia-associated transcription factor gene expression alters skin pigmentation. J Invest Dermatol. 2002;119(6):1330-40.
29. Kim K, Kim J, Kim H, Sung GY. Effect of α-Lipoic Acid on the Development of Human Skin Equivalents Using a Pumpless Skin-on-a-Chip Model. Int J Mol Sci. 2021;22(4):2160.
30. Zhang WJ, Frei B. Alpha-lipoic acid inhibits TNF-alpha-induced NF-kappaB activation and adhesion molecule expression in human aortic endothelial cells. FASEB J. 2001;15(13):2423-32.

Epigallocatechin gallate (EGCG)

28

Polyphenols

✎ Rajesh Mikkilineni

CONTENTS

POLYPHENOLS: NUTRIENT SNAPSHOT

- ▸ REQUIREMENT IN THE INDIAN CONTEXT | **275**
- ▸ ACTIVE FORMS | **276**
- ▸ SAFETY AND DOSAGE | **276**
- ▸ CLINICAL CONDITIONS | **277**
- ▸ SUPPLEMENTATION | **280**

INTRODUCTION | **282**

DIGESTION, ABSORPTION AND STORAGE | **282**

MECHANISM OF ACTION | **282**

KEY TOPICS

- ANTI-AGING
- HAIR GROWTH
- PHOTOPROTECTION
- SKIN HYDRATION

Nutrient Snapshot

▶ **REQUIREMENT IN THE INDIAN CONTEXT**

Polyphenols are naturally occurring, structurally diverse, compounds found largely in the fruits, vegetables, cereals and beverages. In plants, they may contribute to the taste, color, odor and oxidative stability, and are generally involved in defence against ultraviolet radiation and pathogens.[1]

Like for other phytonutrients, there are no recommendations for how much of each polyphenol to consume. We are encouraged to increase our intake of fruit and vegetables to 5–9 servings per day. However, epidemiological studies have consistently shown an inverse association between chronic diseases and the consumption of a polyphenolic-rich diet. In India, the average intake of fruit and vegetables is only 2.3–3.5 servings per day.[2,3]

In skin and hair products, polyphenols like resveratrol, curcumin, proanthocyanidins and catechins, and extracts of grape seed, green tea and berries have become popular ingredients. They exert their benefits on skin and hair due to their antioxidant, anti-inflammatory and photoprotective benefits, and some have shown to promote collagen synthesis and hair growth. However, many supplements may not have a sufficient dose for a clinical effect, while others may be providing higher doses than necessary.

ACTIVE FORMS

ACTIVE FORMS	SUPPLEMENT SOURCES	SALIENT FEATURES
Flavonoids: • Catechins • Epicatechins (like Epigallocatechin gallate; EGCG) • Quercetin	Green tea extract, green tea catechins.[4]	Generally, EGCG bioavailability shows a high interindividual variability related to the GI absorption, the stability of the molecule, the nutritional environment, and when it is administered. Some evidence suggests EGCG may be better absorbed in a fasted state.[5] Bioavailability can be enhanced by nano/microencapsulation of EGCG.[6]
	Quercetin-extracts of citrus fruits, vegetables and other plant sources.[4]	Quercetin has a relatively high bioavailability compared to other phytochemicals.[7]
Anthocyanins-cyanidin, delphinidin	Grapes, berries	Anthocyanins are potent antioxidants, but have extremely low bioavailability as is, but they are often microencapsulated or processed to increase bioavailability. Differing results have been obtained from in vivo and in vitro studies due to the heterogeneity of extracts and gastrointestinal environment.[8]
Tannins	Major sources of tannins are fruits, vegetables, bark, wood, leaves, and seeds such as green tea, apples, cocoa, chocolate, and grapes.	Tannins are sometimes classified as flavonoids (anthocyanins), and can be considered to be a part of these groups.

SAFETY AND DOSAGE

GENERAL REQUIREMENTS	
Indian recommendations	Tea leaves: Upto 10 g per day dried or processed leaf as infusion Black/green tea extract (standardized powder) permitted range: 0.5 g–2 g/day Green tea catechins (epigallocatechin gallate, epicatechin, catechin gallates) permitted range of 0.3–0.7 g per day (in terms of raw herb).[4] Quercetin content (obtained from extracts of citrus fruits, vegetables and other plant sources): Maximum 100 mg/day Anthocyanins or grape seed extract: FSSAI has stated these on the list of permitted ingredients. However, a concentration has not been mentioned. A range of 50–600 mg has only been mentioned for anthocyanins of bilberry extract (as of 2022).[4] Tannins: As of 2022, tannins are not separately stated in the list of permitted ingredients by the FSSAI. However, they are often considered a part of anthocyanins and flavonoids.[4]

▶ SAFETY AND DOSAGE (Continued)

GENERAL REQUIREMENTS	
Global recommendations and limits	Green tea catechins (EFSA): Based on clinical studies, EGCG levels equal to or above 800 mg daily can affect liver function. However, considering that, in some cases, hepatotoxicity has occurred at lower doses, a true safe EGCG dose cannot be established.[9] Quercetin: EFSA does not give any recommendation on the dose but has an opinion paper for the use of quercitin for various health claims (in doses: 20–85 mg). EFSA has not yet established any acceptable intake or upper limit for it.[10] Anthocyanins: • The Joint FAO/WHO Expert Committee on Food Additives has established an acceptable daily intake of 2.5 mg/kg/day for anthocyanins from grape-skin extracts but not for anthocyanins in general.[11] • EFSA panel concluded that the currently available toxicologic database was inadequate to establish a numerically acceptable daily intake for anthocyanins. The majority of toxicologic data are derived from grape skin and blackcurrant extracts, which were considered unlikely to be of safety concern by the EFSA.[12] • China has currently defined a specific proposed level of 50 mg/d for anthocyanins.[11]
Notes:	As per a meta-analysis the dosages of polyphenols used in eight studies were within a range of 15 to 1,400 mg every day over 6 to 12 weeks.[13] Extracts are not standardized for the amount of polyphenols and the effect may depend on the polyphenols present. Polyphenols are considered to be prebiotic, as these compounds could be used by microorganisms, resulting in metabolites with different functional effects compared to the parent molecule. The heterogeneity of gut microbes may therefore result in variable effects.[14] In the absence of reliable information, low doses and clinical trials on ingredients can be encouraged. As a general rule, about 100 mg or less of polyphenols can be consumed in a single dose.

▶ CLINICAL CONDITIONS*

EVIDENCE LEVEL	CONDITION OR USE CASE	DOSAGE	BENEFIT OR MECHANISM OF ACTION
+++	Anti-aging (polyphenols)	Subjects ingested either a supplement containing 258 mg of a resveratrol-procyanidin blend (133 mg grape fruit extract and 125 mg pomegranate extract) or placebo daily for 60 days	After 60 days of treatment, values for systemic oxidative stress, antioxidant capacity, and skin antioxidant power had increased. There was an improvement in skin moisturization and elasticity, while skin roughness and depth of wrinkles and age spots had diminished.[15]

▶ **CLINICAL CONDITIONS*** (*Continued*)

EVIDENCE LEVEL	CONDITION OR USE CASE	DOSAGE	BENEFIT OR MECHANISM OF ACTION
+++++	Anti-aging (Hydrangea serrata leaves)	Subjects either received 300 mg or 600 mg Hydrangea serrata leaves (WHS), or placebo, once daily for 12 weeks	Compared to the placebo, skin wrinkles, and roughness reduced in both WHS groups after 8 and 12 weeks. Skin hydration was enhanced compared to the placebo after 12 weeks. The parameters of skin elasticity improved after 12 weeks of 600 mg WHS administration.[16]
+++++	UV-induced pigmentation (apple polyphenol)	Subjects were randomized to receive tablets containing apple polyphenol (300 or 600 mg/day) or placebo for 12 weeks daily	The intake for 12 weeks prevented UV-induced skin pigmentation (erythema value, melanin value, L value), skin hydration and TEWL. However, a dose-dependent relationship was not clearly observed.[17]
++	UV-induced skin damage (anthocyanins and tannins from pomegranate)	Human reconstituted skin (epiderm) was treated with pomegranate juice, pomegranate extract, and its oil for 1 h prior to UVB irradiation	Pretreatment of epiderm resulted in inhibition of UVB-induced markers of DNA damage and oxidative stress, and enzymes that break down collagen.[18]
++	UV-induced skin damage (delphinidin-anthocyanidin)	Keratinocytes were treated with delphinidin before UV irradiation (1–20 μm for 24 hours) and SKH-1 hairless mouse skin was topically applied with delphinidin (1 mg/0.1 mL m = DMSO/mouse)	The pretreatment of cells protected against UVB mediated decrease in cell viability and induction of apoptosis. It inhibited UVB-mediated increase in lipid peroxidation and oxidative stress. Topical application inhibited UVB-mediated apoptosis and markers of DNA damage such as cyclobutane pyrimidine dimers (photoproduct of DNA) and 8-OHdG.[19]
++	UV induced DNA damage (grape seed proanthocyanidins)	Keratinocytes were treated with grape seed proanthocyanidins (GSPs)	The treatment of inhibited UVB-induced hydrogen peroxide, lipid peroxidation, protein oxidation, and DNA damage. GSPs also inhibited UVB-induced depletion of antioxidant defence components, such as GPx, catalase, SOD, and GSH. This effect was comparable to when cells were treated with other known antioxidants, viz. EGCG, silymarin, ascorbic acid, and N-acetylcysteine. GSPs also inhibited UVB-induced activation of NF-kappaB/p65 (control cell growth and survival).[20]

▶ CLINICAL CONDITIONS* (Continued)

EVIDENCE LEVEL	CONDITION OR USE CASE	DOSAGE	BENEFIT OR MECHANISM OF ACTION
+++++	Pollution-related skin aging (quercetin and many compounds)	Subjects received a (250 mg) dietary supplement capsule containing diterpenes (sum of carnosic acid and carnosol) and quercetin (and some other polyphenols) or placebo daily for 12 weeks	The dietary supplement improved the total antioxidant capacity of saliva, the oxidative damage on skin (lipoperoxides content), skin hydration, TEWL, skin radiance and color, skin elasticity, skin sebum content, skin roughness, and reduced pigmentation of spots in both Caucasian and Asian individuals. Some of these effects were also observed as early as 2 weeks.[21]
+++++	Skin hydration (polyphenols)	N/A (meta-analysis)	Four of nine studies investigated in the meta-analysis showed the influence of polyphenols on skin TEWL. A positive effect on skin hydration was observed for procyanidin, with an unknown effect on TEWL due to insufficient RCTs.[13]
++	Hair growth (EGCG)	The hair follicles of minks were treated with EGCG for 6 days ex vivo and primary dermal papilla cells (DPCs) and outer root sheath cells (ORSCs) were treated with EGCG in vitro	Data from ex vivo culture showed that, in the presence of EGCG, the growth of mink hair follicles was promoted. The proliferation of DPCs and ORSCs was enhanced by EGCG treatment in vitro. More cells entered the S phase, accompanied with upregulation of regulators of cell cycle progression, cyclin D1 and cyclin E1. The sonic hedgehog (Shh) and protein kinase B (AKT) signaling pathways were activated in both hair follicles and primary DPCs and ORSCs on exposure to EGCG.[22]
+++	Hair growth (tea polyphenols)	Mice with hair loss were divided into 2 groups: Group A received 50% fraction of polyphenol extract from green tea in their drinking water Group B received regular drinking water along with their regular rodent diet for 6 months	The results of the study showed that 33% of the mice in Group A, who received polyphenol extract in their drinking water, had hair regrowth during the 6 months treatment while no hair growth was observed among mice in the control group.[23]

▶ CLINICAL CONDITIONS* (Continued)

EVIDENCE LEVEL	CONDITION OR USE CASE	DOSAGE	BENEFIT OR MECHANISM OF ACTION
++	Hair growth (EGCG)	Human scalp hair follicles (ex vivo) and dermal papillae cells (DPC) were treated with EGCG in vitro	EGCG promoted hair growth in hair follicles ex vivo culture and the proliferation of cultured DPCs compared to control. The growth was mediated through the upregulations of phosphorylated Erk (signaling pathway in mitogenesis and cell growth) and Akt (that mediates survival signals) and by an increase in the ratio of Bcl-2/Bax ratio (Bcl-2 has an anti-apoptotic effect, whereas Bax induces apoptosis).[24]
+++++	Hair growth	Subjects first received a placebo for 4 weeks and then a capsule containing: Group 1: 400 mg apple polyphenols Group 2: 400 mg apply polyphenols, biotin (0.20 mg), selenomethionine (80 μg), and zinc acetate (21.0 mg), named AppleMetS twice a day for 8 weeks	No significant changes in hair were seen after placebo. Both supplement groups showed an increase in hair number, hair weight, and the keratin content in 4 weeks. AppleMetS exerted more pronounced effects at the end of the trial period.[25]

*While phytoestrogens (isoflavones, stilbene, coumestan, and lignan) also fall under the umbrella of polyphenols, they have been separately covered in the chapter phytoestrogens.

▶ SUPPLEMENTATION

	BASIS	WHAT TO LOOK OUT FOR
Supplementation form	Green tea extract: Catechins Epicatechins EGCG	The concentration of polyphenols will vary based on the source, its purification and the amount of extract added per serving. This information can be acquired from the manufacturer.

▶ **SUPPLEMENTATION** (*Continued*)

	BASIS	**WHAT TO LOOK OUT FOR**
	Quercetin: The concentration can vary from one plant to another or even in different parts of the same plant.[26] Anthocyanins: The amount of anthocyanin may vary depending on the source.	
Administration form	Capsules, powders, tablets, soft gels, gummies, syrups	N/A
Purity considerations	Purity of polyphenols from extracts is not standardized.	This information can be acquired from the manufacturer.
Patient considerations	As per US pharmacopoeia green tea polyphenols have to be taken with food.[27] Some polyphenols can have a bitter taste and astringency. However, this may not be an issue in capsules and in small doses.	N/A
Safety considerations	Published adverse event case reports associate hepatotoxicity with EGCG intake amounts from 140 mg to ~1,000 mg/day but there could be substantial inter-individual variability in susceptibility, possibly due to genetic factors.[27] Many skin, hair and nail supplements may have one or combinations of these polyphenols. Since there are no recommended ranges available it is best to exercise caution while consuming these supplements. The appropriate dose for specific conditions is not yet established with enough human trials. Polyphenols and their metabolites may have nonspecific interactions with gut microbiota, and drugs or may cause systemic changes. This is under investigation and thus caution must be exercised before taking any compounds.	Clinical studies of safety and efficacy on products.
	Green tea extracts, EGCG, are contraindicated in individuals with liver issues.[27] Individuals who take medications, are recommended to consult a physician prior to the use of isolated quercetin as quercetin is known to interact with many drugs.[28] In toxic doses, quercetin causes emesis, hypertension, nephrotoxicity, and reduction in serum potassium.[29]	Considering all the data it is recommended that individuals with clinical conditions and undergoing medical treatments should seek expert advice before they start any nutritional supplementation.

INTRODUCTION

With over 8000 compounds, polyphenols make up the largest group of phytonutrients, making them the most abundant antioxidants in our diets.[30] All plant phenolic compounds arise from a common intermediate, phenylalanine, or a close precursor, shikimic acid.[31]

Polyphenols are classified into different groups (**Figure 1**) based on the number of phenol rings that they contain and on the structural elements that bind these rings to one another. The main classes include phenolic acids, flavonoids, stilbenes and lignans.[31]

DIGESTION, ABSORPTION AND STORAGE

Digestion and Absorption

- Most polyphenols are present in food in the form of esters, glycosides or polymers that cannot be absorbed in their native form. That's why they are hydrolyzed by intestinal enzymes or by colonic microflora and differ in their site of absorption.[31-33]

- During the course of the absorption, polyphenols undergo extensive modification, by our body and our gut microbes, and their metabolites are biologically active.[31]

- Many polyphenols have poor bioavailability and oxidise easily. However, many manufacturers use encapsulation or structure modification techniques to make them stable and bioavailable.[33,34]

Storage

Polyphenols can be fat and water soluble, so they are stored in various tissue. The form and extent of storage varies with the type and molecular weight of the polyphenol.

MECHANISM OF ACTION

01 | Antioxidant Activity and Photoprotection

Polyphenols are powerful antioxidants that help protect the skin and hair from oxidative stress caused by free radicals. The phenolic groups in polyphenols can accept an electron to form relatively stable phenoxyl radicals, thereby disrupting chain oxidation reactions in cellular components.[31]

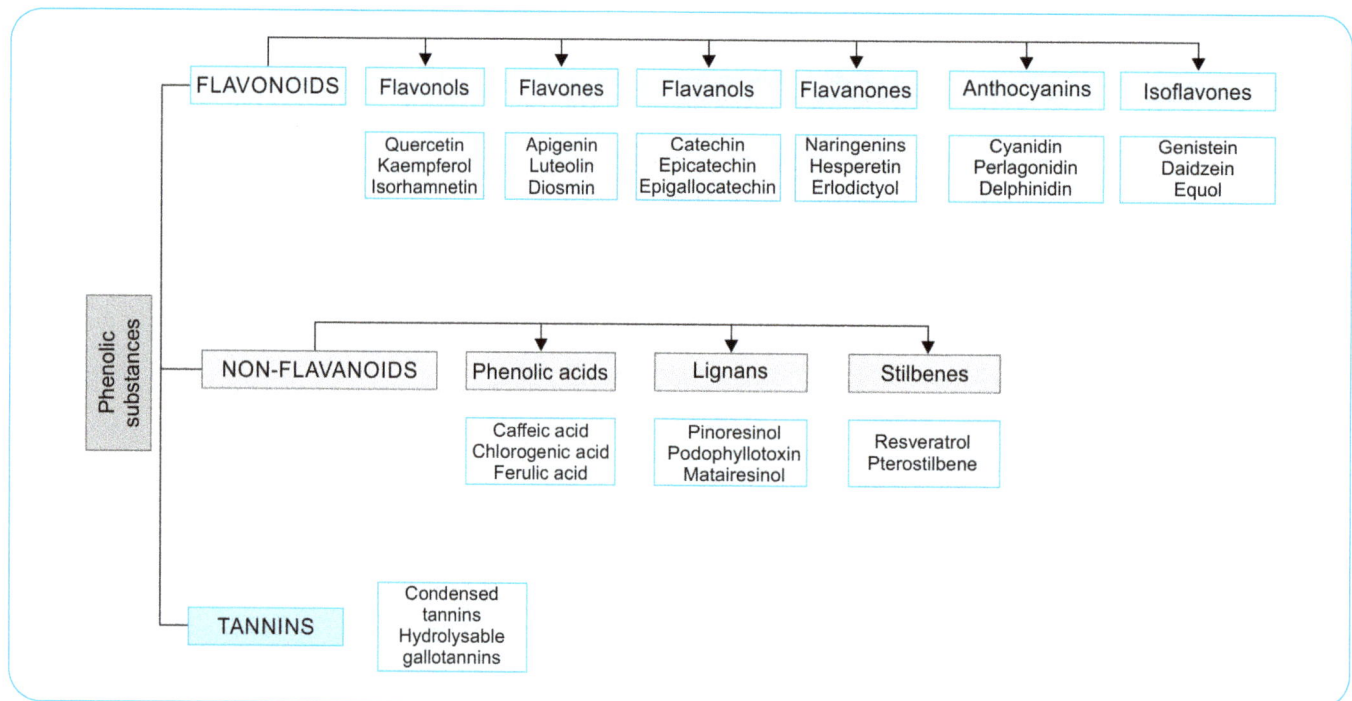

Figure 1: The types of polyphenols.[31] Tannins are often considered as flavonoids.

Polyphenols, particularly those found in green tea and grapes, absorb light in the UV spectra, and can therefore act as sunscreens. Their combination with carotenoids has shown to promote their photoprotective benefits.[35]

02 | Anti-inflammatory Action

By virtue of their antioxidant abilities, polyphenols possess anti-inflammatory properties, which can help reduce inflammation in the skin and the hair follicle.

Most biological effects of polyphenols are attributed to their ability regulate inflammation by a crosstalk between two pathways:[35-37]

- They can upregulate the ARE/Nrf2 signaling pathway that induces genes of antioxidant and detoxifying enzymes that neutralize harmful molecules in the skin.

- They can also upregulate NFκB that induces genes involved in inflammatory processes.

They may also modulate the activities of enzymes involved in proinflammatory arachidonic acid metabolism (phospholipase A2, COX) and arginine metabolism (NOS). Various skin conditions, such as acne, eczema, and psoriasis can therefore benefit from polyphenol intake.[38,39]

03 | Collagen Synthesis

Certain polyphenols, such as those found in green tea and berries, have been shown to stimulate collagen synthesis in the skin. Several in vivo and in vitro studies suggest that green tea supplementation increases the collagen and elastin fiber content, and suppresses collagen degrading enzyme (MMPs) production in the skin.[40,41]

Some polyphenols, like resveratrol, may also act to upregulate the anti-aging, "longevity" gene SIRT1, signaling pathways of which affect cell survival, metabolism, stress resistance, endothelial function, and angiogenesis. Polyphenols are therefore being explored for anti-aging benefits as well as for accelerating wound healing.[42] More on this topic is covered in the Phytoestrogen chapter.

04 | Stimulating Hair Growth

Certain polyphenols, such as those present in green tea, have been associated with promoting hair growth in vitro and with topical application. For example, oligomeric procyanidin, found in apples and grapes, are able to promote hair epithelial cell growth as well as to induce the anagen phase.[25]

In an ex vivo animal model, resveratrol increased the hair shaft length and delayed the entry into catagen.[43] Polyphenols may also regulate the gene expression of telomerase reverse transcriptase and cytokines such as IGF-1 and KGF, which activate the β-catenin pathway, and TGF-β1, which help maintain the niche of hair follicle stem cells.[44]

Polyphenols are believed to improve endothelial function, through its vasodilatory effect,[45] and may improve blood circulation to the hair follicle.

05 | Preventing Androgen Activity

Polyphenols can help inhibit the activity of an enzyme called 5-alpha reductase, which converts testosterone into dihydrotestosterone (DHT), a known contributor to hair loss and thinning. Combining polyphenols with carotenoids, yet again, show a synergy with an improved DHT-blocking ability.[46]

▶ REFERENCES

1. Pandey KB, Rizvi SI. Plant polyphenols as dietary antioxidants in human health and disease. Oxid Med Cell Longev. 2009;2(5):270-8.
2. Mukherjee A, Dutta S, Goyal TM. & Delhi, N. India's Phytonutrient Report A Snapshot of Fruits and Vegetables Consumption, Availability and Implications for Phytonutrient Intake ACADEMIC FOUNDATION.
3. Choudhury S, Shankar B, Aleksandrowicz L, Tak M, Green R, Harris F, et al. What underlies inadequate and unequal fruit and vegetable consumption in India? An exploratory analysis. Glob Food Sec. 2020 Mar;24:100332. doi: 10.1016/j.gfs.2019.100332.
4. Food Safety and Standards (Health supplements, Nutraceuticals, Food for Special Dietary use, Food for Special Medical purpose, Functional Food and Novel Food) Regulations, 2022.
5. Fernández VA, Toledano LA, Pizarro N, Tapia EN, Gómez-Roig MD, Torre RDL, et al. Bioavailability of Epigallocatechin Gallate Administered with Different Nutritional Strategies in Healthy Volunteers. Antioxidants (Basel). 2020;9(5):440.

6. Furniturewalla A, Barve K. Approaches to overcome bioavailability inconsistencies of epigallocatechin gallate, a powerful antioxidant in green tea. Food Chemistry Advances, 100037 (2022).
7. Russo M, Spagnuolo C, Tedesco I, Bilotto S. Russo GL. The flavonoid quercetin in disease prevention and therapy: facts and fancies. Biochem Pharmacol. 2012;83:6-15.
8. Mattioli R, Francioso A, Mosca L, Silva P. Anthocyanins: A Comprehensive Review of Their Chemical Properties and Health Effects on Cardiovascular and Neurodegenerative Diseases. Molecules. 2020;25(17):3809.
9. Younes M, Aggett P, Aguilar F, Crebelli R, Dusemund B, Filipič M, et al. Scientific opinion on the safety of green tea catechins. EFSA J. 2018;16(4):e05239.
10. EFSA Panel on Dietetic Products, Nutrition and Allergies (NDA). Scientific Opinion on the substantiation of health claims related to quercetin and protection of DNA, proteins and lipids from oxidative damage (ID 1647), "cardiovascular system" (ID 1844), "mental state and performance" (ID 1845), and "liver, kidneys" (ID 1846) pursuant to Article 13(1) of Regulation (EC) No 1924/2006. EFSA J. 2011;9(4):2067.
11. Wallace TC, Giusti MM. Anthocyanins. Advances in Nutrition. 2015;6(5):620-2.
12. Scientific Opinion on the re-evaluation of anthocyanins (E 163) as a food additive. EFSA Journal 11, (2013).
13. Sun Q, Wu J, Qian G, Cheng H. Effectiveness of Dietary Supplement for Skin Moisturizing in Healthy Adults: A Systematic Review and Meta-Analysis of Randomized Controlled Trials. Front Nutr. 2022;9:895192.
14. Molino S, Lerma-Aguilera A, Jiménez-Hernández N, Gosalbes MJ, Rufián-Henares JA, Francino MP. Enrichment of Food with Tannin Extracts Promotes Healthy Changes in the Human Gut Microbiota. Front Microbiol Front Microbiol. 202;12:625782.
15. Buonocore D, Lazzeretti A, Tocabens P, Nobile V, Cestone E, Santin G, et al. Clinical, Cosmetic and Investigational Dermatology Resveratrol-procyanidin blend: nutraceutical and antiaging efficacy evaluated in a placebo-controlled, double-blind study. Clin Cosmet Investig Dermatol. 2012;5:159-65.
16. Myung DB, Lee JH, Han H-S, Lee K-Y, Ahn HS, Shin Y-K, et al. Oral Intake of Hydrangea serrata (Thunb.) Ser. Leaves Extract Improves Wrinkles, Hydration, Elasticity, Texture, and Roughness in Human Skin: A Randomized, Double-Blind, Placebo-Controlled Study. Nutrients. 2020;12(6):1588.
17. Shoji T, Masumoto S, Moriichi N, Ohtake Y, Kanda T. Administration of Apple Polyphenol Supplements for Skin Conditions in Healthy Women: A Randomized, Double-Blind, Placebo-Controlled Clinical Trial. Nutrients. 2020;12(4):1071.
18. Afaq F, Zaid MA, Khan N, Dreher M, Mukhtar H. Protective effect of pomegranate derived products on UVB-mediated damage in human reconstituted skin. Exp Dermatol. 2009;18(6):553-61.
19. Afaq F, Syed DN, Malik A, Hadi N, Sarfaraz S, Kweon M-H, et al. Delphinidin, an anthocyanidin in pigmented fruits and vegetables, protects human HaCaT keratinocytes and mouse skin against UVB-mediated oxidative stress and apoptosis. J Invest Dermatol. 2007;127(1):222-32.
20. Mantena SK, Katiyar SK. Grape seed proanthocyanidins inhibit UV-radiation-induced oxidative stress and activation of MAPK and NF-kappaB signaling in human epidermal keratinocytes. Free Radic Biol Med. 2006;40(9):1603-14.
21. Nobile, V Schiano I, Peral A, Giardina S, Spartà E, Caturla N. Antioxidant and reduced skin-ageing effects of a polyphenol-enriched dietary supplement in response to air pollution: a randomized, double-blind, placebo-controlled study. Food Nutr Res. 2021;65.
22. Zhang H, Nan W, Wang S, Song X, Si H, Li T, et al. Epigallocatechin-3-Gallate promotes the growth of mink hair follicles through sonic hedgehog and protein kinase B signaling pathways. Front Pharmacol. 2018:9:674.
23. Esfandiari A, Kelley P. The Effects of Tea Polyphenolic Compounds on Hair Loss among Rodents. J Natl Med Assoc. 2005;97(6):816-8.
24. Kwon OS, Han JH, Yoo HG, Chung JH, Cho KH, Eun HC, et al. Human hair growth enhancement in vitro by green tea epigallocatechin-3-gallate (EGCG). Phytomedicine. 2007;14(7-8):551-5.
25. Tenore GC, Caruso D, Buonomo G, D'Avino M, Santamaria R, Irace C, et al. Annurca Apple Nutraceutical Formulation Enhances Keratin Expression in a Human Model of Skin and Promotes Hair Growth and Tropism in a Randomized Clinical Trial. J Med Food. 2018;21(1):90-103.
26. Salehi B, Machin L, Monzote L, Sharifi-Rad J, Ezzat SM, Mohamed AS, et al. Therapeutic Potential of Quercetin: New Insights and Perspectives for Human Health. ACS Omega. 2020;5(20):11849-72.
27. Oketch-Rabah HA, Roe AL, Rider CV, Bonkovsky HL, Giancaspro GI, Navarro V, et al. United States Pharmacopeia (USP) comprehensive review of the hepatotoxicity of green tea extracts. Toxicol Rep. 2020:7:386-402.
28. Andres S, Pevny S, Ziegenhagen R, Bakhiya N, Schäfer B, Hirsch-Ernst KI, et al. Safety Aspects of the Use of Quercetin as a Dietary Supplement. Mol Nutr Food Res. 2018;62(1).
29. Anand David, AV, Arulmoli R, Parasuraman S. Overviews of Biological Importance of Quercetin: A Bioactive Flavonoid. Pharmacogn Rev. 2016;10(20):84-9.
30. Scalbert A, Williamson G. Dietary Intake and Bioavailability of Polyphenols. J Nutr. 2000;130(8S Suppl):2073S-85S.
31. Pandey KB, Rizvi SI. Plant polyphenols as dietary antioxidants in human health and disease. Oxid Med Cell Longev. 2009;2(5):270-8.
32. Serra V, Salvatori G, Pastorelli G. Dietary Polyphenol Supplementation in Food Producing Animals: Effects on the Quality of Derived Products. Animals (Basel). 2021;11(2):401.
33. Gonçalves AC, Nunes AR, Falcão A, Alves G, Silva LR. Dietary Effects of Anthocyanins in Human Health: A Comprehensive Review. Pharmaceuticals (Basel). 2021;14(7):690.
34. Tian Y, Mao X, Sun R, Zhang M, Xia Q. Enhanced oral bioavailability of oligomeric proanthocyanidins by a self-double-emulsifying drug delivery system. Food Sci Nutr. 2020;8(7):3814-25.
35. Calniquer G, Khanin M, Ovadia H, Linnewiel-Hermoni K, Stepensky D, Trachtenberg A, et al. Combined Effects of Carotenoids and Polyphenols in Balancing the Response of Skin Cells to UV Irradiation. Molecules. 2021;26(7):1931.
36. Stranieri C, Guzzo F, Gambini S, Cominacini L, Fratta Pasini AM. Intracellular Polyphenol Wine Metabolites Oppose Oxidative Stress and Upregulate Nrf2/ARE Pathway. Antioxidants (Basel). 2022;11(10):2055.
37. Zhou Y, Jiang Z, Lu H, Xu Z, Tong R, Shi J, et al. Recent Advances of Natural Polyphenols Activators for Keap1-Nrf2 Signaling Pathway. Chem Biodivers. 2019;16(11):e1900400.
38. Hussain T, Tan B, Yin Y, Blachier F, Tossou MCB, Rahu N. Oxidative Stress and Inflammation: What Polyphenols Can Do for Us? Oxid Med Cell Longev. 2016:2016:7432797.
39. Seeram NP, Cichewicz RH, Chandra A, Nair MG. Cyclooxygenase inhibitory and antioxidant compounds from crabapple fruits. J Agric Food Chem. 2003;51(7):1948-51.

40. Prasanth MI, Sivamaruthi BS, Chaiyasut C, Tencomnao T. A Review of the Role of Green Tea (Camellia sinensis) in Antiphotoaging, Stress Resistance, Neuroprotection, and Autophagy. Nutrients. 2019;11(2):474.

41. Roh E, Kim J-E, Kwon J-Y, Park J-S, Bode AM, Dong Z, et al. Molecular mechanisms of green tea polyphenols with protective effects against skin photoaging. Crit Rev Food Sci Nutr. 2017;57(8):1631-7.

42. Pignet AL, Schellnegger M, Hecker A, Kohlhauser M, Kotzbeck P, Kamolz LP. Resveratrol-Induced Signal Transduction in Wound Healing. Int J Mol Sci. 2021;22(23):12614.

43. Zhang Y, Ni C, Huang Y, Tang Y, Yang K, Shi X, et al. Hair Growth-Promoting Effect of Resveratrol in Mice, Human Hair Follicles and Dermal Papilla Cells. Clin Cosmet Investig Dermatol. 2021:14:1805-14.

44. Kubo C, Ogawa M, Uehara N, Katakura Y. Fisetin Promotes Hair Growth by Augmenting TERT Expression. Front Cell Dev Biol. 2020:8:566617.

45. Ahmad A, Khan RMA, Alkharfy KM. Effects of selected bioactive natural products on the vascular endothelium. J Cardiovasc Pharmacol. 2013;62(2):111-21.

46. Linnewiel-Hermoni K, Khanin M, Danilenko M, Zango G, Amosi Y, Levy J, et al. The anti-cancer effects of carotenoids and other phytonutrients resides in their combined activity. Arch Biochem Biophys. 2015:572:28-35.

Trans-resveratrol

Phytoestrogens

✍ Rajesh Mikkilineni

CONTENTS

PHYTOESTROGENS: NUTRIENT SNAPSHOT
- REQUIREMENT IN THE INDIAN CONTEXT | 287
- ACTIVE FORMS | 288
- SAFETY AND DOSAGE | 288
- CLINICAL CONDITIONS | 289
- SUPPLEMENTATION | 291

INTRODUCTION | 293

DIGESTION, ABSORPTION AND STORAGE | 293

MECHANISM OF ACTION | 293

KEY TOPICS
- ANTI-AGING
- ATOPIC DERMATITIS
- HAIR GROWTH
- VASCULARITY
- WOUND HEALING
- WRINKLES

Nutrient Snapshot

▶ REQUIREMENT IN THE INDIAN CONTEXT

Phytoestrogens are plant-derived compounds that have a chemical structure similar to the hormone estrogen, but are weakly estrogenic. They can interact with estrogen receptors in the body, leading to various effects. Four phenolic compounds classified as phytoestrogens are isoflavones, stilbene, coumestan, and lignan.[1,2]

The source of phytoestrogens are nuts, seeds, fruits and vegetables. Food sources of phytoestrogens that frequent the Indian diet include soybeans, garlic, carrots, potatoes, rice, wheat, fenugreek, lentils and legumes. The average daily intake of phytoestrogens in East and Southeast Asia is estimated to be between 20–50 mg per day.[2]

Recently, scepticism has developed concerning the effects of phytoestrogens on hormonal dysregulation, leading to some people avoiding soy products. However, studies have not shown endocrine disruption, perhaps because phytoestrogens exert a weak estrogen-like effect by binding to estrogen receptors with low affinity.[3]

Resveratrol is a phytoestrogen that has attracted increasing research attention to understand its properties and benefits for various diseases and conditions associated with aging, including skin health.[3]

While there are benefits to supplementing with phytoestrogens, further research is required to establish clear outcomes and safety with long-term use.

▶ ACTIVE FORMS

ACTIVE FORMS	SUPPLEMENT SOURCES	SALIENT FEATURES
Soy isoflavones- genistein, daidzein	Soy Isoflavones	The systemic bioavailability of genistein is much greater than that of daidzein.[4]
Lignans	Flaxseed oil, vitexin	Flaxseed has a high content of lignan. Lignans are normally used for promoting cardiovascular and immune health. Lignan bioavailability is characterized by marked inter-individuals differences,[5] as it may be associated with gut microbiota metabolism.[6]
Stilbenes- resveratrol	Saccharomyces cerevisiae, synthetic	Resveratrol has low bioavailability, poor solubility, limited stability, a high rate of metabolic breakdown, and low target specificity. In order to tackle these challenges, the synthetic derivatives are generated by modifying the chemical structure of resveratrol or it is nano/microencapsulated.[7]

▶ SAFETY AND DOSAGE

GENERAL REQUIREMENTS	
Indian recommendations	RDA or upper limit is not established for isoflavones and resveratrol. FSSAI allows the use of various soy products, isoflavones (genistein, daidzein) and resveratrol in nutraceutical supplements but has not stated any permitted range for the same.[8]
Global recommendations and limits	The NOAEL of soy isoflavones (rat model) is considered to be 0.2 g/kg body weight.[9] *Isoflavones*: The FDA recommends an intake of 50 mg per day from all sources, which is considered to be safe.[10] *EFSA*: Soy isoflavones: Isoflavone intake is safe, and the doses should be used as per studies.[11] Resveratrol: The intended intake level of 150 mg/day for adults does not raise safety concerns.[12]
Notes:	Extracts are not standardized for the amount of polyphenols and the effect may depend on heterogeneity of gut microbes and metabolic factors. In the absence of reliable information, known safe doses and clinical trials on ingredients can be encouraged.

▶ CLINICAL CONDITIONS

EVIDENCE LEVEL	CONDITION OR USE CASE	DOSAGE	BENEFIT OR MECHANISM OF ACTION
+++++	Aging-related skin changes and vascularity (soy isoflavones)	Subjects received 100 mg/day of an isoflavones-rich, concentrated soy extract for 6 months	The use of a concentrated, isoflavone-rich soy extract during six consecutive months caused increases in epithelial thickness, the number of elastic and collagen fibers, as well as the blood vessels.[13]
+++++	Aging related skin changes (soy isoflavones)	Subjects received either test food (40 mg of soy isoflavone aglycone) daily or placebo for 12 weeks	The test food group showed an improvement of fine wrinkles at week 12 and of malar skin elasticity at week 8, compared with the control group.[14]
+++	Anti-aging (genistein and daidzein mixture)	Male rats administered the soy isoflavone mixture (daidzein and genistein) in a dose of 2 or 20 mg/kg body weight/day for 5 days weekly (given to pups until sexual maturity)	The thickness of the skin epidermis and collagen fibers in the dermis and amount of elastic fibers were greater in the isoflavone-treated groups, compared to the group not treated. Isoflavones decreased catalase activity in the skin and at a higher dose inhibited lipid peroxides formation.[15]
++	Aging related skin pathologies (Resveratrol)	Mice were randomly divided into 4 groups and fed diets for 12 weeks: control diet, control diet containing 0.04% (w/w) trans-resveratrol (RSV) and control diets containing 0.1% or 0.5% (w/w) Melinjo seed extract (MSE)	Orally MSE and RSV treatment reversed the skin thinning associated with increased oxidative damage in the mice. MSE and RSV also normalized gene expression of Col1a1 (gene regulating collagen synthesis) and p53 (age-related genes) and upregulated gene expression of Sirt1 (protects various organs against aging) in skin tissues.[16]
+++	Wrinkles (Resveratrol)	Mice were orally fed with either 2 g grape peel extract (GPE) or 2 mg resveratrol per kg body weight	The oral supplementation of GPE and resveratrol attenuated UVB-induced epidermal thickening compared to the only UVB-treated group and had marginally protective effects on wrinkle formation of skin exposed to UVB. This photoaging was mitigated possibly through activation of Nrf2/HO-1 (antioxidant enzyme) signaling pathway.[17]

▶ **CLINICAL CONDITIONS** (*Continued*)

EVIDENCE LEVEL	CONDITION OR USE CASE	DOSAGE	BENEFIT OR MECHANISM OF ACTION
+++	Wound healing (genistein)	Mice were divided into three groups: control, 0.025% genistein, and 0.1% genistein for two weeks	This study suggested that genistein supplementation reduced oxidative stress by increasing antioxidant capacity and modulated proinflammatory cytokine expression during the early stage of wound healing.[18]
+++	Atopic dermatitis (AD; Resveratrol)	AD-like lesions were induced in mice. Mice were divided into three groups: group I (control), group II (vehicle control), and group III/ resveratrol (30 mg/kg body weight/day) was administered for 6 weeks	There was an improvement in epithelial thickness in group III compared with group II mice. The numbers of IL-25, IL-33, and TSLP-positive cells in the epithelium were lower in group III than in group II mice. The number of caspase-3-positive cells, as an indicator of apoptosis, in the epithelium was lower in group III than in group II mice.[19]
+++	Atopic dermatitis (AD; Resveratrol)	Mice were fed with 0, 5 or 25 mg/kg body weight resveratrol (duration not available)	Resveratrol ameliorated the onset of AD-like skin lesions and improved the 2,4-dinitrochlorobenzene (DNCB)-induced dermal destruction in mice. It also reduced the levels of chemokines, downregulated the expression of the proinflammatory cytokine, kallikrein 7 (KLK7), and upregulated the expression of barrier proteins, such as envoplakin (EVPL), filaggrin (FLG), and transglutaminase (TG).[20]
++	Hair growth (lignans-vitexin)	Human dermal papilla cells (hDPCs) were treated with vitexin compound 1 (VB-1) in vitro	The study demonstrated that VB-1 promotes the proliferation of hDPCs in a concentration-dependent manner. The hair growth-related gene, dkk1 (a paracrine factor involved in androgen receptor signaling) was clearly down-regulated in hDPCs treated with VB-1. Gene regulatory activity of VB-1 led to the activation of Wnt/β-catenin signaling, which is essential for hair morphogenesis and cycling.[21]

▶ SUPPLEMENTATION

	BASIS	WHAT TO LOOK OUT FOR
Supplementation form	Genistine: • Glycosylated (genistin) • Aglycone (genistein) The genistein is readily bioavailable, while the glycoside derivative (genistin) is poorly absorbed in the small intestine due to the higher molecular weight and hydrophilicity[22] Resveratrol: • Cis-resveratrol • Trans-resveratrol • Various other analogues are used in supplementation Structural changes, lipid nanoparticles and nanostructured lipid carriers are used to enhance bioavailability.[23-25]	Soy isoflavone types may not be mentioned on the product packaging. Various hair supplements or protein blends may contain soy isoflavones in them. The form of resveratrol may be given in then ingredients list of the product packaging. The manufacturer can provide the information not provided on the packaging.
Administration form	Capsules, powders, tablets, soft gels, gummies, syrups	
Purity considerations	Purity of these extracts is not standardized.	This information can be acquired from the manufacturer.
Patient considerations	Some of these nutrients can have a bitter taste and astringency. However, this may not be an issue in capsules and in small doses with established safety.	Gummies and syrups can be avoided.

▶ SUPPLEMENTATION (Continued)

	BASIS	WHAT TO LOOK OUT FOR
Safety considerations	A study done in older men and women suggests that 100 mg/day of soy isoflavones are safe and well-tolerated.[26] 600 mg of flaxseed lignans supplementation on older adults did not had any adverse effects.[27] Resveratrol does not appear to have side effects at short-term doses (1.0 g). Side effects may occur for 2.5 g/day dose or more like nausea, vomiting, diarrhea and liver dysfunction in patients with nonalcoholic fatty liver disease. But there are other studies evaluating multiple dosing, and have found resveratrol to be safe and reasonably well-tolerated at doses of up to 5 g/day.[23,28,29] There is no conclusive data available on the role of soy isoflavones in the incidence of breast cancer so it is best to exercise caution for those at risk of it.[30] Resveratrol may interact with drugs given for any treatment including anticoagulants, and chemotherapy. Thus, individuals on any medication should exercise caution before taking resveratrol supplementation as it may negatively affect the treatment.[23] Many skin, hair and nail supplements may have one or combinations of polyphenols and phytoestrogens. Since there is no recommended range available it is best to exercise caution while consuming these supplements and avoid high doses as their effects are subjective and high doses may lead to toxicity.	It is recommended that individuals with clinical conditions and undergoing medical treatments should seek expert advice before they start any nutritional supplementation. It is recommended to keep an eye on liver and kidney function (blood tests) when taking phytoestrogens over a period of months.

INTRODUCTION

Research suggests that phytoestrogens can affect a number of physiological and pathological processes related to reproduction, bone remodeling, and skin health, as well as cardiovascular, nervous, immune systems and metabolism.[31]

Phytoestrogens may be divided in chalcones, isoflavonoids (isoflavones, pterocarpans, and coumestans), lignans, stilbenoids, and miscellaneous other classes. Particular attention has been paid to isoflavonoids and stilbenoids in recent times due to their varied effects on cell signaling pathways **(Figure 1)**, and perhaps on the gut microbiome as well.[3]

DIGESTION, ABSORPTION AND STORAGE

Digestion and Absorption

- Phytoestrogens are metabolized by intestinal bacteria, and their metabolites are absorbed, conjugated in the liver, and circulated in plasma.[31,32]

- The amount of active metabolites created by a given dose of phytoestrogens may therefore vary considerably, dependant on the microflora of the gut.[31]

Storage

Polyphenols can be fat and water soluble, so their storage in the body varies considerably.

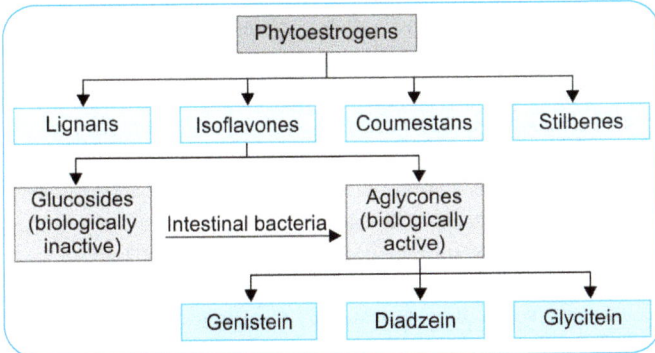

Figure 1: The types of phytoestrogens
Source: Adapted from Soni (2014).[35]

MECHANISM OF ACTION

Being part of the polyphenol group, phytoestrogens have antioxidant and anti-inflammatory actions in the skin (as covered in the Polyphenol chapter). Further to this, phytoestrogens exert other benefits:

01 | Anti-aging Activity

Estrogens significantly modulate skin physiology by targeting keratinocytes, fibroblasts, melanocytes, hair follicles, sebaceous glands, and immune cells. Its protective functions get compromised as we age, causing hair loss, impaired wound healing, pigmentary changes and an increased incidence of skin cancer. Phytoestrogens like daidzein, genistein and resveratrol may have anti-aging effects on the skin via estrogen receptors, as they have been shown to increase hyaluronic acid, collagen and elastin synthesis and reduce collagen degrading enzymes (MMPs) and melanin synthesis.[3,31,33,34]

Most phytoestrogens have a preference for estrogen receptor beta (over alpha receptors), which mainly promotes cellular apoptosis. Therefore it is possible that these changes occur due to mechanisms that do not involve estrogen receptors. A number of other mechanisms have been reported including their activity of serotoninergic and IGF-1 receptors, and their effects on DNA and RNA.[31]

02 | Cell Protection

Resveratrol can ameliorate the aging of human skin by stimulating the "longevity" gene sirtuin (silent mating type information regulation 2 homolog) 1 (SIRT1). SIRT1 signaling pathways affect cell survival, metabolism, stress resistance, endothelial function, and angiogenesis. Both UV and H_2O_2, two major factors of skin cell damage, down-regulate SIRT1 in a time- and dose-dependent manner. Resveratrol therefore protects against UV- and H_2O_2-induced apoptotic cell death.[3]

Resveratrol has shown to downregulate free radical-induced increases in AP-1 and NF-κB and therefore help in preserving dermal collagen and reducing skin inflammation.[3]

Furthermore, phytoestrogens offer protection against UV induced senescence by significantly upregulating intracellular activity of superoxide dismutases (SODs), an important antioxidant defence against oxidative stress in the body.[31]

03 | Probiotic Effect

Phytoestrogens may also exert antimicrobial activity and can interact with the pathogen strains. As a result, they might modulate the diversity of the microflora in the colon by inhibiting pathogen growth, or by increasing the beneficial bacterial populations, thus contributing to the improved health of the individual.[32]

▶ REFERENCES

1. Desmawati D, Sulastri D. Phytoestrogens and Their Health Effect. Open Access Maced J Med Sci. 2019;7(3):495-9.
2. Sirtori CR, Arnoldi A, Johnson SK. Phytoestrogens: end of a tale? Ann Med. 2005;37(6):423-38.
3. Liu T, Li N, Yan Y qi, Liu Y, Xiong K, Liu Y, et al. Recent advances in the anti-aging effects of phytoestrogens on collagen, water content, and oxidative stress. Phytotherapy Research. 2020;34(3):435-47.
4. Setchell KD, Brown NM, Desai P, Zimmer-Nechemias L, Wolfe BE, Brashear WT, et al. Bioavailability of pure isoflavones in healthy humans and analysis of commercial soy isoflavone supplements. J Nutr. 2001;131(4 Suppl):1362S-75S.
5. Clavel T, Doré J, Blaut M. Bioavailability of lignans in human subjects. Nutr Res Rev. 2006;19(2):187-96.
6. Senizza A, Rocchetti G, Mosele JI, Patrone V, Callegari ML, Morelli L, et al. Lignans and Gut Microbiota: An Interplay Revealing Potential Health Implications. Molecules. 2020;25(23):5709.
7. Reinisalo M, Kårlund A, Koskela A, Kaarniranta K, Karjalainen RO. Polyphenol Stilbenes: Molecular Mechanisms of Defence against Oxidative Stress and Aging-Related Diseases. Oxid Med Cell Longev. 2015;2015:340520.
8. Food Safety and Standards Authority of India. Direction under section 16(5) of the Food Safety and Standards Act, 2006 regarding operationalization of FSS(Health Supplements, Nutraceuticals, Food for Special Dietary Use, Food for Special Medical Purpose and Prebiotic and Probiotic Food) Regulations, 2022. [FSS (Nutra) Regulations, 2022)
9. Zhang WZ, Cui WM, Zhang X, Wang W, et al. Subchronic Toxicity Study on Soy Isoflavones in Rats. Biomed Environ Sci. 2009;22(3):259-64.
10. Kim IS. Current Perspectives on the Beneficial Effects of Soybean Isoflavones and Their Metabolites for Humans. Antioxidants (Basel). 2021;10(7):1064.
11. EFSA Panel on Food Additives and Nutrient Sources added to Food (ANS). Risk assessment for peri- and post-menopausal women taking food supplements containing isolated isoflavones. EFSA Journal. 2015;13(10):4246.
12. EFSA Panel on Dietetic Products, Nutrition and Allergies (NDA). Safety of synthetic trans-resveratrol as a novel food pursuant to Regulation (EC) No 258/97. EFSA Journal. 2016;14(1):4368.
13. Accorsi-Neto A, Haidar M, Simões R, Simões M, Soares-Jr J, Baracat E. Effects of Isoflavones on the Skin of Postmenopausal Women: A Pilot Study. Clinics (Sao Paulo). 2009;64(6):505-10.
14. Izumi T, Saito M, Obata A, Arii M, Yamaguchi H, Matsuyama A. Oral intake of soy isoflavone aglycone improves the aged skin of adult women. J Nutr Sci Vitaminol (Tokyo). 2007;53(1):57-62.
15. Duchnik E, Kruk J, Baranowska-Bosiacka I, Pilutin A, Maleszka R, Marchlewicz M. Effects of the soy isoflavones, genistein and daidzein, on male rats' skin. Postepy Dermatol Alergol. 2019;36(6):760-6.
16. Watanabe K, Shibuya S, Ozawa Y, Izuo N, Shimizu T. Resveratrol Derivative-Rich Melinjo Seed Extract Attenuates Skin Atrophy in Sod1-Deficient Mice. Oxid Med Cell Longev. 2015;2015:391075.
17. Kim J, Oh J, Averilla JN, Kim HJ, Kim JS, Kim JS. Grape Peel Extract and Resveratrol Inhibit Wrinkle Formation in Mice Model Through Activation of Nrf2/HO-1 Signaling Pathway. J Food Sci. 2019;84(6):1600-8.
18. Park E, Lee SM, Jung IK, Lim Y, Kim JH. Effects of genistein on early-stage cutaneous wound healing. Biochem Biophys Res Commun. 2011;410(3):514-9.
19. Caglayan Sozmen S, Karaman M, Cilaker Micili S, Isik S, Arikan Ayyildiz Z, Bagriyanik A, et al. Resveratrol ameliorates 2,4-dinitrofluorobenzene-induced atopic dermatitis-like lesions through effects on the epithelium. PeerJ. 2016;4:e1889.
20. Shen Y, Xu J. Resveratrol Exerts Therapeutic Effects on Mice With Atopic Dermatitis. Wounds. 2019;31(11):279-84.
21. Luo J, Chen M, Liu Y, Xie H, Yuan J, Zhou Y, et al. Nature-derived lignan compound VB-1 exerts hair growth-promoting effects by augmenting Wnt/β-catenin signaling in human dermal papilla cells. PeerJ. 2018;6:e4737.
22. Irrera N, Pizzino G, D'Anna R, Vaccaro M, Arcoraci V, Squadrito F, et al. Dietary Management of Skin Health: The Role of Genistein. Nutrients. 2017;9(6):622.
23. Salehi B, Mishra AP, Nigam M, Sener B, Kilic M, Sharifi-Rad M, et al. Resveratrol: A Double-Edged Sword in Health Benefits. Biomedicines. 2018;6(3):91.
24. Montenegro L, Parenti C, Turnaturi R, Pasquinucci L. Resveratrol-Loaded Lipid Nanocarriers: Correlation between In Vitro Occlusion Factor and In Vivo Skin Hydrating Effect. Pharmaceutics. 2017;9(4):58.
25. Lephart ED, Andrus MB. Human skin gene expression: Natural (trans) resveratrol versus five resveratrol analogs for dermal applications. Exp Biol Med (Maywood). 2017;242(15):1482-9.
26. Gleason CE, Carlsson CM, Barnet JH, Meade SA, Setchell KDR, Atwood CS, et al. A preliminary study of the safety, feasibility and cognitive efficacy of soy isoflavone supplements in older men and women. Age Ageing. 2009;38(1):86-93.
27. Di Y, Jones J, Mansell K, Whiting S, Fowler S, Thorpe L, et al. Influence of Flaxseed Lignan Supplementation to Older Adults on Biochemical and Functional Outcome Measures of Inflammation. J Am Coll Nutr. 2017;36(8):646-53.
28. Brown VA, Patel KR, Viskaduraki M, Crowell JA, Perloff M, Booth TD, et al. Repeat Dose Study of the Cancer Chemopreventive Agent Resveratrol in Healthy Volunteers: Safety, Pharmacokinetics and Effect on the Insulin-like Growth Factor Axis. Cancer Res. 2010;70(22):9003-11.
29. Patel KR, Scott E, Brown VA, Gescher AJ, Steward WP, Brown K. Clinical trials of resveratrol. Ann N Y Acad Sci. 2011;1215:161-9.
30. Gómez-Zorita S, González-Arceo M, Fernández-Quintela A, Eseberri I, Trepiana J, Portillo MP. Scientific Evidence Supporting the Beneficial Effects of Isoflavones on Human Health. Nutrients. 2020;12(12):3853.
31. Sirotkin AV, Harrath AH. Phytoestrogens and their effects. Eur J Pharmacol. 2014;741:230-6.
32. Ionescu VS, Popa A, Alexandru A, Manole E, Neagu M, Pop S. Dietary Phytoestrogens and Their Metabolites as Epigenetic Modulators with Impact on Human Health. Antioxidants. 2021;10(12):1893.

33. Pignet AL, Schellnegger M, Hecker A, Kohlhauser M, Kotzbeck P, Kamolz LP. Resveratrol-Induced Signal Transduction in Wound Healing. Int J Mol Sci. 2021;22(23):12614.

34. Boo YC. Human Skin Lightening Efficacy of Resveratrol and Its Analogs: From in Vitro Studies to Cosmetic Applications. Antioxidants (Basel). 2019;8(9):332.

35. Soni M, Rahardjo TBW, Soekardi R, Sulistyowati Y, Lestariningsih, Yesufu-Udechuku A, et al. Phytoestrogens and cognitive function: a review. Maturitas. 2014;77(3):209-20.

SECTION 06

Probiotics and Prebiotics

30. Prebiotics and Synbiotics — *Jaishree Sharad*
31. Probiotics — *Jaishree Sharad*

30

Galactooligosaccarides (GOS), Fructooligosaccarides (FOS)

Prebiotics and Synbiotics

✎ Jaishree Sharad

CONTENTS

PREBIOTICS AND SYNBIOTICS: NUTRIENT SNAPSHOT

- ▶ REQUIREMENT IN THE INDIAN CONTEXT | 299
- ▶ ACTIVE FORMS | 300
- ▶ SAFETY AND DOSAGE | 300
- ▶ CLINICAL CONDITIONS | 301
- ▶ SUPPLEMENTATION | 304

INTRODUCTION | 305

DIGESTION, ABSORPTION AND STORAGE | 305

MECHANISM OF ACTION | 305

KEY TOPICS

- GENERAL SKIN HEALTH
- MELASMA
- PHOTOPROTECTION
- PRURITUS IN ATOPIC DERMATITIS
- SKIN DRYNESS AND QUALITY
- SKIN AGING

Nutrient Snapshot

▶ **REQUIREMENT IN THE INDIAN CONTEXT**

- Host-microbe interactions occur primarily along mucosal surfaces, and the human intestinal mucosa is one of its largest interfaces.[1] There are emerging links between the commensal microbes of the human body and their effects on our brain and skin homeostasis, referred to as the gut-brain-skin axis.[2] An alteration in gut microbial diversity (dysbiosis) can disrupt mucosal immunological tolerance and increase host vulnerability to several diseases. These include dermatologic conditions, such as acne, atopic dermatitis (AD), psoriasis, and rosacea.[3,4]

- Our diet is the chief source of energy for the growth of commensal microbes. Prebiotics describe those nutrients that are fermented by gut microbiota and benefit the host. These include various types of fiber (and other compounds), fermentation of which produces metabolites like short-chain fatty acids (SCFAs), such as acetate, lactate, butyrate, and propionate, essential for intestinal integrity, and have anti-inflammatory benefits amongst others. The term synbiotics is attributed to the products that provide the combinational benefits of both, prebiotics and probiotics.[1]

- While there is considerable interest in India for probiotic foods, they have some disadvantages: (a) most bacteria cannot withstand the harsh environment of the upper gastrointestinal tract; (b) probiotics must compete with commensals for attachment to the intestinal mucosa; (c) effects are not only phyla, but also strain specific; (d) the host may mount an immune response; (e) shelf life and (f) the diversity in our diet, and thereby our commensals, can make it difficult to provide a one-size-fits-all approach.[5,6] Prebiotics can bypass many of these limitations by easily reaching the intestine and simultaneously promoting multiple commensal strains.

- Whilst promoting healthy faecal clearance, prebiotics also aim to balance the ratio of the phyla Firmicutes/Bacteroidetes (F/B), which is a major contributor in maintaining intestinal homeostasis.[7] They are also used to increase number of healthy-promoting genera like Bifidobacteria and Lactobacilli, which are low in the Western diet, which have an increasing impression on urban India.[8]

▶ ACTIVE FORMS

ACTIVE FORMS	SUPPLEMENT SOURCES	SALIENT FEATURES
Fructans-inulin, fructooligosaccharides (FOS)	Natural sources such as onion, chicory, garlic, asparagus, banana, artichoke	FOS are subtly sweet and low-calorie. The number of fructose units ranges from 2 to 60.[9]
Galactooligosaccharides (GOS)	Derived form lactose from cow's milk and bioidentical human breast milk	GOS consist of 3–10 molecules of galactose and glucose. Commercial GOS contain complex mixtures of oligosaccharides.[10]
Human milk oligosaccarides Eg. 2'-fucosyllactose (2'-FL)	Derived from bacterial cultures	Normally added to infant formula, 2-FL is the most abundant human milk oligosaccharide with multiple functions including acting as a prebiotic, protecting against infections and inflammation, and modulating the immune system.
Other dietary fiber	Resistant starch, galactomannan from fenugreek seeds and many more	Many types of dietary fiber are classified as prebiotic if they are fermentable by colonic bacteria.[11]
Noncarbohydrate prebiotics	Polyphenols such as those found in grape seed extract and other plant sources	Various phytonutrients and other compounds can serve as prebiotics, but they are normally used for metabolic issues.

▶ SAFETY AND DOSAGE

GENERAL REQUIREMENTS	
Indian recommendations	Currently, the FSSAI has only stated the list of permitted prebiotics.[12] The ICMR-NIN recommends 40 g of dietary fiber per 2000 kcal/day for adults.[13]
Global recommendations and limits	Currently, there are no standard guidelines for prebiotics. The EFSA panel considers dietary fiber intakes of 25 g/day to be adequate for normal laxation in adults. Recommendations for dietary dietary fiber in most European countries and in the US are between 30–35 g per day for men and between 25–32 g/day for women.[14]
	A daily dose of prebiotics required to exert their beneficial functions on human health: 2.5–10 g/day.[15]
	A FOS dose of 4–15 g/day can be given to healthy subjects to reduce constipation.[9]
	2-FL has been given Generally Recognized As Safe (GRAS) status by the FDA and the European Union has approved the use.
Notes:	The selective properties of prebiotics may relate to the growth of bifidobacteria and lactobacilli at the expense of other groups of bacteria in the gut. Caution must be exercised for long-term use, i.e., longer than the period of the desired effect, to avoid dysbiosis.[16]

▶ **CLINICAL CONDITIONS**

EVIDENCE LEVEL	CONDITION OR USE CASE	DOSAGE	BENEFIT OR MECHANISM OF ACTION
++++	Melasma	Oral synbiotics, TS6, sachet containing a combination of 50 billion CFUs of 6 probiotics strains – (*Lactococcus lactis, Lactobacillus acidophilus, Lactobacillus casei, Bifidobacterium longum, Bifidobacterium infantis, Bifidobacterium bifidum*) along with an unknown amount of FOS, skim milk powder, lactose, maltodextrin, and citric acid for 12 weeks or placebo for 12 weeks	Daily supplementation showed a reduction in the severity of melasma score from baseline to week 4, week 8 and week 12. At week 12, melasma score in the synbiotics group was significantly lower than that of the placebo group.[17]
+++	Pruritus in AD	Capsules containing Bifidobacterium animalis subsp lactis LKM512 powder approx. 6×10^9 CFU and an excipient of skim milk, glucose, inulin, dextrin, and silicon dioxide or placebo for 4 weeks	The treatment group showed alleviation in itching and an improvement in dermatology specific quality of life. The treatment increased the expression of the antipruritic and antinociceptive metabolite kynurenic acid (KYNA) in patients whose itch score had improved.[18]
+++	General skin health	Fermented milk containing 6×10^{10} and 5×10^{10} CFU of B. breve and other lactic acid bacteria 0.6 g GOS and 3.1g polydextrose, [Strains–Bifidobacterium breve strain Yakult (YIT 12272), *Lactococcus lactis* YIT 2027 and *Streptococcus thermophilus* YIT 2021], or placebo for a duration of 4 weeks	There was a significant increase in cathepsin L-like activity in the stratum corneum, an indicator of keratinocyte differentiation, and a decrease in serum and urine phenol levels. The latter helps to prevent skin from drying.[19]
+++	Photoprotection	In a mouse model, 4 groups received either UV control group, 100 mg GOS-treated group (HC-GOS), *Bifidobacterium longum* 10^9 CFU group, and a combination of the probiotic and prebiotic for 12 weeks	GOS administration with or without Bifidobacteria increased the water-holding capacity of the skin and reduced TEWL compared to the control. There was a reduction in the erythema formation of 16.8% in the GOS-only treated group compared with the control.

▶ **CLINICAL CONDITIONS** (*Continued*)

EVIDENCE LEVEL	CONDITION OR USE CASE	DOSAGE	BENEFIT OR MECHANISM OF ACTION
			CD44 gene expression was significantly increased in GOS with or without Bifidobacterium. CD44 gene expression plays an important role in keratinocyte functions. Oral administration of GOS and/or Bifidobacterium significantly increased TIMP-1, an inhibitor of MMP, and collagen type 1 (Col1) mRNA expression compared with the control.[20]
+++	Photoprotection	Mice were randomly divided into four groups of unirradiated mice (NOR), UVB irradiated control (CON), collagen tripeptide intake at 200 mg/kg (CTP) and GOS intake at 200 mg/kg (GOS) for 8 weeks	The GOS or CTP group showed a higher water holding capacity compared to the control group. The wrinkle area and mean wrinkle length in the GOS and CTP groups significantly decreased. Skin aging-related genes, MMP, had significantly lower expression in the CTP and GOS groups. Oral administration of GOS and CTP significantly lowered the tissue cytokine (IL-6 and -12, and TNF-α) levels. The GOS group had a significantly lower amount of UVB-induced phosphorylation of JNK, p38, and ERK, which activate the MAPK pathway leading to an inflammatory response.[21]
+++	Photoprotection	The mice were divided into 9 groups: Groups 1 and 2 were control, groups 3 and 4 received UVB +collagen (200 mg/ kg BW) with or without B.longum (10^9 CFU), group 5 received UV B radiation with only B. longum (10^9 CFU), group 6 and 7 received UVB radiation with either GOS 50 mg or 100 mg/kg BW, group 8 and 9 received UVB radiation plus B. longum (10^9 CFU) with either 50 mg or 100 mg of GOS per kg BW for 6 weeks	Dietary supplementation with B. longum and GOS, individually and in combination, exerted protective effects against UVB-induced photoaging, showing anti-inflammatory and antioxidative effects. The supplementation with the combination of B. longum and GOS showed stronger protective effects than supplementation with the probiotic or prebiotic alone. The serum levels of SCFAs and acetate were increased following dietary supplementation with B. longum and GOS, especially in combination.[22]

▶ CLINICAL CONDITIONS *(Continued)*

EVIDENCE LEVEL	CONDITION OR USE CASE	DOSAGE	BENEFIT OR MECHANISM OF ACTION
+++	Skin dryness and quality	Fermented milk containing 1 g GOS, 2.5 g polydextrose, *B. breve* strain Yakult (YIT 12272): >1 × 10^{10} CFU, *Lactococcus lactis* YIT 2027: >1 × 10^{10} CFU and *Streptococcus thermophilus* YIT 2021 for 4 weeks	Skin hydration of the stratum corneum significantly increased, and urinary phenol and p-cresol levels significantly decreased after intake compared to baseline values. As per previous studies, phenol negatively affects in vitro keratinocyte differentiation, and a reduced serum phenol levels improves skin conditions.[23] The treatment group showed clearness of the skin as assessed by a visual analogue scale.
+++++	Skin aging	Capsule containing 1g of GOS or placebo twice a day for 12 weeks	The results showed an increase in epidermal hydration at week 12 from baseline, compared to placebo. Wrinkle area and TEWL in the GOS group were reduced significantly after 12 weeks of GOS treatment.[24]
++	Hyperpigmentation (2-FL)	Human melanocytes (MNT-1) and mouse melanoma cells (B16) were treated with 2'-FL (10 or 20 g/L) for 24 hours. This was followed by a human skin model containing human primary melanocytes being treated with 2'-FL (20 or 40 g/L).	Melanin in MNT-1 cells and B16 cells significantly decreased after 2'-FL treatment compared to untreated controls. In a human skin equivalent model, 2'-FL treatment led to significant recovery from skin pigmentation. The study suggested that 2'-FL activates autophagy via the AMPK-ULK1 axis, leading to melanosome degradation and reduced melanin levels.[25]
+++	Acne vulgaris (FOS + GOS)	A food supplement containing 100 mg FOS, and 500 mg GOS was administered as one sachet daily for 3 months	FOS + GOS supplementation in women with adult mild-to-moderate acne led to significant improvements in metabolic parameters. Fasting blood glucose decreased by 10% and total cholesterol by 13% after 3 months. In subjects with higher baseline insulin levels, a 45% reduction was observed. Triglycerides also decreased slightly. A general improvement in acne lesion count was noted.[26]

▶ SUPPLEMENTATION

	BASIS	**WHAT TO LOOK OUT FOR**
Supplementation form	Dietary fiber (galactomannan, psyllium, etc.) FOS GOS Human milk oligosaccharides (e.g., 2-FL)	Clinical studies of the dose for the specific benefit.
Administration form	Capsule, liquid, powder, gummies, effervescent tablet	Administration form is stated on the packaging.
Purity considerations	Varies with source and may be affected with the presence of probiotics.	Information available on the nutrition table.
Patient considerations	Prebiotic supplements are generally to be taken before meals. Prebiotic supplements should ideally be taken at a different time of the day as a vitamin or mineral-containing supplement.	Directions for use are normally given on the packaging.
Safety considerations	Prebiotic supplementation could lead to gastrointestinal-related symptoms such as osmotic diarrhea, bloating, cramping, and flatulence.[15] Side effects of the prebiotics may depend on chain length. Shorter chain length may have more effects.[15] Adverse effects may also be dose dependent. Low dose (2.5–10 g/day) can cause flatulence while high dose (40–50 g/day) may cause diarrhea.[15] Another study said that excessive intake of prebiotics especially oligosaccharides like FOS, GOS, etc. may cause abdominal discomfort like bloating and distension or flatulence but ≤12 g per day of GOS is normally well-tolerated.[27,28] Safety data for administration of synbiotics is scanty and inconclusive, and depends on the strain and prebiotic used.	The prebiotic dosage is given nutritional information on the back label. If a patient follows a fiber-rich diet, a lower dose of prebiotics can be recommended. This information can be acquired from the manufacturing company.
Other considerations	Caution needs to be exercised for certain types of irritable bowel syndrome (IBS) as it may aggravate the condition depending on IBS subtype or specific diets.[29]	N/A
	The effects of synbiotics may be caused by the prebiotic alone. Very few bacteria survive the harsh environment of the gut, unless they are microencapsulated or form spores.	Information about the bacteria administration form can be procured from the company.

▶ INTRODUCTION

The gut-skin axis is not just a bidirectional interaction between these organs, but jointly forms two microbial barriers to protect the host. It is no wonder that gut issues manifest on the skin as well.

The term pharmabiotic encompasses any form of therapeutic exploitation of the commensal flora, which is becoming increasingly popular in the dermatology space.[1] While the mechanisms through which the gut microbiome affects skin health are still uncertain, their metabolic activities and immune regulation can have lasting effects on our skin, as is seen by outcomes of clinical trials.[3] However, as mentioned previously, delivering microbes to the colon might be a bigger challenge than simply providing an energy source to commensal bacteria.

The main source of energy for our gut bacteria is dietary fiber, composed of indigestible carbohydrates. However, not all are fermented in the same manner. For example, bulking agents, such as lignin and psyllium, are nonfermentable by colonic bacteria.[30] Supplements commonly contain fructans – like fructooligosaccharides (FOS) and inulin, and galactans like galactooligosaccharides (GOS), both of which are fermented by Bifidobacteria and Lactobacillus, and increase their growth in the gut when consumed at relatively small amounts (< 20 g/day).[1,30]

The main SCFA-producing bacteria belong to the phylum Firmicutes, including the genera *Bacillus*, *Clostridium*, *Enterococcus*, *Lactobacillus*, and *Ruminicoccus*. Anaerobes from other phyla may also produce SCFAs.[31] Other than SCFA synthesis, the phylum Bacteroidetes are associated with immunomodulation via cytokine synthesis.[7] Together, the gut microbes protect the intestinal barrier as well as extra intestinal tissue.

Recommendations of prebiotics should take into consideration the ability of the prebiotic to enhance the growth of the specific species of intestinal bacteria and the effective doses.

▶ DIGESTION, ABSORPTION AND STORAGE

Digestion and Absorption

- Indigestible carbohydrates are resistant to breakdown and pass through our gastrointestinal tract relatively unchanged until they are fermented by the gut microbes, mainly in the large intestine.[16]

- Dietary fiber can be soluble and insoluble. Insoluble fiber promotes fecal bulking, and passes unchanged through the gut. Soluble fiber can have a prebiotic effect, provided they are fermentable. For example, psyllium is mostly non-fermentable, while others are partially fermentable (like galactomannan).[30]

Storage

Fibre fermentation produces SCFA and gas. The rest is eliminated in stool.

▶ MECHANISM OF ACTION

01 | Promoting Intestinal Integrity

Prebiotics feed the beneficial bacteria in our gut, to boost their number. They aim to balance the intestinal ecosystem. A healthy microbiome can limit the growth of harmful and opportunistic pathogens and also prevent their attachment to the intestinal mucosa.[3,7]

Dietary fiber can help with fecal bulking, which has a laxative effect. It decreases intracolonic pressure and affects colonic transit time, which helps prevent the formation of colonic diverticula and minimizes colonic exposure to toxins.[30]

Maintaining the integrity of the intestinal wall prevents the passage of microbes, toxic products, neurotransmitters, and immune cells through the circulatory system to the skin, which can otherwise lead to skin inflammation and pathogen overgrowth.[3]

02 | Anti-inflammatory Action and Nutrient Availability

Metabolites of prebiotic fermentation can confer many health benefits that translate directly or indirectly to the skin. SCFAs produced in the colon maintain colonic health and are also transported to distant tissues through the peripheral circulation. SCFAs bind to G protein-coupled receptors (GPCRs) that are expressed on skin cells, leukocytes, neutrophils, and other types of cells. SCFAs mitigate inflammation by a range of mechanisms (Figure 1):[32]

- Acetate, propionate and butyrate can modulate the immune response of dendritic cells (DCs), neutrophils, macrophages and regulatory T (Treg) cells.[4,32]

- Butyrate is metabolized by epidermal keratinocytes, which enhances the synthesis of keratinocyte-derived long-chain fatty acids (LCFAs) and very long-chain fatty acids (VLCFAs), a key event in the generation of ceramides that are critical to skin barrier function.[32]

- Butyrate enhances the expression of filaggrin (FLG) and transglutaminase-1 (TGM1) and promotes normal human epidermal keratinocytes (NHEKs) terminal differentiation to maintain skin homeostasis.[32]

- SFCAs markedly reduce IL-6 and ICAM-1 mRNA levels in human keratinocytes (HaCaT cells) stimulated with TNF-α and INF-γ in vitro, which have been shown to be involved in the pathophysiology of atopic dermatitis.[32]

3 | Affecting Nutrient Availability

Prebiotics in our food may also promote skin and hair, and overall health by increasing nutrient availability.

- They improve the overall absorption of calcium, iron, vitamin D, magnesium, vitamin E and β-carotene.[33] Taking the example of iron, prebiotics may lower the pH of the luminal content, boost reduction of Fe (III) to Fe (II), and stimulate expression of mineral-transport proteins in epithelial cells, to enhance iron absorption.[34]

- Prebiotics feed commensal bacteria, such as Lactobacillus and Bifidobacterium, which can de novo synthesize and supply vitamins to the host. For example, it has been estimated that up to half of the daily vitamin K requirement is provided by gut bacteria.[35]

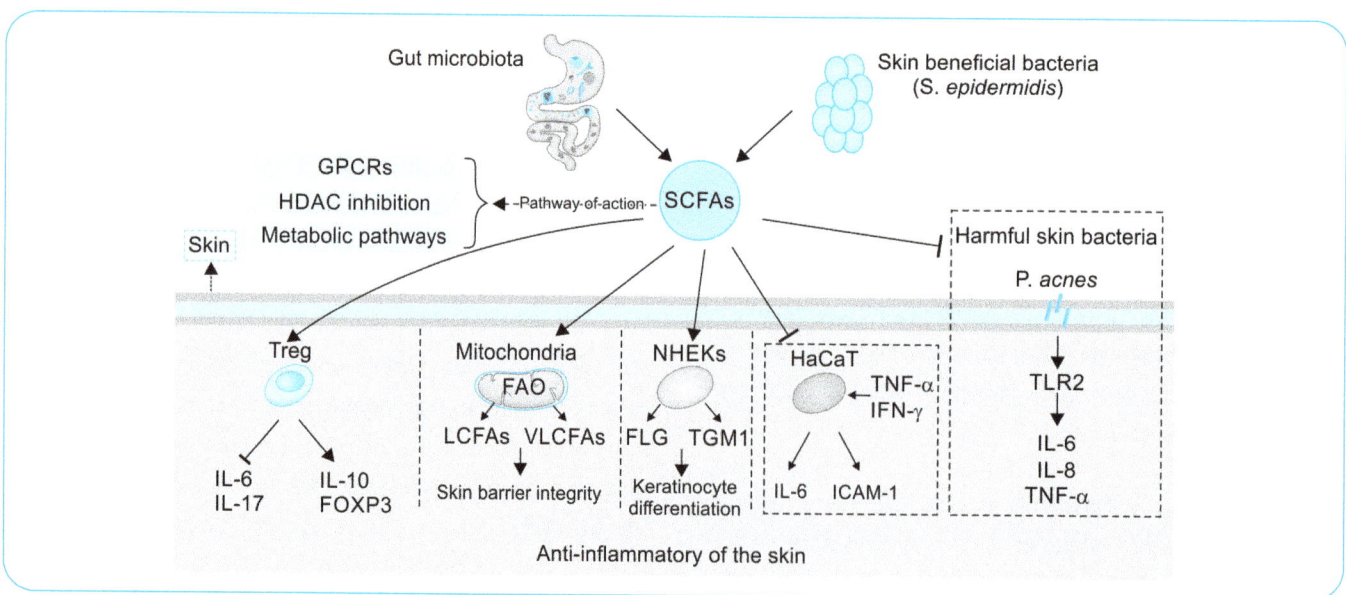

Figure 1: Schematic representation of the roles of SCFAs in inflammatory skin diseases.[32]

REFERENCES

1. O'Hara AM, Shanahan F. The gut flora as a forgotten organ. EMBO reports. 2006;7(7):688-93.
2. Navarro-López V, Núñez-Delegido E, Ruzafa-Costas B, Sánchez-Pellicer P, Agüera-Santos J, Navarro-Moratalla L. Probiotics in the Therapeutic Arsenal of Dermatologists. Microorganisms. 2021;9(7):1513.
3. Mahmud MdR, Akter S, Tamanna SK, Mazumder L, Esti IZ, Banerjee S, et al. Impact of gut microbiome on skin health: gut-skin axis observed through the lenses of therapeutics and skin diseases. Gut Microbes. 2022;14(1):2096995.
4. Lee SY, Lee E, Park YM, Hong SJ. Microbiome in the Gut-Skin Axis in Atopic Dermatitis. Allergy Asthma Immunol Res. 2018;10(4):354-62.
5. Hajela N, Nair GB, Ramakrishna BS, Ganguly NK. Probiotic foods: Can their increasing use in India ameliorate the burden of chronic lifestyle disorders? Indian J Med Res. 2014;139(1):19-26.
6. Han S, Lu Y, Xie J, Fei Y, Zheng G, Wang Z, et al. Probiotic Gastrointestinal Transit and Colonization After Oral Administration: A Long Journey. Front Cell Infect Microbiol. 2021;11:609722.
7. Stojanov S, Berlec A, Štrukelj B. The Influence of Probiotics on the Firmicutes/Bacteroidetes Ratio in the Treatment of Obesity and Inflammatory Bowel disease. Microorganisms. 2020;8(11):1715.
8. Hassan NE, El Shebini SM, El-Masry SA, Ahmed NH, Kamal AN, Ismail AS, et al. Brief overview of dietary intake, some types of gut microbiota, metabolic markers and research opportunities in sample of Egyptian women. Sci Rep. 2022;12(1):17291.
9. Sabater-Molina M, Larqué E, Torrella F, Zamora S. Dietary fructooligosaccharides and potential benefits on health. J Physiol Biochem. 2009;65(3):315-28.
10. Hong KB, Kim JH, Kwon HK, Han SH, Park Y, Suh HJ. Evaluation of Prebiotic Effects of High-Purity Galactooligosaccharides in vitro and in vivo. Food Technol Biotechnol. 2016;54(2):156-63.
11. Fuentes-Zaragoza E, Sánchez-Zapata E, Sendra E, Sayas E, Navarro C, Fernández-López J, et al. Resistant starch as prebiotic: A review. Starch - Stärke. 2011;63(7):406-15.
12. Food Safety and Standards Authority of India. Direction under section 16(5) of the Food Safety and Standards Act, 2006 regarding operationalization of FSS (Health Supplements, Nutraceuticals, Food for Special Dietary Use, Food for Special Medical Purpose and Prebiotic and Probiotic Food) Regulations, 2022. [FSS (Nutra) Regulations, 2022].
13. National Institute of Nutrition Indian Council of Medical Research. Recommended Dietary Allowances and Estimated Average Requirements for Indians - 2020. RDA Full Report 2020.
14. Stephen AM, Champ MMJ, Cloran SJ, Fleith M, van Lieshout L, Mejborn H, et al. Dietary fibre in Europe: current state of knowledge on definitions, sources, recommendations, intakes and relationships to health. Nutr Res Rev. 2017;30(2):149-90.
15. Davani-Davari D, Negahdaripour M, Karimzadeh I, Seifan M, Mohkam M, Masoumi SJ, et al. Prebiotics: Definition, Types, Sources, Mechanisms, and Clinical Applications. Foods. 2019;8(3):92.
16. Macfarlane S, Macfarlane GT, Cummings JH. Review article: prebiotics in the gastrointestinal tract. Alimentary Pharmacology and Therapeutic. 2006;24(5):701-14.
17. Piyavatin P, Chaichalotornkul S, Nararatwanchai T, Bumrungpert A, Saiwichai T. Synbiotics supplement is effective for Melasma improvement. J Cosmet Dermatol. 2021;20(9):2841-50.
18. Matsumoto M, Ebata T, Hirooka J, Hosoya R, Inoue N, Itami S, et al. Antipruritic effects of the probiotic strain LKM512 in adults with atopic dermatitis. Ann Allergy Asthma Immunol. 2014;113(2):209-16.e7.
19. Kano M, Masuoka N, Kaga C, Sugimoto S, Iizuka R, Manabe K, et al. Consecutive Intake of Fermented Milk Containing Bifidobacterium breve Strain Yakult and Galacto-oligosaccharides Benefits Skin Condition in Healthy Adult Women. Biosci Microbiota Food Health. 2013;32(1):33-9.
20. Hong KB, Jeong M, Han KS, Hwan Kim J, Park Y, Suh HJ. Photoprotective effects of galacto-oligosaccharide and/or Bifidobacterium longum supplementation against skin damage induced by ultraviolet irradiation in hairless mice. Int J Food Sci Nutr. 2015;66(8):923-30.
21. Suh MG, Bae GY, Jo K, Kim JM, Hong KB, Suh HJ. Photoprotective Effect of Dietary Galacto-Oligosaccharide (GOS) in Hairless Mice via Regulation of the MAPK Signaling Pathway. Molecules. 2020;25(7):1679.
22. Kim D, Lee KR, Kim NR, Park SJ, Lee M, Kim OK. Combination of Bifidobacterium longum and Galacto-Oligosaccharide Protects the Skin from Photoaging. J Med Food. 2021;24(6):606-16.
23. Mori N, Kano M, Masuoka N, Konno T, Suzuki Y, Miyazaki K, et al. Effect of probiotic and prebiotic fermented milk on skin and intestinal conditions in healthy young female students. Biosci Microbiota Food Health. 2016;35(3):105-12.
24. Hong YH, Chang UJ, Kim YS, Jung EY, Suh HJ. Dietary galacto-oligosaccharides improve skin health: a randomized double blind clinical trial. Asia Pac J Clin Nutr 2017;26(4):613-8
25. Lei K, Wang D, Lin L, Zeng J, Li Y, Zhang L, Lane JA, et al. 2'-fucosyllactose inhibits imiquimod-induced psoriasis in mice by regulating Th17 cell response via the STAT3 signaling pathway. Int Immunopharmacol. 2020;85:106659.
26. Dall'Oglio F, Milani M, Micali G. Effects of oral supplementation with FOS and GOS prebiotics in women with adult acne: the "S.O. Sweet" study: a proof-of-concept pilot trial. Clin Cosmet Investig Dermatol. 2018;11:445-9.
27. Pandey KR, Naik SR, Vakil BV. Probiotics, prebiotics and synbiotics- a review. J Food Sci Technol. 2015;52(12):7577-87.
28. Niittynen L, Kajander K, Korpela R. Galacto-oligosaccharides and bowel function. Scand J Food Nutr. 2007;51(2):62-6.
29. Chlebicz-Wójcik A, Śliżewska K. Probiotics, Prebiotics, and Synbiotics in the Irritable Bowel Syndrome Treatment: A Review. Biomolecules. 2021;11(8):1154.
30. ScienceDirect. Short Chain Fatty Acid - an overview.
31. Parada Venegas D, De la Fuente MK, Landskron G, González MJ, Quera R, Dijkstra G, et al. Short Chain Fatty Acids (SCFAs)-Mediated Gut Epithelial and Immune Regulation and Its Relevance for Inflammatory Bowel Diseases. Front Immunol. 2019;10:277.
32. Xiao X, Hu X, Yao J, Cao W, Zou Z, Wang L, et al. The role of short-chain fatty acids in inflammatory skin diseases. Front Microbiol. 2022;13:1083432.
33. Costa G, Vasconcelos Q, Abreu G, Albuquerque A, Vilarejo J, Aragão G. Changes in nutrient absorption in children and adolescents caused by fructans, especially fructooligosaccharides and inulin. Arch Pediatr. 2020;27(3):166-9.
34. Ahmad AMR, Ahmed W, Iqbal S, Javed M. Prebiotics and iron bioavailability? Unveiling the hidden association - A review. Trends in Food Science & Technology. 2021;110:584-90.
35. Morowitz MJ, Carlisle E, Alverdy JC. Contributions of Intestinal Bacteria to Nutrition and Metabolism in the Critically Ill. Surg Clin North Am. 2011;91(4):771-85.

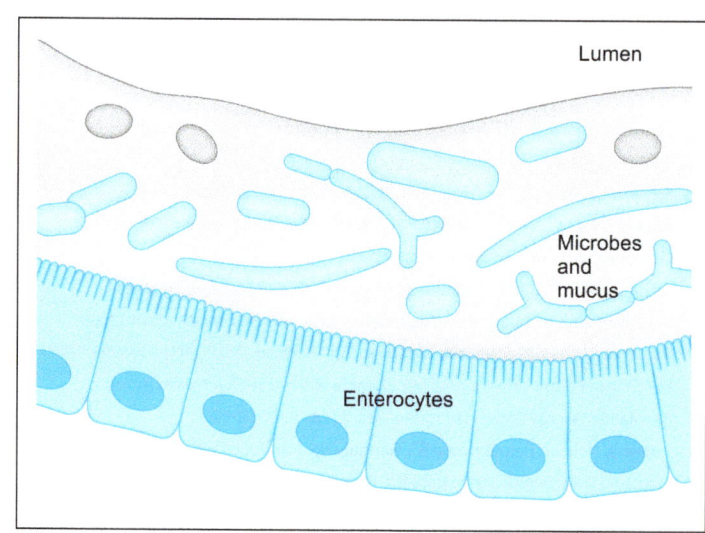

The gastrointestinal barrier

Probiotics

✍ Jaishree Sharad

CONTENTS

PROBIOTICS: NUTRIENT SNAPSHOT

▸ REQUIREMENT IN THE INDIAN CONTEXT | **309**

▸ ACTIVE FORMS | **310**

▸ SAFETY AND DOSAGE | **310**

▸ CLINICAL CONDITIONS | **310**

▸ SUPPLEMENTATION | **312**

INTRODUCTION | **314**

DIGESTION, ABSORPTION AND STORAGE | **314**

MECHANISM OF ACTION | **314**

KEY TOPICS

- ACNE VULGARIS
- ATOPIC DERMATITIS
- DRY SKIN
- PSORIASIS
- WOUND HEALING
- WRINKLES

Nutrient Snapshot

▶ **REQUIREMENT IN THE INDIAN CONTEXT**

Oral probiotics are used in managing and treating a variety of disease states. They are live microorganisms that are known to help improve health, by unifying with the commensal bacteria in our gut.[1] There is emerging research on the skin microbiome and its connection with the gut, referred to as the gut-skin axis and its effects on skin health and dermatoses.[2]

While the mechanisms through which the gut microbiome affects skin health are still unclear, it is reasonable to accept that the metabolic activities, protection from microbes and immune regulation of the gut can affect our skin.[3] An alteration among gut microbial diversity (dysbiosis) can disrupt mucosal immunological tolerance and increase host vulnerability. Several dermatologic conditions, such as acne, atopic dermatitis, psoriasis, and rosacea are linked with intestinal dysbiosis.[3,4]

The phyla Firmicutes and Bacteroidetes largely dominate the adult microbiome, followed by Actinobacteria, Proteobacteria, Fusobacteria, and Verrucomicrobia.[5] Indians are thought to harbor far lesser numbers of Bacteroidetes than North American counterparts.[6,7] The Firmicutes/Bacteroidetes (F/B) ratio is widely accepted to influence in maintaining intestinal homeostasis. Increased or decreased F/B ratio, or low numbers of beneficial genera like Bifidobacteria and Lactobacilli, is regarded as dysbiosis.[5,8]

Since the inception of the Human Microbiome Project in 2007, there is considerable public interest in India in probiotic foods, due to the burden of lifestyle disorders, uncontrolled use of antibiotics, and poor nutrient intake. While consumption of yogurt and other fermented products is associated with improved health outcomes, they may not be part of all diets. The large spectrum of diet and cultural diversity, can make it harder to provide clear solutions for the general public.[6]

With probiotics being both strain and disease-specific, it is crucial to identify the strains that produce the best outcome for different ailments to achieve the most optimal results.[1] For less explored disorders, it may be better to recommend prebiotics or foods that help the growth of beneficial bacteria. This is especially true for supplements that do not provide evidence of probiotic survival through the harsh environment of the gastrointestinal tract, or those with low count i.e., very few colony forming units (CFUs).[9]

▶ ACTIVE FORMS

ACTIVE FORMS	SUPPLEMENT SOURCES	SALIENT FEATURES
Lactobacillus strains[10,11] Bifidobacterium strains[11]	N/A	Lactobacillus and bifidobacterium are the most used and well-researched microorganisms for probiotic supplements.
Other strains	N/A	Various microbes are used in supplements and their effects are strain-dependant

▶ SAFETY AND DOSAGE

GENERAL REQUIREMENTS	
Indian recommendations	The FSSAI has stated the list of bacteria that are approved for the use in supplements: Lactobacillus, Limosilactobacillus, Ligilactobacillus, Lacticaseibacillus, Levilactobacillus, Bacillus, Bifidobacterium, Streptococcus, and Saccharomyces. The minimum viable number shall be $\geq 10^8$ CFU in the recommended serving size per day.[12]
Global recommendations and limits	As per World Gastroenterology Organisation practice guidelines for pre and probiotics, it is not possible to recommend general dose needed for probiotics rather it should be based on human studies that are effective.[13]
Notes:	Probiotics are capable of causing local and systemic side effects so risk-benefit should be considered before recommending it.[14] The selective growth of a type of bacteria is at the expense of other groups of bacteria in the gut. Caution must be exercised for long-term use, i.e., longer than the period of the desired effect, to avoid dysbiosis.[15] The FAO-WHO stated that the so-called 'minimum therapeutic' level of viable probiotic microorganisms should be at least 10^6 CFU/g of viable cells throughout the product shelf-life.[16]

▶ CLINICAL CONDITIONS

EVIDENCE LEVEL	CONDITION OR USE CASE	DOSAGE	BENEFIT OR MECHANISM OF ACTION
+++++	Atopic dermatitis	Mixture- 1×10^9 CFU *Lactobacillus plantarum* PBS067, 1×10^9 CFU *Lactobacillus reuteri* PBS072 and 1×10^9 CFU *Lactobacillus rhamnosus* LRH020, (1 mg) or placebo was given for 56 days	Patients receiving treatment showed improvement in skin smoothness, skin moisturization, self-perception, and a decrease in SCORAD index as well as in the levels of inflammatory markers associated with AD on 28th day which was maintained at 84th day (after washout of 1 month)[17]

▶ **CLINICAL CONDITIONS** (*Continued*)

EVIDENCE LEVEL	CONDITION OR USE CASE	DOSAGE	BENEFIT OR MECHANISM OF ACTION
+++++	Atopic dermatitis	N/A (meta-analysis of variable strains and doses)	According to the meta-analysis, there was a significant reduction in the SCORAD index of atopic dermatitis patients receiving the probiotic supplement.[18]
+++++	Wrinkles and dryness	Capsule of 1.75×10^9 CFU BI-04 (ATCC SD5219) or placebo for 12 weeks.	Treatment significantly improved facial skin wrinkle parameters (total wrinkle area and volume, average depth of wrinkles, and arithmetic average roughness) versus placebo at 4 weeks, but there were no differences at week 8 or 12 between groups. Skin hydration, TEWL, elasticity, and gloss were similar between groups.[19]
+++++	Wrinkles and dryness	Probiotic powder containing either 1×10^{10} CFU/day of *L. plantarum* HY7714 or placebo for 12 weeks.	There was a significant increase in the skin water content in the face and hands at week 12 in the probiotic group. TEWL decreased significantly in both probiotic and placebo groups at weeks 4, 8, and 12. Volunteers in the probiotic group had a significant reduction in wrinkle depth at week 12, and skin gloss was also improved by week 12. Skin elasticity improved by 13.17% after 4 weeks and by 21.73% after 12 weeks.[20]
++++	Mild-to-moderate acne vulgaris	Subjects received either probiotic supplement (group A) containing a combination of *Lactobacillus acidophilus* (NAS super-strain, 5 billion CFU, *Lactobacillus delbrueckii* subspecies *bulgaricus* (LB-51 super-strain, 5 billion CFU) and Bifidobacterium bifidum (Malyoth superstrain, 20 billion CFU); or minocycline alone (group B) or combination of probiotic supplement and minocycline (group C) for 12 weeks.	There was a significant improvement in total lesion count after 4 weeks of treatment in all 3 groups with continued improvement till the follow-up week. At 8- and 12-week visits, group C had a significant decrease in total lesion count as compared to groups A and B.[21]

▶ **CLINICAL CONDITIONS** (*Continued*)

EVIDENCE LEVEL	CONDITION OR USE CASE	DOSAGE	BENEFIT OR MECHANISM OF ACTION
+++	Acne vulgaris	A liquid supplement containing *Lactobacillus rhamnosus* SP1 at a dose of 3×10^9 CFU/day or placebo was given for 12 weeks	Compared with the placebo the probiotic group showed a 32% reduction in insulin-like growth factor 1 (IGF1) while 65% increase in forkhead box protein O1 (*FOXO1*) gene expression (nuclear transcription factor which normalizes the pathogenesis of acne) in the skin, thus improving the appearance of adult acne.[22]
+++	Wound healing	In a rodent model, the probiotic group was supplemented with *Lactobacillus paracasei* LPC-37, Bifidobacterium lactis HN0019, *Lactobacillus rhamnosus* HN001, *Lactobacillus acidophilus* NCFM® at a dose of 200,000 to 210,000 CFU given orally daily for 15 days.	Wound contraction was faster in the probiotic group when compared to the controls, resulting in a smaller wound area in the 7th postoperative day. This group also showed increased fibrosis from 3rd to 7th postoperative day. This group also showed an increase in type III collagen at the 7th day and type I collagen on the 10th day.[23]
+++++	Psoriasis	Capsule containing a mixture of Bifidobacterium longum CECT 7347, B. lactis CECT 8145 and *Lactobacillus rhamnosus* CECT 8361 with a total of 1×10^9 CFU per capsule, formulated on maltodextrin for 12 weeks.	66.7% of patients in the probiotic group and and 41.9% in the placebo group showed reduction in Psoriasis Area and Severity Index of up to 75%. A clinically relevant difference was observed in the Physician Global Assessment index: 48.9% in the probiotic group achieved a score of 0 or 1.[24]

▶ **SUPPLEMENTATION**

	BASIS	WHAT TO LOOK OUT FOR
Supplementation form	Microencapsulated probiotics (both live microorganism and spores) have better gut viability. The viability of spore-based probiotics is better than live microorganisms as many of these spore based probiotics can resist the stomach acids unlike the live microorganisms.[25]	Majority of the products available in the market are microencapsulated but if this information is not available on the label it can be obtained from the company. Whether the probiotic is spore-based or not is often not mentioned on the packaging. The company can provide this information.

▶ **SUPPLEMENTATION** (*Continued*)

	BASIS	**WHAT TO LOOK OUT FOR**
Administration form	Liquids, capsules, gummies and powders. Administration frequency may vary for different probiotics.	Administration form and frequency is stated on the packaging.
Purity considerations	Viability of bacteria may vary considerably, especially for live, non spore-forming microbes.[15] Bacterial viability may be lower closer to the expiry date.	Microorganisms dose is given on the nutritional table, but shelf-life information can be procured from the manufacturer.
Patient considerations	Best time to take probiotic supplements is based on the strains and their role in the body. Some have to be taken empty stomach in the morning or 30 minutes before the meal while some have to be taken post-meal or at bedtime.[26] Gas and bloating may occur, but are typically transient.	Consider the usage instructions given on the packaging.
Safety considerations	Immediate side effects of probiotics are usually minor and consist of gastrointestinal symptoms, such as gas.[27] But it should not be given to elderly individuals, critically ill patients, immunocompromised individuals and those with chronic diseases without doctor's consultations.[1,28] Bacterial LPS, also known as endotoxin, is not normally toxic upon oral intake. However, the use of bolus doses of gram negative bacteria should be avoided by severely ill patients, as well as immunosuppressed or immunocompromised individuals.[29] Horizontal gene transfer is a possibility in certain probiotics. Serious concerns are of genes conferring resistance to antibiotics.[30,31]	N/A Endotoxemia can induce inflammation, fever, and in severe cases, septic shock.[29] Risk assessment of antibiotic resistance or genetic screening of the probiotic strains can be acquired. In the absence of this data, risk-benefit must be considered.[30]
Other considerations	Storage conditions: Specific strains of probiotics have to be stored in cold temperatures. Our commensal microbes may prohibit colonization of the probiotic. This may be an issue especially with spore-forming bacteria.	Consider the storage instruction given on the packaging. A clinical study of the effects of the specific strains can be useful. However, colonization resistance may vary among individuals.

▶ INTRODUCTION

Skin and gut are active, complex immunological and neuroendocrine organs that are exposed to the outside environment on a frequent basis and host a wide range of microbes.[3] These commensal microbes outnumber the cells in our body, and form the first line of defence from invading pathogens. The gut microbiota of a healthy individual differs in different parts of the gastrointestinal tract and changes with time due to aging, dietary habits, lifestyle, and antibiotic consumption. The gut microbiota is typically dominated by bacteria and mostly by members of the phyla Bacteroidetes and Firmicutes.[6]

The phylum Firmicutes includes gram-positive bacteria with rigid cell walls that are predominantly from the genera *Bacillus, Clostridium, Enterococcus, Lactobacillus,* and *Ruminococcus*. They play a key role in the nutrition and metabolism of the host through short-chain fatty acid (SCFA) synthesis. In contrast, the phylum Bacteroidetes includes species of gram-negative bacteria that are predominantly from the genera *Bacteroides, Alistipes, Parabacteroides, and Prevotella*. They are associated with immunomodulation, as their components, lipopolysaccharides (LPS) and flagellin, interact with cell receptors and enhance immune reactions through cytokine synthesis.[5,8]

The United Nations Food and Agricultural Organization defines probiotics as "live microorganisms, which, once administered in adequate amounts, confer a health benefit to the host." The most commonly used bacteria as probiotics are the *Lactobacillus* and *Bifidobacteria*. Current limitations with the use of probiotics include strain-specific outcomes, shelf-life, survival in the gut, and poor attachment of probiotics to intestinal mucosa, amongst others. However, many suppliers are employing technologies to bypass these limitations.[6,9]

▶ DIGESTION, ABSORPTION AND STORAGE

Digestion and Absorption

- Most probiotics survive the saliva, which is applicable to powders and drinks.[9]

- The acidic environment in the stomach is extremely lethal to most bacteria, which is compounded by mechanical churning. Pancreatic juices and bile further hinder bacterial survival. Therefore, spore-forming bacteria[32] or techniques like microencapsulation are used to improve probiotic viability through the gut.[9,16]

- Probiotics must compete with the host microbiota for adhesion sites to be able to colonize the colonic mucosa and proliferate. This 'colonization resistance', which normally protects against pathogens, can backfire as the biggest challenge for probiotics. Furthermore, the composition of the gut microbiota is highly variable, making probiotic effects variable on the host.[9]

- *Enterococcus* and *Saccharomyces* species are thought to survive at a range of pH and attach to the colon.[33]

- Regardless of microbial survival, probiotic foods may be beneficial due to the metabolites produced in the food.[16]

Storage

- Acid, bile and pancreatic secretions limit bacterial colonization of the stomach and proximal small intestine by most bacteria.[34]

- The majority of microorganisms in the gut inhabit the distal small intestine and the colon, where bacterial density ranges from 10^{11} to 10^{12} CFU/mL.[34]

▶ MECHANISM OF ACTION

The microbes in our gut help break down fiber and other nutrients from our diet and transform it into beneficial nutrients needed for our health, like SCFAs (specifically butyrate and propionate) and vitamins (specifically K and B12). They also antagonize harmful microbes by several mechanisms; however, producing antibacterial peptides (bacteriocins) is among the most common.[3,8] The gut microbiome can modulate the gut-skin axis through direct and indirect pathways.[4]

Dysbiosis in the gut can decrease the gut mucus layer, resulting in the passage of microbes through the intestinal barrier, causing the production of toxic products, inducing harmful effects by neurotransmitters, producing B cell hyperresponsiveness, impairing T cell differentiation, and creating low levels of IgA secretion. Dysbiotic gut microbes, toxic products, neurotransmitters, and altered immune cells pass through the circulatory system to the skin, leading to pathogen overgrowth and skin inflammation amongst other issues.[3]

01 | Immunomodulatory Effects

Probiotics can interact with gastrointestinal mucosa and gut-associated lymphoid tissue (GALT), where >70% of immune cells are located, specifically with epithelial cells, mucosal dendritic cells (DCs), and macrophages. Depending on the probiotic strain, they can either induce immune activation signaling by producing interleukin (IL)-12, IL-18, and tumor necrosis factor alpha (TNF-α) or trigger tolerance signaling by stimulating anti-inflammatory cytokines, IL-10 and transforming growth factor-beta (TGF-β). In the IL-10/TGF-β-enriched cytokine milieu, macrophages and DCs can enhance the generation of induced regulatory T (Treg) cells that suppress an immune response, thereby maintaining homeostasis and self-tolerance.[4] Increase in circulating TGF-β has also been shown to affect barrier integrity since it has a dual proliferation-inhibition effect on keratinocytes **(Figure 1)**.[35]

02 | Effects by Probiotic Metabolites

The metabolites and neurotransmitters produced from the gut microbiome such as SCFAs, γ-aminobutyric acid (GABA), acetylcholine, serotonin and tryptophan can affect our skin (and brain function) directly. That's why the gut-skin axis is often also referred to as the gut-brain-skin axis.[4] Further to their countless, complex physiological roles, these metabolites play important roles in skin health:

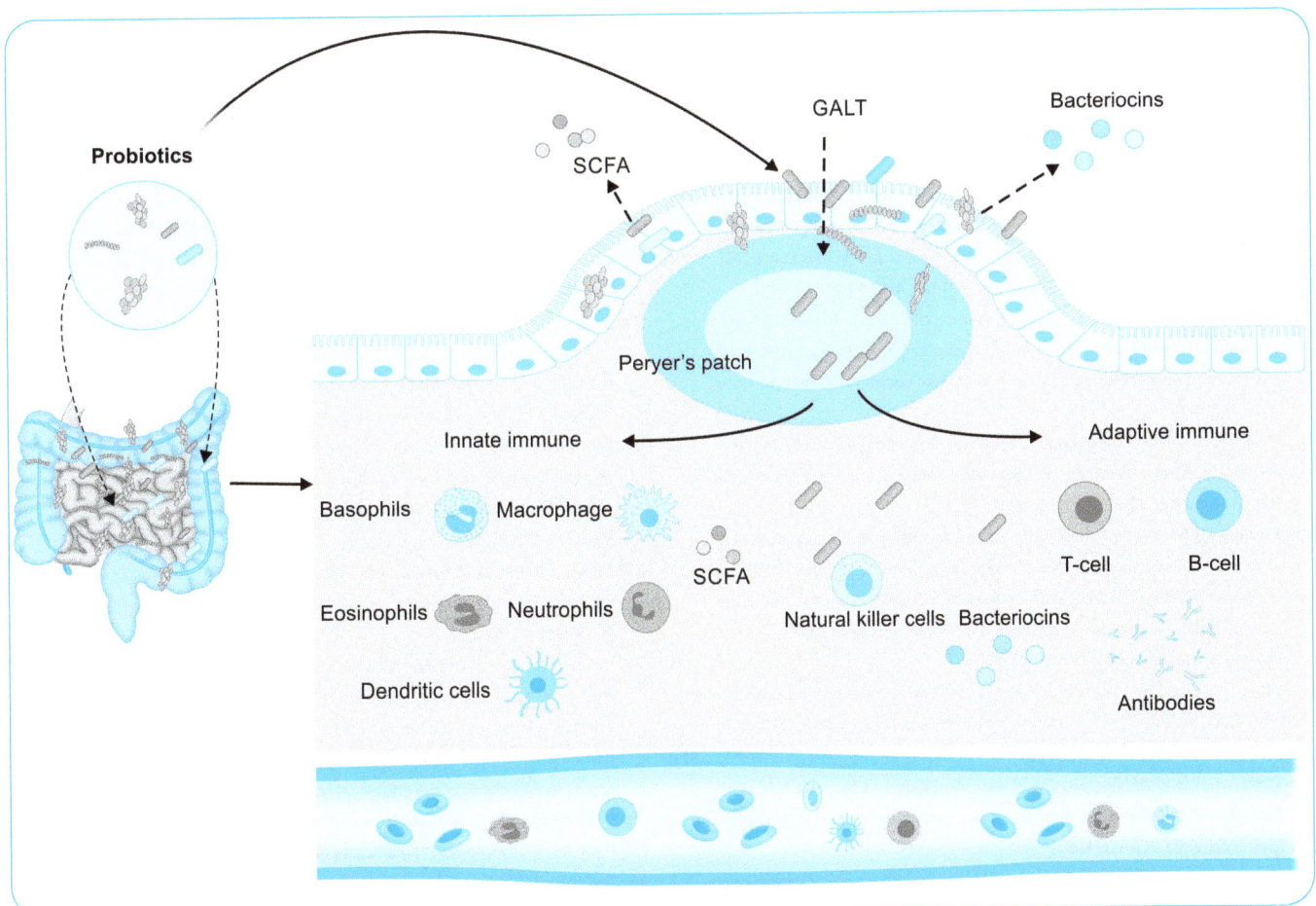

Figure 1: Microbes travel through Peyer's patches, small masses of lymphatic tissue, leading to an immune response.[36]

- GABA increases T helper cell type 1 (Th1), balancing the Th1 and T helper cell type 2 (Th2) levels, which effectively wanes AD-like skin lesions. GABA also suppresses matrix metalloproteinase-1 (MMP-1) and increases the expression of collagen type I to maintain skin elasticity.[3]

- SCFAs and acetylcholine are involved in the maintenance of barrier function. SCFAs can enhance the activity of Treg, improve mitochondrial metabolism, promote keratinocyte differentiation and reduce the expression of inflammatory factors. SCFAs can also inhibit the inflammatory response induced by UV radiation[37] and *P. acnes*.[38]

- Via the modulation of melatonin, serotonin and its precursor, tryptophan, are involved in skin pigmentation, wound healing, thermoregulation and hair growth.[3,39]

▶ REFERENCES

1. Shahrokhi M, Nagalli S. Probiotics. StatPearls, StatPearls Publishing, 3 July 2023.
2. Navarro-López V, Núñez-Delegido E, Ruzafa-Costas B, Sánchez-Pellicer P, Agüera-Santos J, Navarro-Moratalla L. Probiotics in the Therapeutic Arsenal of Dermatologists. Microorganisms. 2021;9(7):1513.
3. Mahmud MdR, Akter S, Tamanna SK, Mazumder L, Esti IZ, Banerjee S, et al. Impact of gut microbiome on skin health: gut-skin axis observed through the lenses of therapeutics and skin diseases. Gut Microbes. 2022;14(1):2096995.
4. Lee SY, Lee E, Park YM, Hong SJ. Microbiome in the Gut-Skin Axis in Atopic Dermatitis. Allergy Asthma Immunol Res. 2018;10(4):354-62.
5. Hassan NE, El Shebini SM, El-Masry SA, Ahmed NH, Kamal AN, Ismail AS, et al. Brief overview of dietary intake, some types of gut microbiota, metabolic markers and research opportunities in sample of Egyptian women. Sci Rep. 2022;12(1):17291.
6. Hajela N, Nair GB, Ramakrishna BS, Ganguly NK. Probiotic foods: Can their increasing use in India ameliorate the burden of chronic lifestyle disorders? Indian J Med Res. 2014;139(1):19-26.
7. Eckburg PB, Bik EM, Bernstein CN, Purdom E, Dethlefsen L, Sargent M, et al. Diversity of the Human Intestinal Microbial Flora. Science. 2005;308(5728):1635-8.
8. Stojanov S, Berlec A, Štrukelj B. The Influence of Probiotics on the Firmicutes/Bacteroidetes Ratio in the Treatment of Obesity and Inflammatory Bowel disease. Microorganisms. 2020;8(11):1715.
9. Han S, Lu Y, Xie J, Fei Y, Zheng G, Wang Z, et al. Probiotic Gastrointestinal Transit and Colonization After Oral Administration: A Long Journey. Front Cell Infect Microbiol. 2021;11:609722.
10. Dolan KE, Pizano JM, Gossard CM, Williamson CB, Burns CM, Gasta MG, et al. Probiotics and Disease: A Comprehensive Summary—Part 6, Skin Health. Integr Med (Encinitas). 2017;16(4):32-41.
11. Kimoto-Nira H. New lactic acid bacteria for skin health via oral intake of heat-killed or live cells. Anim Sci J. 2018;89(6):835-42.
12. Food Safety and Standards Authority of India. Direction under section 16(5) of the Food Safety and Standards Act, 2006 regarding operationalization of FSS (Health Supplements, Nutraceuticals, Food for Special Dietary Use, Food for Special Medical Purpose and Prebiotic and Probiotic Food) Regulations, 2022. [FSS (Nutra) Regulations, 2022].
13. Guarner F, Sanders ME, Eliakim R, Fedorak R, et al. Probiotics and prebiotics. World Gastroenterology Organisation Global Guidelines, February 2017.
14. Lerner A, Shoenfeld Y, Matthias T. Probiotics: If It Does Not Help It Does Not Do Any Harm. Really? Microorganisms. 2019;7(4):104.
15. Ciorba MA. A Gastroenterologist's Guide to Probiotics. Clin Gastroenterol Hepatol. 2012;10(9):960-8.
16. Terpou A, Papadaki A, Lappa IK, Kachrimanidou V, Bosnea LA, Kopsahelis N. Probiotics in Food Systems: Significance and Emerging Strategies Towards Improved Viability and Delivery of Enhanced Beneficial Value. Nutrients. 2019;11(7):1591.
17. Michelotti A, Cestone E, Ponti ID, Giardina S, Pisati M, Spartà E, et al. Efficacy of a probiotic supplement in patients with atopic dermatitis: a randomized, double-blind, placebo-controlled clinical trial. European Journal of Dermatology. 2021;31(2):225-32.
18. Umborowati MA, Damayanti D, Anggraeni S, Endaryanto A, Surono IS, Effendy I, et al. The role of probiotics in the treatment of adult atopic dermatitis: a meta-analysis of randomized controlled trials. Journal of Health, Population and Nutrition. 2022;41(1):37.
19. Huuskonen L, Lyra A, Lee E, Ryu J, Jeong H, Baek J, et al. Effects of Bifidobacterium animalis subsp. lactis Bl-04 on Skin Wrinkles and Dryness: A Randomized, Triple-Blinded, Placebo-Controlled Clinical Trial. Dermato. 2022;2(2):30-52.
20. Lee DE, Huh CS, Ra J, Choi ID, Jeong JW, Kim SH, et al. Clinical Evidence of Effects of Lactobacillus plantarum HY7714 on Skin Aging: A Randomized, Double Blind, Placebo-Controlled Study. 2015;25(12):2160-8.
21. Jung GW, Tse JE, Guiha I, Rao J. Prospective, randomized, open-label trial comparing the safety, efficacy, and tolerability of an acne treatment regimen with and without a probiotic supplement and minocycline in subjects with mild to moderate acne. J Cutan Med Surg. 2013;17(2):114-22.
22. Fabbrocini G, Bertona M, Picazo Ó, Pareja-Galeano H, Monfrecola G, Emanuele E. Supplementation with Lactobacillus rhamnosus SP1 normalises skin expression of genes implicated in insulin signalling and improves adult acne. Benef Microbes. 2016;7(5):625-30.
23. Tagliari E, Campos LF, Campos AC, Costa-Casagrande TA, De Noronha L. Effect of Probiotic Oral Administration on Skin Wound Healing In Rats. Arq Bras Cir Dig. 2019;32(3):e1457.
24. Navarro-López V, Martínez-Andrés A, Ramírez-Boscá A, Ruzafa-Costas B, Núñez-Delegido E, Carrión-Gutiérrez MA, et al. Efficacy and Safety of Oral Administration of a Mixture of Probiotic Strains in Patients with Psoriasis: A Randomized Controlled Clinical Trial. Acta Derm Venereol. 2019;99(12):1078-84.
25. Neag MA, Melincovici CS, Catinean A, Muntean DM, Pop RM, Bocsan IC, et al. The Role of Probiotic Bacillus Spores and Amino Acids with Immunoglobulins on a Rat Enteropathy Model. Biomedicines. 2022;10(10):2508.
26. Tompkins TA, Mainville I, Arcand Y. The impact of meals on a probiotic during transit through a model of the human upper gastrointestinal tract. Benef Microbes. 2011;2(4):295-303.

27. Fact Sheet for Health Professionals. Probiotics [Online]. Available from: https://ods.od.nih.gov/factsheets/Probiotics-HealthProfessional/
28. Katkowska M, Garbacz K, Kusiak A. Probiotics: Should All Patients Take Them? Microorganisms. 2021;9(12):2620.
29. Wassenaar TM, Zimmermann K. Lipopolysaccharides in Food, Food Supplements, and Probiotics: Should We be Worried? Eur J Microbiol Immunol (Bp). 2018;8(3):63-9.
30. Lerner A, Matthias T, Aminov R. Potential Effects of Horizontal Gene Exchange in the Human Gut. Front Immunol. 2017;8:1630.
31. Tóth AG, Csabai I, Judge MF, Maróti G, Becsei Á, Spisák S, et al. Mobile Antimicrobial Resistance Genes in Probiotics. Antibiotics (Basel). 2021;10(11):1287.
32. Elshaghabee Fouad M F, Rokana N, Gulhane R D, Sharma C, Panwar H. Bacillus as Potential Probiotics: Status, Concerns, and Future Perspectives Front Microbiol. 2017:8:1490.
33. You S, Ma Y, Yan B, Pei W, Wu Q, Ding C, et al. The promotion mechanism of prebiotics for probiotics: A review. Front Nutr. 2022;9:1000517.
34. O'Hara AM, Shanahan F. The gut flora as a forgotten organ. EMBO reports. 2006;7(7):688-93.
35. Hashimoto K. Regulation of keratinocyte function by growth factors. J Dermatol Sci. 2000;24(Suppl 1):S46-50.
36. Youssef M, Ahmed HY, Zongo A, Korin A, Zhan F, Hady E, et al. Probiotic Supplements: Their Strategies in the Therapeutic and Prophylactic of Human Life-Threatening Diseases. International Journal of Molecular Sciences. 2021;22(20):11290.
37. Teng Y, Huang Y, Danfeng X, Tao X, Fan Y. The Role of Probiotics in Skin Photoaging and Related Mechanisms: A Review. Clin Cosmet Investig Dermatol. 2022;15:2455-64.
38. Xiao X, Hu X, Yao J, Cao W, Zou Z, Wang L, et al. The role of short-chain fatty acids in inflammatory skin diseases. Front Microbiol. 2023:13:1083432.
39. Slominski AT, Hardeland R, Zmijewski MA, Slominski RM, Reiter RJ, Paus R. Melatonin: A Cutaneous Perspective on its Production, Metabolism, and Functions. J Invest Dermatol. 2018;138(3):490-9.

Index

Page numbers followed by *f* refer to figure.

A

Absorption
  dose-dependent 61
  fractional 113
Acetate 306
Acne 77, 114, 224
  blemishes 16
Acne vulgaris 16, 28, 50, 108, 109, 119, 120, 135, 139, 200, 203, 204, 212, 215, 221, 223, 224, 236, 240, 303, 308, 312
  alongside isotretinoin for 215
  isotretinoin treatment for 212, 221
  mild-to-moderate 311
Acquired perforating dermatosis 148, 150
Actinobacteria 309
Adenosine monophosphate kinase 218
Adenosylcobalamin 34, 40
Aging 254, 270
Aglycone 291
Algal calcium 129
Alistipes 314
Alopecia 75, 135, 138, 142
  areata 39, 108, 135, 138
  universalis 148, 150
Alpha-linolenic acid 213, 214, 217f, 225
Alpha-lipoic acid 267-269
Alpha-tocopherol 76, 83
  transfer protein 76, 83
Alpha-tocotrienol 82, 83
Amino acid 103, 172, 173
  catabolism of branched-chain 52
  chelated form 122
  roles of 173f
  sulfur-containing 172
Anabolic pathways 30
Androgen activity, preventing 283
Androgenetic alopecia areata 114
Angiogenesis 283
Anthocyanins 276

Anti-ageing 148, 150, 176, 179, 181-184, 192, 195, 228, 231, 236, 242, 244, 251, 259, 267, 270, 274, 277, 278, 286
Anti-inflammation 236
Anti-inflammatory
  action 20, 218, 265, 272, 283, 306
  long-chain polyunsaturated fatty acids, biosynthesis of 44
  property 226, 244
Antimelanogenic activity 256
Antioxidant
  activity 62, 84, 94, 115, 145, 247, 256, 271, 282
    increasing 189
  defence systems 44
  enzyme 189, 289
  properties 265
  role 114
Apoptotic cell death 293
Arachidonic acid 223, 225
Arginine 167, 173
Ascorbic acid 103
  acts 61
Astaxanthin 238, 239, 243-245
Athlete's foot 200, 205
Atopic dermatitis 38, 57, 68, 77, 114, 121, 135, 139, 140, 164, 168, 176, 186, 200, 205, 221, 223, 228, 231, 236, 245, 286, 290, 308, 310, 311
  patients, platelets of 140
  pediatric 91
  pruritus in 298
Atopic eczema 121
Autoantibody production 81
Avidin 52

B

Bacteria, spore-forming 314
Bacterial fermentation synthetic 89

Barrier function 72, 233
Behcet's disease 110
Beta-carotene 02, 05, 06
Betaine 43
Bifidobacteria 314
Bifidobacterium
  bifidum 301
  infantis 301
  longum 301
  strains 310
Biomolecules protecting, sulfhydryl groups of 114
Biotin 47, 48, 51, 52
  dependent carboxylases 52
  doses of 51
  functions 52
  in dermatology, role of 48
  in food 52
  tolerability of 51
Biotinidase deficiency 50
Biotinylation 52
Blood clotting 94
Body tissue 84
Boosting cell metabolism 62
Branched-chain amino acids 173

C

Caffeine 133
Calcium 124, 127-129, 133
  absorption 129
  accumulation 90
  carbonate 129
  competitor 125
  homeostasis 133
  in cells and tissue, level of 125f
  ion 133
  oxalate 133
  supplementation 133
Canities, premature 37, 50

Capsules 51
Carbohydrate
　diets, low 75
　indigestible 305
Carboxylases 52
Carotenoids 237
　function 247
　mix 241
Casein 166
Catabolic pathways 30
Catalase 189
Catechins 275, 276, 280
Cell
　differentiation and migration, regulating 128
　growth and
　　differentiation 08
　　signaling 145, 160
　metabolism 257
　proliferation of 124
　protection 293
　receptors 209
　signaling 233
　　pathways 293
　　role in 114
Cellular activity 133, 197, 226
　role in 113
Cellular antioxidant network, central role in 257f
Cellular changes, aging-related 27
Cellular components 282
Cellular energy metabolism 30
Cellular function, regulation of 94
Cellular redox homeostasis 83
Cellulitis 176, 186
Ceramide 228-230, 233
　production 58
　role of 234f
　synthesis 84
Chewable capsules 59
Chewable tablets 51
Chloasma 80
Chloric acne 139
　vulgaris 135
Choline 43
Chylomicrons 83
Citrate, absorption of 111
Coenzyme Q10 94, 259, 260
Collagen 152, 177, 188
　deposition 236, 242
　metabolism 90
　peptide 176, 177, 188
　　protective mechanism of 189f
　　supplements 188
　synthesis 15, 35, 62, 283
Colony forming units 309
Colostrum 200, 202
Copper 148-150, 152
　absorption 152
　oxide 151
　transport protein 152
Coral calcium 129
C-reactive protein 124
Cupric
　carbonate 151
　citrate 151
　gluconate 151
　sulphate 151
Curcumin 275
Cutaneous adaptive immunity 72
Cutaneous inflammatory disorders 154, 158
Cutaneous leishmaniasis 110
Cutaneous lesions 39
Cutaneous pigmentation 28
Cutaneous sporotrichosis 154
Cyanidin 276
Cyanocobalamin hydroxocobalamin 40
Cyclic adenosine monophosphate 189
Cyclic nucleotide phosphodiesterase, inhibitor of 114
Cyclooxygenases 218, 218f, 225f, 226
Cysteine, tripeptide of 252
Cytokines 125, 283

D

Daidzein 288
Dairy protein 166
D-biotin 51
Deficiency, degree of 125
Dehydroascorbic acid 55
Delphinidin 276
Depigmentation 228
Dermal density 242
Dermal papilla cells 38
Dermatitis 212, 215
　syndrome 121
Detoxification 256
Diabetes
　skin damage related to 139
　wound healing in 39
Dietary fiber 300, 305
Dietary iron 103
Digestion and absorption 145, 152, 160, 172, 188, 197, 208, 217, 225, 233, 247, 256, 264, 271, 314
　and storage 145, 152, 160, 172, 188, 197, 208, 217, 225, 233, 247, 256, 264, 271, 305, 314
Dihomo-gamma linolenic acid 223
Dihydroceramide 232
Dihydrofolate 44
Dihydrolipoic acid 271
Dihydrotestosterone
　activity, preventing 248
　inhibition 245
　production, role in 114
Distant tissues 306
Dithiolane-3-pentanoic acid 268
DNA
　protection 209
　repair 30
Docosahexaenoic acid 214, 217
Dry skin 192, 194, 195, 212, 215, 221, 223, 228, 230, 231, 308
Dysbiosis 309
Dysbiotic gut microbes 315

E

Eicosanoids 225f
Eicosapentaenoic acid 214, 217, 225f
Eicosatetraenoic acid 225f
Elastin
　fibers 90
　formation 152
Endothelial function 283
Enterococcus 314
Enterocytes 83
Enzymatic hydroxylation 62
Enzymatic reactions, role in 113
Enzymes 218f, 225f
　inhibiting 189
　ten-eleven translocation family of 63
Epicatechins 276, 280
Epidermal proliferation, processes of 72
Epidermis 133
　metabolites in 234f
Epigallocatechin gallate 276
Epigenetic regulation 63
Erythema 236, 240, 241
　dose, minimal 261
　induced MMP-1 production 236
　UV induced 78
Erythromycin-resistant acne vulgaris 109

Estrogen receptors 287
Extracellular matrix 09

F

Facial skin esthetics 192, 195
Fat soluble vitamin 66, 71, 83, 84
Fatty acid 211, 217f
   long-chain 306
   oxidation, regulating 52
   roles of short chain 306f
Ferric polymaltose complex 100
Ferric state 100
Ferrous
   ascorbate 101
   bisglycinate 101
   form, chelated 100
   fumarate 101
   gluconate 101
   polymaltose complex 100
   salts 101
   state 100
   sulphate 101
Fibroblasts 293
   cells 27
   senescence 120
Filaggrin 133
Flavin-adenine dinucleotide 20
Flavonoids 282f
Flaxseed oil 288
Folate 44f
   deficiencies of 43
   shortage 44f
Folic acid 40, 42
   supplementation 41
   synthetic 34
Free biotin, absorption of 52
Fructans-inulin 300
Fructooligosaccharides 300, 305
Fusobacteria 309

G

Galactooligosaccharides 300, 305
Gamma-glutamylcysteine 253
Gamma-linolenic acid 222, 223, 225
Gastric acid production 103
Gastrointestinal system 152
Genistein 288, 290, 291
Genital warts 58
Gluconeogenesis 52
Glucosylceramide 232
   content 228, 230

Glutamic acid 252
Glutamine 167, 173
Glutathione 75, 83, 251, 252, 256, 257, 257f, 271
   levels 252
   peroxidase 140, 145, 189
   reduced 253
   reductase, cofactor for 83
Glycine 173, 252
Glycosaminoglycans 209
Glycosylated 291
Glycosylceramides 232
Granulation tissue formation 209f
Green tea extract 280
Growth factor beta, expression of transforming 94
Gummies 51, 59
Gut
   bacteria 305
   microflora of 293
Gut-skin axis 305

H

Hair
   aging 259, 262
      related changes in 17
   and nail growth 169
   and skin quality 192, 195
   cycle, modulation of 09
   cycling and pigmentation, regulating 160
   epithelial cell growth 283
   greying of 37, 50
   issues 50
   pigmentation 43
   premature graying of 127, 130
   promote growth of 85
   supplements 165
   temporary thinning 186
   thinning 176, 185, 186
Hair follicle 124, 262, 293
   cycle 134
   development 38
   growth 17
   stem cells 283
Hair growth 43, 164, 169, 176, 186, 200, 203, 209, 212, 215, 274, 279, 280, 286, 290
   promoting 21, 134
   stimulating 283
Hair loss 17, 50, 80, 164, 168
   excessive 100
   female pattern 101, 221, 224

Heme iron 103
Hemostasis 209f
Hidradenitis suppurativa 110, 114
Hormones 128
Human dermal
   fibroblast 262
   keratinocytes 262
Human embryonic kidney cells 90
Human epidermal
   keratinocytes 38
   melanocytes 36
Hyaluronic acid 192-194, 197
Hydrangea serrata leaves 278
Hydrolyzed collagen peptides 178
Hydroxycobalamin 40
Hydroxyeicosatetraenoic acids 225
Hyperpigmentation 37, 228, 231, 303
Hypothalamic-pituitary-thyroid axis 160

I

Immune
   cells 293, 305
   function, regulating 146, 160
   response 315f
Immunity, regulating 44
Immunomodulation 72
Immunomodulatory effects 315
Immunoregulation 63, 84, 94, 208
Infections, prevalence of 128
Inflammation 209f
   regulating 44
Inflammatory dermatoses 118
Inflammatory diseases 118
Inflammatory long-chain polyunsaturated fatty acids, biosynthesis of 44
Inflammatory neuropeptides 125
Inflammatory skin diseases 306f
Inorganic copper salts 150
Inorganic ferric salts 100
Inorganic ferrous salts 100
Inorganic salts 129
Inorganic zinc 107
   salts 111
Intestinal dysbiosis 309
Intestinal enzymes 282
Intestinal integrity, promoting 305
Inulin 305
Involucrin 133
Iodine 154-156, 160
   from sea kelp 159
Iodothyronine deiodinases 145

Iron 99
  chelation 208
  deficiency 43, 99
    clinical features of 103
    elemental form of 102
    inorganic form of 102
    polymaltose complex 101
    supplementation, doses of 107
Isoflavones 288
Isoleucine 52
Isotretinoin treatment, side effect of 224
Itchiness 231

J

Jejunum 43

K

Keratinocyte 278, 293, 315
  regulation 71
Keratins 133
Ketogenic diet 75

L

Lactobacillus 314
  acidophilus 301
  casei 301
  rhamnosus 310, 312
  strains 310
Lactococcus lactis 301
Lactoferrin 200-202, 209f
Lactotransferrin 201
L-ascorbic acid 56
  ingestion of 55
Leprosy 81
Leucine 52, 167
Leukotrienes 125, 226
Lifestyle disorders, burden of 309
Lignans 288
Lignans-vitexin 290
Linoleic acid 217f, 222, 223, 225
Lipoic acid 268, 271
Lipopolysaccharide 209
Liposomal iron 102
Lipoteichoic acid 209
Lipoxygenases 218, 218f, 225f, 226
Loricrin 133
Lozenges 59
Lupus erythematous 81
Lutein 238, 244
Lycopene 238-240, 243, 246

Lymphatic tissue, small masses of 315f
Lysine 172
  complex, chelated 150
Lysozyme 209

M

Macronutrients, oxidation of 30
Magnesium 118, 119, 124, 125f, 133
  absorption 124
  ascorbate 122
  aspartate 122
  citrate 122
  deficit diets 118
  doses of 123
  fumarate 122
  gluconate 122
  hydroxide 122
  lactate 122
  malate 122
  orotate 122
  oxide 122
  phosphate dibasic 122
  status, low 125f
  sulfate 122
  supplementation, adverse effects of 123
  transport system 124
Mammalian cells, histones in 63
Matrix protein synthesis, promoting 188
Melanin synthesis 153
Melanocytes 293
Melanogenesis 57
  inhibition of 271
Melasma 114, 298, 301
Menadione 89
Menaquinones 89, 91
Metabolism 283
Metal ion 118
  chelation of 271
Metal-binding protein metallothionein 114
Metalloproteinases 09
Metal-response element 114
Metformin 42
Methionine 43, 52
Methotrexate, toxicity of 42
Methylcobalamin 34, 40
Methyltetrahydrofolate 34
Methyltetrahydrofolic acid glucosamine salt 40
Microbes 305
Microcirculatory dysfunction 125
Microvascular lumen 125
Migraine 118

Minerals 97
Mitochondria 52
Mitochondrial activity 94
Mitochondrial ATP synthesis 264
Molecular targets 114
Mononucleotide 20

N

Nail quality 164, 168
Natural lycopene 242
Natural methylcobalamin 34
Neurotransmitters 305, 315
Niacin 23
Niacinamide 29
Nicotinamide 26, 29, 30
  in vitro 27
  inhibits cytokines 30
  mononucleotide 29
Nicotinic acid 29
  absorption of 30
Noncarbohydrate prebiotics 300
Nonmelanoma skin cancers 26, 127, 130
Non-provitamin A carotenoids 236
N-pteroyl-l-glutamic acid 40
Nucleic acids 209
Nutrient availability 306
Nutritional biotin deficiency 48

O

Oligosaccharides, human milk 300
Omega-3
  fats 44
  fatty acids 212, 213, 222
Omega-6 fats 44
  acids 213, 221, 222
One-carbon metabolism 43, 44f
Oral probiotics 309
Osteogenic cells 94
Oxidative damage 236, 243
Oxidative stress 56, 90, 293
Oxidized glutathione 253

P

Palm oil 76
Panthenol 18
Pantothenic acid 20
  doses of 52
Papulopustular rosacea 38
Parabacteroides 314
Peptides 163
Peroxyl radicals react 84

Peyer's patches 315f
Phosphorylated 43
Photoaging 164, 176, 236, 243
   skin 189f
Photoimmunosuppresion 26
Photoprotection 62, 71, 78, 84, 135, 154, 218, 247, 259, 274, 282, 298, 301, 302
   UV radiation induced 242
Phylloquinone 89, 91
Phylum firmicutes 314
Phytoceramides 228, 229, 233
Phytoene 238, 241, 243, 244
Phytoestrogens 286, 287, 293, 294
   source of 287
   types of 293f
Phytofluene 238, 241, 243, 244
Phytonutrients 275
Pigmentation 267, 269
   reducing 62
Pigmented contact dermatitis 80
Pigmented purpuric dermatosis 59
Pityriasis alba 114
Plant proteins 166
Plasma 84, 124
   concentrations 264, 271
   iron homeostasis, role in 103
   membrane 124, 133
Platelet derived growth factor 94
Poliosis 135, 138
Polymorphic light eruption photodermatosis 236, 241
Polyphenol group, part of 293
Polyphenolic-rich diet 275
Polyphenols 274, 275, 277, 279, 282, 283
   certain 283
   types of 282f
Polyunsaturated fatty acids 213, 217, 257
Potassium
   hyaluronate 195
   iodate 159
Prebiotic 298, 306
   effect 198
Prevotella 314
Proanthocyanidins 275
Probiotic 308
   effect 294
   metabolites, effects by 315
   survival, evidence of 309
Proinflammatory factors, aging-related 91
Proliferation-inhibition effect 315
Proline 172

Promoting barrier
   function 160
   properties 219
Propionate 306
Prostaglandins 125, 218, 225, 226
Protein 163, 164, 172
   functional roles of 172
   intake
      benefits of 174
      improves iron status 103
   P53 26
   structural roles of 172
Proteobacteria 309
Proton pump inhibitors 42
Pseudoalbinism 135, 142
Pseudoxanthoma elasticum 90
Psoriasis 36, 57, 67, 77, 79, 108, 114, 130, 135, 139, 200, 206, 212, 215, 308, 312
Psychological stress 118
Psyllium 305
Pustular psoriasis 127, 130
   generalized 130
Pyridoxal-5-phosphate 34
Pyridoxine hydrochloride pyridoxal 5′-phosphate 40

Q

Quercetin 276, 281

R

Radical concentrations low 83
Reactive oxygen species 188, 208, 257, 264, 268, 271
   protection from 153
Re-epithelialization 209f
Resveratrol 275, 288, 291, 293
Retinoic acid X receptor 71
Retinyl esters 08
Riboflavin 18, 20
Rosacea 28, 109

S

Saccharomyces species 314
S-adenosylhomocysteine 44f
S-adenosylmethionine 44f
Scalp hair follicles 280
Sebaceous glands 293
   modulation of 09
Seborrheic dermatitis 44, 109, 114
Sebum production 44

Selenious acid 144
Selenium 43, 135-137, 145
   enrich yeast 144
   nanoparticles 144
Selenocysteine 144
Selenomethionine 144
Selenoprotein 145
Serum 124
Sesbania grandiflora 49
   extracts 51
Severe acute respiratory syndrome coronavirus 2 136
Sirtuins 30
Skim milk powder 166
Skin 35, 56, 62, 228, 230
   allergy 135, 141
   and gut 314
   cancer 26, 142
   cell apoptosis, protection of 143
   color 251, 254
   damage, diabetes-related 135
   dehydration, UV radiation-induced 185
   deterioration, UV radiation induced 243
   development 135, 141
   diseases 139
   dryness and quality 298, 303
   elasticity 176, 180, 184
   flushing 29
   hydration 197, 228, 231, 274, 279
   hypersensitivity 135, 143
   immunity, modulation of 09
   lightening 254
   lipid barrier 226
   moisture 176, 179, 192, 194, 200, 205, 231
   photoaging 168
   profile 195
   texture 164, 167, 200, 205
   whitening 200, 206, 251, 254
Skin aging 164, 180, 182, 242, 243, 298, 303
   pollution-related 279
   signs of 261
Skin and hair
   health 173f
   products 275
Skin appearance 154, 157
   enhancing 248
Skin barrier
   function 27, 58, 228, 231, 306
   promoting 20
   properties 133f

Skin changes
    age-related 167
    UV irradiated 244
Skin health 287
    general 298, 301
Skin inflammation 267, 270, 305
    UV induced 78
Sodium
    hyaluronate 195
    hydrogen selenite 144
    iodate 159
    selenate 144
    selenite 144
Soft gels 51, 82
Soy isoflavones 288
Sphingosine 232
Sporotrichosis 154, 158
Squamous cell carcinoma 127, 130
Staphylococcus aureus 68
Stilbenes 288
Stress resistance 283
Sunburn 69, 78
Sunflower oil 76
Sunshine vitamin 66
Superoxide dismutase 152, 189
    activity of 293
Synbiotics 298
Synthetic cyanocobalamin 34
Synthetic forms 29
Synthetic hydroxocobalamin 34
Synthetic methylcobalamin 34
Synthetic tetrahydrofolate 34

T

T cell function 84
    modulate 94
T helper cells 72, 316
Tablets 51
Tannins 276
Tea polyphenols 279
Telogen effluvium 16, 67, 108, 114, 164, 168, 176, 185
    chronic 101
Tetrahydrofolate 44
Thermal stress 81
Thiamine 20
    mononitrate 18
Thioctic acid 268
Threonine 52
Thromboxanes 226
Thyroglobulin, iodination of 104

Thyroid
    gland 104
    hormones 146, 160
        production of 104
    metabolism 104
    peroxidase catalyzes, heme-containing 104
Tinea pedis 200, 205
Tissue remodeling 209f
Tocopherol 76
Tocotrienols 76
    accumulated 84
Toll-like receptors 198
Tomato
    carotenoids 240
    paste 242
Toxic products 305, 315
Transcription processes, regulation of 30
Transepidermal water loss 118, 133, 219
    reducing 189
Transforming growth factor-beta 315
Tristetraprolin 114
Tumor necrosis factor alpha 209
Tyrosinase 62

U

Ubiquinol 261, 263
Ubiquinone 261, 263
Ulcerative colitis 42
Ultraviolet A protection 262
Ultraviolet B
    induced sunburn 57
    irradiated photoprotection 157
    protection 262
Ultraviolet-induced
    DNA damage 26
    erythema 236, 240, 241
    photoaging 27
Uncombable hair syndrome 49
Undereye dark circles 236
Urticaria 68, 69

V

Valine 52
Verrucomicrobia 309
Viral warts 109
Vitamin 01
    B complex 16
    B1 11, 14, 16, 20
    B2 11, 14, 20
    B3 23
    B5 11, 15-17, 20, 21, 52

    B7 47
    D2 67, 70
    D3 67, 70, 71
    K1 89, 91, 93
    K2 89
    K2-MK7 91
    K3 89
    synthetic 40
Vitamin A 02, 05
    compounds 08
Vitamin B12 32, 34, 36-41, 44f
    absorption of 40
    deficiencies of 43
    role of 44f
Vitamin B6 32, 34, 35, 38-44
    human body absorbs 43
    role of 44f
Vitamin B9 32, 34, 36, 38-42
    role of 44f
Vitamin B-complex 18, 37, 39
    levels of 43
Vitamin C 43, 54, 61, 62, 75, 83, 103, 271
    capacity 61
    circulates 61
    deficiency 55
    forms of 61
    intakes of 61
    promotes 62
    stimulates 63
    synthesizing species 61
    topical application of 55
Vitamin D 65, 71, 128, 133
    absorption 71
    deficiencies of 43, 118
    doses of 70, 118
    mediates 72
    regulates biochemical steps 71
    role in cell division 71
    signaling 71
    treatment 72
Vitamin E 74-76, 84, 271
    concentration of 83
    deficiency 75
    derivatives 85
    modulates 84
    prevents 84
    supplemental 75
    synthetic 82
Vitamin K 87
    deficiency of 88
    dependent signaling pathways 94
    requirement 306

Vitexin 288
Vitiligo 36, 67, 77, 79, 110, 114, 135, 140, 267, 269
   non-segmental 267, 269
von Zumbusch psoriasis 127, 130

W

Wound healing 14, 15, 18, 28, 39, 72, 90, 94, 108, 164, 168, 200, 206, 209, 209f, 212, 286, 290, 308, 312
   chronic 215
   process 209f
Wrinkles 57, 192, 194, 286, 308

X

Xerotic cheilitis 224

Z

Zeaxanthin 238, 244
Zinc 105-107, 114
   absorption 113
   acetate 111
   binds 114
   chelated 107, 111
   citrate 111
   competes 114
   deficiency 108
   doses of 107
   finger motifs 113, 114
   for various dermatosis, use of 114
   gluconate 110, 111
      absorption of 111
   glycine 111
   metalloproteins 113
   methionine 111
   oxide 111
   plays, role in 113
   sulfate 110, 111
   supplementation 115, 152

EU GSPR Authorised Reprsentative
Logos Europe, 9 rue Nicolas Poussin
1700, La Rochelle, France
Phone: +33 (0) 6 67 93 73 78
E-mail: contact@logoseurope.eu